Canadian Immunization Guide

Seventh Edition – 2006

Published by the
Public Health Agency of Canada
Infectious Disease and Emergency Preparedness Branch
Centre for Infectious Disease Prevention and Control
under the authority of the Minister of Public Works and
Government Services Canada

Également disponible en français sous le titre
Guide canadien d'immunisation

Text prepared by the
National Advisory Committee on Immunization

Chief Public Health Officer
Public Health Agency of Canada

The seventh edition of the *Canadian Immunization Guide* was developed by the National Advisory Committee on Immunization (NACI), with the support of the Immunization and Respiratory Infections Division, Public Health Agency of Canada, to provide updated information and recommendations on the use of vaccines in Canada. The Public Health Agency of Canada conducted a survey in 2004, which confirmed that the *Canadian Immunization Guide* is a very useful and reliable resource of information on immunization.

The seventh edition of the *Guide* will also be available on the NACI Web site at www.naci.gc.ca. New or updated recommendations from NACI are published in the Canada Communicable Disease Report (CCDR) and are also available on the NACI Web site.

If you have suggestions or comments on the *Guide* please send them to us at NACI@phac-aspc.gc.ca.

To promote health and protect Canadians from vaccine-preventable disease, I encourage parents, guardians, and adults to maintain their children's immunizations up to date and all adults to be immunized according to NACI recommendations.

Producing such a publication was possible through the dedication and voluntary time commitment on the part of those involved. I would like to extend my sincere thanks to the members, liaison members, and ex-officio members of NACI for completing this very important resource. I would also like to take this opportunity to acknowledge their invaluable contribution and continued commitment in providing ongoing advice and recommendations on vaccine use in Canada.

Dr. David Butler-Jones, MD
Chief Public Health Officer of Canada

Preface

The seventh edition of the *Canadian Immunization Guide* contains numerous changes from the 2002 version. Every chapter has been thoroughly reviewed and updated as required, taking into consideration the input received from the user survey conducted in 2004.

Three new chapters have been added: *Principles of Combination Vaccines, Principles of Vaccine Interchangeability*, and *Immunization of Persons New to Canada*.

Some key changes from the 2002 *Canadian Immunization Guide* are:

- Each disease-specific vaccine chapter is prefaced with a notation about major changes.

- The *Vaccine Safety* chapter replaces the *Adverse Events* chapter and includes more information.

- The *Vaccine Administration Practices* chapter replaces the *Immunization Techniques* chapter and incorporates more detail.

- The *Communicating Effectively About Immunization* chapter replaces *Talking with Patients About Immunization*, focusing on the principles of risk communication.

- The *Benefits of Vaccines* chapter replaces the *Cost Benefit* chapter and covers the benefits of vaccines to health.

- The *General Considerations* chapter includes a table listing all vaccines approved for use in Canada, based on product availability as of May 2006.

- The *Immunization of Patients in Health Care Institutions* chapter incorporates the recommendations for acute-care and long-term care institutions.

- The *Immunization for Adults* chapter has been expanded to include recommendations for health care workers and specific risk situations.

- The chapter on *Immunization of Persons with Neurologic Disorders* has been expanded with recommendations related to adults.

- The recommendations for travellers are integrated into one chapter.

- The *Lyme Disease Vaccine* chapter was discarded, since there is currently no vaccine available against this disease in Canada.

In an effort to keep the *Guide* user friendly, we developed a standard template to present the information in the Active Immunizing Agents sections with a summary of key changes since the publication of the previous edition. We also used different colors for each part of the *Guide* and included a condensed version of the Table of Contents on the back cover for easier reference. Look for a new and improved on-line version available in HTML format with direct links to updates in each section of the *Guide*.

As we publish this seventh edition of the *Guide* some information is already outdated, which reflects the rapidly expanding environment in the immunization field. This continues to be a challenge for the National Advisory Committee on Immunization (NACI) as more new vaccines are approved for use, new vaccine combinations are developed, the data to be analyzed become more complex, and additional data are available on the immunogenicity and efficacy of vaccines. Updates and new recommendations are published in the Canada Communicable Disease Report and are available at the NACI Web site at www. naci.gc.ca.

As the Chair of the Committee, I would like to gratefully acknowledge the expert contributions of my member, liaison, and ex-officio representative colleagues on the Committee and the support from the Immunization and Respiratory Infections Division, Public Health Agency of Canada. It has been an honor and privilege to work with such a committed group of professionals on an activity that results in guidelines that are so widely incorporated into practice in Canada.

On behalf of the Committee, I would also like to acknowledge the contribution of Dr. Monique Landry and the *Groupe sur l'acte vaccinal du Québec* for the final editing of the Guide's French version.

Dr. Monika Naus
Chair
National Advisory Committee on Immunization

Preamble

The National Advisory Committee on Immunization (NACI) provides the Public Health Agency of Canada with ongoing and timely medical, scientific, and public health advice relating to immunization. The Public Health Agency of Canada acknowledges that the advice and recommendations set out in this *Guide* are based upon the best current available scientific knowledge and is disseminating this document for information purposes. People administering the vaccine should also be aware of the contents of the relevant package insert(s) or product monograph(s). Recommendations for use and other information set out herein may differ from that set out in the product monograph(s) of the Canadian manufacturer(s) of the vaccine(s). Manufacturer(s) have sought approval of the vaccine(s) and provided evidence as to its safety and efficacy only when it is used in accordance with the product monographs. NACI members and liaison members conduct themselves within the context of the Public Health Agency of Canada's Policy on Conflict of Interest, including yearly declaration of potential conflict of interest.

National Advisory Committee on Immunization
Membership List

Chair

M. Naus
BC Centre for Disease Control
Vancouver, British Columbia

Vice-Chair

J. Langley
IWK Health Centre
Halifax, Nova Scotia

Members

S. Dobson
Vaccine Evaluation Center
Vancouver, British Columbia

B. Duval
Institut National de Santé Publique
  du Québec
Beauport, Quebec

J. Embree
University of Manitoba
Winnipeg, Manitoba

A. Hanrahan
Capital Health Region
Edmonton, Alberta

K. Laupland
University of Calgary
Calgary, Alberta

A. McGeer
Mount Sinai/Toronto Medical Laboratories
Toronto, Ontario

S. McNeil
Division of Infectious Diseases
Dalhousie University
Halifax, Nova Scotia

M.-N. Primeau
Université de Montréal
Montreal, Quebec

B. Tan
Royal University Hospital
Saskatoon, Saskatchewan

B. Warshawsky
Middlesex-London Health Unit
London, Ontario

Executive Secretary

S. Deeks
Immunization and Respiratory
  Infections Division
Centre for Infectious Disease Prevention
  and Control
Public Health Agency of Canada
Ottawa, Ontario

T. Tam (2004-2006)
Immunization and Respiratory
  Infections Division
Centre for Infectious Disease Prevention
  and Control
Public Health Agency of Canada
Ottawa, Ontario

Advisory Committee Secretariat

N. Groleau
Immunization and Respiratory
  Infections Division
Centre for Infectious Disease Prevention
  and Control
Public Health Agency of Canada
Ottawa, Ontario

S. Laforest
Immunization and Respiratory
  Infections Division
Centre for Infectious Disease Prevention
  and Control
Public Health Agency of Canada
Ottawa, Ontario

J. Rendall
Immunization and Respiratory
  Infections Division
Centre for Infectious Disease Prevention
  and Control
Public Health Agency of Canada
Ottawa, Ontario

Liaison Representatives

Advisory Committee on Causality
Assessment
B. Law
Ottawa, Ontario

Centres for Disease Control and
  Prevention
L. Chapman
Atlanta, Georgia

Association of Medical Microbiology and
  Infectious Disease Canada
P. Orr
Winnipeg, Manitoba

College of Family Physicians of Canada
S. Rechner
Hamilton, Ontario

Canadian Association for Immunization
  Research and Evaluation
D. Scheifele
Vancouver, British Columbia

Committee to Advise on Tropical
  Medicine and Travel
J. Salzman
Vancouver, British Columbia

Canadian Nursing Coalition for
  Immunization
A. Honish
Edmonton, Alberta

Community and Hospital Infection
  Control Association
S. Callery
Toronto, Ontario

Canadian Paediatric Society
M. Salvadori
London, Ontario

Council of Chief Medical Officers of Health
B. Larke
Whitehorse, Yukon Territory

Canadian Public Health Association
J. Carsley
Montreal, Quebec

Society of Obstetricians and Gynaecologists
  of Canada
D. Money
Vancouver, British Columbia

Ex-Officio Representatives

Biologics and Genetic Therapies
Directorate
Health Canada
F. Hindieh
H. Rode
Ottawa, Ontario

First Nations and Inuit Health Branch
Health Canada
M. Lem
Ottawa, Ontario

Department of National Defence
M. Tepper
Ottawa, Ontario

Public Health Agency of Canada
J. Sciberras
P. Varughese
Ottawa, Ontario

Other contributors

Previous Members, Liaison Members and Ex-Officio representatives who worked on this edition of the Guide while they were active on the committee:

I. Bowmer, Health Sciences Centre, St. John's Newfoundland

G. De Serres, Centre de santé publique de Québec, Beauport, Québec

I. Gemmill, Kingston, Frontenac and Lennox & Addington Health Unit, Kingston Ontario

A. Gruslin, Ottawa Hospital, Ottawa, Ontario (SOGC)

V. Lentini, Department of National Defence, Ottawa, Ontario (DND)

A. McCarthy, Department of National Defence, Ottawa, Ontario (AMMI Canada)

L. Samson, Children's Hospital of Eastern Ontario, Ottawa, Ontario (CPS)

A. Zierler, Safe Kids Canada, Toronto, Ontario

Table of Contents

Part 1
General Guidelines

General Considerations.. 3
The Benefits of Vaccines... 17
National Guidelines for Immunization Practices................... 22
Communicating Effectively about Immunization.................... 29
Principles of Combination Vaccines............................... 33
Principles of Vaccine Interchangeability 36
Vaccine Administration Practices................................. 38
Storage and Handling of Immunizing Agents 45
Timing of Vaccine Administration 51
Recent Administration of Human Immune Globulin Products 53
Immunization Records... 55

Part 2
Vaccine Safety and Adverse Events Following Immunization

Vaccine Safety... 59
General Contraindications and Precautions 73
Anaphylaxis: Initial Management in Non-Hospital Settings......... 80
Anaphylactic Hypersensitivity to Egg and Egg-Related Antigens... 85

Part 3
Recommended Immunization

Recommended Immunization Schedules.............................. 93
Immunization of Adults.. 96
Immunization of Children and Adults with Inadequate
    Immunization Records 105
Immunization in Pregnancy and Breast-Feeding 107
Immunization of Infants Born Prematurely 113
Immunization of Patients in Health Care Institutions............ 115
Immunization of Immunocompromised Persons 117
Immunization of Persons with Neurologic Disorders 131
Immunization of Persons with Bleeding Disorders................. 134
Immunization of Travellers 136
Immunization of Persons New to Canada........................... 144

Part 4
Active Immunizing Agents

Bacille Calmette-Guérin (BCG) Vaccine 149
Cholera Vaccine.. 158
Diphtheria Toxoid 166
Haemophilus Vaccine... 172
Hepatitis A Vaccine 179
Hepatitis B Vaccine... 189
Hepatitis Vaccines Combined... 205
Influenza Vaccine 209
Japanese Encephalitis Vaccine.. 221
Measles Vaccine.. 228
Meningococcal Vaccine 237
Mumps Vaccine 251
Pertussis Vaccine 257
Pneumococcal Vaccine 267
Poliomyelitis Vaccine 277
Rabies Vaccine.. 285
Rubella Vaccine 298
Smallpox Vaccine 308
Tetanus Toxoid 309
Typhoid Vaccine 317
Varicella Vaccine... 327
Yellow Fever Vaccine... 343

Part 5
Passive Immunization

Passive Immunizing Agents 353
Immune Globulin (Human)... 354
Recommended Usage 354
    Measles.. 354
    Hepatitis A 355
    Rubella 355
    Hepatitis C 355
Safety of Immunoglobulin Preparations... 355
Adverse Reactions 356
Contraindications and Precautions 356

Specific Immune Globulins 356
    Botulism antitoxin (equine) 357
    Diphtheria antitoxin (equine) 357
    Hepatitis B immune globulin (HBIg) 357
    Rabies immune globulin (RabIg) 358
    Palivizumab (RSVAb) 358
    Tetanus immune globulin (TIg) 359
    Varicella-zoster immune globulin (VarIg) 360

Appendix
Abbreviations for Products Available in Canada 365

Index 367

Comparison of Effects of Diseases and Vaccines

Part 1

General Guidelines

General Considerations

The goal of those concerned with immunization is the elimination of vaccine-preventable diseases. Eradication of smallpox has been achieved. Currently, global efforts are directed at the eradication of polio and the elimination of measles. Ongoing immunization programs with high vaccine coverage are needed to maintain low levels of other vaccine-preventable diseases. When the incidence of a communicable disease decreases to low levels because of successful vaccination programs, there is a potential for people to question the need to continue the programs, and this may lead to lower vaccine coverage and, inevitably, resurgence of the disease. Therefore, immunization providers must advocate for the continuation of successful programs.

An ideal vaccine would confer lifelong protection against a disease after a single dose. It would be inexpensive, stable during shipping and storage, easy to administer and without adverse effects. Researchers and vaccine manufacturers continue to work to improve vaccines; in the meantime, our existing vaccines save lives. The diseases against which vaccines protect may also change over time for reasons unrelated to vaccine programs. These factors mean that the efficacy, effectiveness and safety of vaccines and vaccination programs must be evaluated continually to ensure that Canadians achieve the greatest possible benefit.

In this *Guide*, information is presented on the immunizing agents available in Canada and their use in the prevention of communicable diseases. Recommendations on routine immunizations are discussed in some detail, and an attempt is made to answer most of the day-to-day queries from providers regarding immunization.

Because of variation in manufacturers' products, precise details of the dosage and route of administration of individual products are not usually given. Readers are referred to manufacturers' labelling and package inserts for this information. As well, the manufacturer has sought approval of the vaccine and provided evidence as to its safety and efficacy only when it is used in accordance with the product monograph. Some information in the *Guide* may differ from that in product monograph(s) and package inserts. Information in the *Guide* is based upon the best and most current publicly available scientific knowledge.

What's in a vaccine?

Vaccines are highly regulated, complex biologic products designed to induce a protective immune response both effectively and safely. The main vaccine types as well as the derivation, purpose and potential risk of vaccine constituents are summarized below. See Table 1 (page 7) for specific information on the type and key constituents of each vaccine marketed in Canada.

Part 1 — General Guidelines

3

Immunogen: The part of the vaccine that stimulates an immune response is also the basis for classification of vaccine type, as follows:

- *Live attenuated:* The vaccine contains whole, living bacteria or viruses that induce immunity by actively replicating within the host. Since the agent replicates within the recipient, the stimulus more closely resembles that associated with natural infection, resulting in longer lasting and broader immunity than can be achieved with other vaccine types. Attenuated means the vaccine strains are weakened so that infection is usually inapparent or very mild, in marked contrast to the natural infection (see inside back cover). Live vaccines require careful storage and handling to avoid inadvertent inactivation and are contraindicated for pregnant women and people with immunodeficiencies.

- *Inactivated:* The vaccine contains killed bacteria or virus. Such vaccines pose no risk for immunocompromised persons and may induce a broad immunity since multiple antigens are present. Disadvantages include the usual need for multiple doses because the response may be weaker than that induced by live organisms and potential toxicity associated with unwanted portions of the killed organism (as was true for the whole-cell pertussis vaccine).

- *Subunit:* The vaccine contains purified products that usually come from the bacteria or virus that causes natural infection but may also be synthesized in the laboratory using recombinant technology (e.g., hepatitis B surface antigen). These products may require inactivation to prevent toxic side effects, and all are purified through a variety of steps in the manufacturing process. The end products include proteins, polysaccharides and protein-polysaccharide conjugates. Subunit vaccines have excellent safety profiles and facilitate the preparation of a variety of combination products. Disadvantages include lower immunogenicity, which sometimes requires the presence of an adjuvant and/or multiple doses.

Adjuvant: A substance added to a vaccine to enhance the immune response by degree and/or duration, making it possible to reduce the amount of immunogen per dose or the total number of doses needed to achieve immunity. The only adjuvants used in vaccines currently marketed in Canada are aluminum salts (aluminum hydroxide, aluminum phosphate or potassium aluminum sulfate), which primarily enhance the immune response to proteins. They have been shown to be safe over seven decades of use. Rarely, they may cause injection site reactions, including subcutaneous nodules, granulomatous inflammation or contact hypersensitivity. Subcutaneous rather than intramuscular deposition, as occurs when using too short a needle, may increase the risk of such reactions. After oxygen and silicon, aluminum is the third most abundant element in the environment and daily exposure occurs, primarily through food. Infant formula contains from 0.2 to 1.1 mg aluminum/litre whereas vaccines contain from 0.2 to 0.85 mg per dose. Both exposures are considered to be within the limits of safety (see Keith et al. for a more detailed discussion).

Preservatives: Chemicals (e.g., thimerosal, phenol, 2 phenoxyethanol) added to multidose, killed or subunit vaccines in order to prevent serious secondary infections as a result of bacterial or fungal contamination. In recent years there has been a great deal of opposition to the use of thimerosal, an ethyl mercury derivative, because of a theoretical risk of brain damage. Scientific evidence has refuted this risk, and it is no longer necessary for health care providers to raise this as a concern before administering influenza or hepatitis B vaccines, which may contain thimerosal. Thimerosal-free versions of both vaccines are available for use in select circumstances (see the relevant chapters in this *Guide*).

Additives: Substances other than those already mentioned may be added to vaccines for two different purposes:

◆ **to support the growth and purification of specific immunogens and/or the inactivation of toxins.** These include antibiotics added to prevent contamination during viral cell culture; substances needed for the growth of viruses, such as egg or yeast proteins, glycerol, serum, amino acids and enzymes; and formaldehyde used to inactivate viruses and protein toxins. Most of these reagents are removed in subsequent manufacturing steps, but minute "trace" amounts may remain in the final product. The amounts present are only of consequence for individuals who are allergic to them (see Table 1 for a listing of potential allergens in vaccines authorized for marketing in Canada). Concern has been expressed about formaldehyde because of its use as an embalming agent. However formaldehyde is also an intermediate in human metabolism, and the amount normally found in blood, even of a young infant, exceeds by 10 fold or more what is found in a dose of vaccine.

◆ **to confirm product quality or stability.** Compounds may be added to vaccines for a variety of manufacture-related issues: controlling acidity (pH); stabilizing immunogens through necessary steps in the manufacturing process, such as freeze drying; and preventing immunogens from adhering to the sides of glass vials with a resultant loss in immunogenicity. Examples of such additives include potassium or sodium salts, lactose, polysorbate 20 or 80, human serum albumin and a variety of animal proteins, such as gelatin and bovine serum albumin. Concerns have been expressed regarding the following:

  ◦ Human serum albumin: There is a theoretical risk of infectious agents being present in products made from human blood. However, steps in the manufacturing process of both human albumin and vaccines that contain it greatly reduce the possibility of transmission of these agents. To date, there have been no documented cases of transmission of infectious agents by human serum albumin.

  ◦ Gelatin: This protein may be the cause of rare hypersensitivity reactions to gelatin-containing vaccines (approximately 1 event per 2 million doses). Table 1 identifies which of the vaccines currently marketed in Canada contain gelatin. All individuals who have had an anaphylactic reaction to one of these products should be referred to an allergist, as should individuals with a history of immediate allergic reactions to foods containing gelatin.

* Bovine reagents: The risk of transmitting variant Creutzfeld Jakob disease from vaccines containing bovine-derived material is theoretical, estimated to be 1 in 40 billion or less (see http://www.fda.gov/cber/BSE/risk.htm). In Canada, the bovine-derived reagents commonly added to vaccines included in the routine schedule are manufactured from animals considered to be free of bovine spongiform encephalopathy.

Selected references

Keith LS, Jones DE, Chou C. *Aluminum toxicokinetics regarding infant diet and vaccinations.* Vaccine 2002;20:S13-17.

Offit PA, Jew RK. *Addressing parents' concerns: Do vaccines contain harmful preservatives, adjuvants, additives, or residuals?* Pediatrics 2003;112:1394-1397. URL: <www.pediatrics.org/cgi/content/full/112/6/1394>.

Table 1. Type and Contents of Vaccines Currently Approved for Use in Canada

Brand name	Mfr/distr.	Route	Vaccine type	Immunogen +	Products	Adjuvant	Preservative	Potential allergens (egg, antibiotic, gelatin, latex, trace of thimerosal)	Other materials
Act-HIB®	SP	IM	Subunit	Hib	Conjugate				
Actacel™*	SP	IM	Subunit	D, T, aP + (Hib)	Proteins + conjugate	Alum	PE		
Adacel®	SP	IM	Subunit	T, d, ap	Proteins	Alum	PE		
Avaxim®	SP	IM	Inactivated	HA	Killed virus	Alum	PE	Neomycin	Formaldehyde
Avaxim® – Pediatric	SP	IM	Inactivated	HA	Killed virus	Alum	PE	Neomycin	Formaldehyde
BCG Vaccine (Freeze-Dried)	SP	Intra-dermal	Live attenuated	BCG	Live bacteria				Polysorbate 80
Boostrix®*	GSK	IM	Subunit	D, T, aP	Proteins	Alum	PE		Formaldehyde
DT Polio Adsorbed	SP	IM	Subunit + inactivated	D, T, IPV	Proteins + killed virus	Alum	PE	Polymyxin B, Neomycin	Formaldehyde
Dukoral™	SBL/SP	Oral	Subunit + inactivated	Chol-Ecol-O	Proteins + killed bacteria				Saccharin
Engerix®-B Multi dose vial Single dose vial	GSK	IM	Subunit	HB	Recombinant protein	Alum	PE None	Trace thimerosal	Yeast proteins

Part 1 — General Guidelines

Table 1. Type and Contents of Vaccines Currently Approved for Use in Canada

Brand name	Mfr/ distr.	Route	Vaccine type			Adjuvant	Preservative	Potentiel allergens (egg, antibiotic, gelatin, latex, trace of thimerosal)	Other materials
			Vaccine type	Immunogen +	Products				
Eolarix™ *	GSK	SC	Live	M,R	Live virus			Neomycin	Human albumin Lactose, Dextran
Epaxal®**	BERN	IM	Inactivated	HA in Inf virosome	Killed virus		Tm		Formaldehyde
Fluviral® S/F	IDB	IM	Inactivated	Inf	Killed virus		Tm	Egg proteins	Formaldehyde
FSME - IMMUN	BAX	IM	Inactivated	TBE	Inactivated whole virus	Alum		Neomycin Gentamycin Egg Protamine sulfate Chick protein	Formaldehyde Human serum albumin Sucrose
Havrix®	GSK	IM	Inactivated	HA	Killed virus	Alum	PE	Neomycin Latex in stopper pre-filled syringes	Formaldehyde Polysorbate 20
Hiberix®*	GSK	IM	Subunit	Hib	Conjugate				Lactose
Imovax® Polio*	SP	SC	Inactivated	IPV	Killed virus		PE	Polymyxin B Neomycin, Streptomycin	Bovine serum Formaldehyde Polysorbate 80
Imovax® Rabies	SP	IM	Inactivated	Rab	Killed virus			Neomycin	Human albumin

Table 1. Type and Contents of Vaccines Currently Approved for Use in Canada

Brand name	Mfr/distr.	Route	Vaccine type	Immunogen+	Products	Adjuvant	Preservative	Potentiel allergens (egg, antibiotic, gelatin, latex, trace of thimerosal)	Other materials
Inactived Poliomyelitis Vaccine – IPV	SP	SC	Inactivated	IPV	Killed virus		PE	Polymyxin B Neomycin	Bovine serum Formaldehyde Polysorbate 80
Infanrix™*	GSK	IM	Subunit	D, T, aP	Proteins	Alum	PE		Formaldehyde Polysorbate 80
Infanrix™-hexa*	GSK	IM	Subunit + inactivated	D, T, aP, HB IPV + (Hib)	Proteins + killed viruses + conjugate	Alum	PE	Polymyxin B Neomycin Trace thimerosal	Yeast protein Formaldehyde Lactose Polysorbate 20 and 80 Bovine serum albumin
Infanrix™/Hib*	GSK	IM	Subunit	D, T, aP + (Hib)	Proteins + conjugate	Alum	PE		Formaldehyde Lactose Polysorbate 80
Infanrix™-IPV*	GSK	IM	Subunit + inactivated	D, T, aP IPV	Proteins + killed virus	Alum	PE	Polymyxin B Neomycin	Bovine serum Formaldehyde Polysorbate 80

Table 1. Type and Contents of Vaccines Currently Approved for Use in Canada

Brand name	Mfr/distr.	Route	Vaccine type	Immunogen +	Products	Adjuvant	Preservative	Potential allergens (egg, antibiotic, gelatin, latex, trace of thimerosal)	Other materials
				Vaccine type					
Infanrix™ - IPV/Hib*	GSK	IM	Subunit + inactivated	D, T, aP, IPV + (Hib)	Protein + killed virus + conjugate	Alum	PE	Polymyxin B Neomycin	Formaldehyde Polysorbate 80 Lactose Bovine serum albumin
Influvac™	SOLV	IM/SC	Inactivated	Inf	Killed virus			Gentamicin Egg protein	Chicken protein Formaldehyde Polysorbate 80
JE-VAX®	BIKEN/SP	SC	Inactivated	JE	Killed virus		Tm	Gelatin	Mouse serum Protein Formaldehyde
Liquid Pedvax HIB®	MF	IM	Subunit	Hib	Conjugate	Alum		Latex in stopper	
Meningitec™	BERN/WA	IM	Subunit	Men	Conjugate	Alum			
Meningococcal Polysaccharide Vaccine, Groups A and C, Menomune® A/C	SP	SC	Subunit	Men	Polysaccharide				Lactose
Menjugate®	CHIR	IM	Subunit	Men	Conjugate	Alum			

Table 1. Type and Contents of Vaccines Currently Approved for Use in Canada

Brand name	Mfr/ distr.	Route	Vaccine type	Immunogen +	Products	Adjuvant	Preservative	Potential allergens (egg, antibiotic, gelatin, latex, trace of thimerosal)	Other materials
Multidose vial Menomune® A/C/Y/W-135 Single dose vial	SP	SC	Subunit	Men	Polysaccharide		Tm† None	Latex in stopper	Lactose
M-M-R® II	MF	SC	Live	M, M, R	Live virus			Gelatine Neomycin Residual components of chick embryo cell cultures	Bovine Serum Glutamate Human albumin Residual protein from cell culture Sorbitol Sucrose
Mutacol™**	BERN	Oral	Live	Chol	Live bacteria				Yeast extract Lactose Aspartame
Neisvac-C™	BAX/ GSK	IM	Subunit	Men	Conjugate	Alum			
Pediacel®*	SP	IM	Subunit + inactivated	D, T, aP, IPV, Hib	Protein, killed virus + conjugate	Alum	PE	Neomycin Polymyxin B Streptomycin Latex in stopper	Bovine serum Formaldehyde Polysorbate 80

Part 1 — General Guidelines

11

Table 1. Type and Contents of Vaccines Currently Approved for Use in Canada

Brand name	Mfr/ distr.	Route	Vaccine type	Immunogen+	Products	Adjuvant	Preservative	Potential allergens (egg, antibiotic, gelatin, latex, trace of thimerosal)	Other materials
				Vaccine type					
Pediarix™*	GSK	IM	Subunit + inactivated	D, T, aP, HB, IPV	Protein + killed virus	Alum	PE	Polymyxin B Neomycin	Yeast protein Formaldehyde Polysorbate 80 Bovine serum albumin
Pentacel®	SP	IM	Subunit + inactivated	D, T, aP, IPV + (Hib)	Protein + killed virus + (conjugate)	Alum	PE	Polymyxin B Neomycin Latex in stopper	Bovine albumin Formaldehyde Polysorbate 80
Pneumo 23®	SP	IM/SC	Subunit	Pneu	Polysaccharide		P		
Multidose vial* Pneumovax® 23 Single dose vial	MF	IM/SC	Subunit	Pneu	Polysaccharide		P		
Prevnar®	WA	IM	Subunit	Pneu	Conjugate	Alum		Latex in stopper	
Priorix®	GSK	SC	Live	M, M, R	Live virus			Neomycin	Lactose
Quadracel®	SP	IM	Subunit + inactivated	D, T, aP, IPV	Protein + killed virus	Alum	PE	Polymyxin B Neomycin Latex in stopper	Bovine albumin Formaldehyde Polysorbate 80

Table 1. Type and Contents of Vaccines Currently Approved for Use in Canada

Brand name	Mfr/distr.	Route	Vaccine type			Adjuvant	Preservative	Potential allergens (egg, antibiotic, gelatin, latex, trace of thimerosal)	Other materials
			Vaccine type	Immunogen+	Products				
RabAvert®	CHIR/MF	IM	Inactivated	Rab	Killed virus			Neomycin Chlortetracycline Amphotericin B Processed gelatin	Human albumin Ovalbumin Bovine serum
Multidose vial Recombivax HB® Single dose vials	MF	IM	Subunit	HB	Recombinant protein	Alum	Tm† None	Latex in stopper	Yeast proteins Formaldehyde
Td Adsorbed	SP	IM	Subunit	T, d	Protein	Alum			Formaldehyde
Td Polio Adsorbed	SP	IM	Subunit + inactivated	T, d, IPV	Protein + killed virus	Alum	PE	Polymyxin B Neomycin	Bovine albumin Formaldehyde Polysorbate 80
Tetanus Toxoid Adsorbed	SP	IM	Subunit	T	Protein	Alum	Tm		
Tripacel®	SP	IM	Subunit	D, T, aP	Protein	Alum	PE	Latex instopper	Formaldehyde Glutaraldehyde
Twinrix®	GSK	IM	Subunit + inactivated	HB, HA	Recombinant protein + killed virus		PE	Neomycin Trace thimerosal Latex in stopper pre-filled syringes	Yeast proteins Formaldehyde Polysorbate 20

Table 1. Type and Contents of Vaccines Currently Approved for Use in Canada

Brand name	Mfr/distr.	Route	Vaccine type			Adjuvant	Preservative	Potential allergens (egg, antibiotic, gelatin, latex, trace of thimerosal)	Other materials
			Vaccine type	Immunogen+	Products				
Twinrix® Junior	GSK	IM	Subunit + inactivated	HB, HA	Recombinant protein + killed virus		PE	Neomycin Trace thimerosal Latex in stopper pre-filled syringes	Yeast proteins Formaldehyde Polysorbate 20
Typherix®	GSK	IM	Subunit	Typh-I	Polysaccharide		P	Latex in stopper pre-filled syringes	
Typhim Vi®	SP	IM	Subunit	Typh-I	Polysaccharide		P		
Vaqta®	MF	IM	Inactivated	HA	Killed virus	Alum		Neomycin Latex in stopper	Bovine albumin Formaldehyde Residual protein from cell culture
Varilrix®	GSK	SC	Live	Var	Live virus			Neomycin Latex in stopper pre-filled syringes for diluent	Human albumin Lactose
Varivax® III	MF	SC	Live	Var	Live virus			Gelatin Neomycin	Bovine serum Glutamate Residual protein from cell culture Sucrose Urea

Table 1. Type and Contents of Vaccines Currently Approved for Use in Canada

Brand name	Mfr/ distr.	Route	Vaccine type	Immunogen+	Products	Adjuvant	Preservative	Potential allergens (egg, antibiotic, gelatin, latex, trace of thimerosal)	Other materials
Multidose vial Vaxigrip® Single dose vial	SP	IM	Inactivated	Inf	Killed virus		Tm†	Neomycin Egg protein	Formaldehyde
ViVaxim™	SP	IM	Subunit + inactivated	Typh-I + (HA)	Polysaccharide + killed virus	Alum	PE	Neomycin	Formaldehyde
Vivotif® L	BERN	Oral	Live	Typh-O	Live virus				Lactose Aspartame
Vivotif®	BERN	Oral	Live	Typh-I	Live virus			Gelatin	Lactose
YF-VAX®	SP	SC	Live	YF	Live virus			Gelatin Egg protein Latex in stopper	Chicken protein

Empty boxes indicate a lack of the specified component.

* Drug Identification Number assigned (approved for use but not currently marketed)

** Product is on the market but not currently available

† Thimerosal in multidose vial only

Notes and Abbreviations

The information in this table is based on the product's availability as of May 2006. Please consult the manufacturer for complete and up-to-date information. The National Advisory Committee on Immunization (NACI) will publish updated information as required, which will be available at www.naci.gc.ca.

Part 1 — General Guidelines

Part 1 — General Guidelines

Manufacturer (Mfr) and Distributor (Distr.): For some products, the distributor could be different from the manufacturer.

BAX, Baxter Healthcare Corporation; *BERN*, Berna Biotech; *BIKEN*, Biken; *CHIR*, Chiron; *GSK*, GlaxoSmithKline; *IDB*, ID Biomedical Corporation; *MF*, Merck Frosst; *SBL*, SBL Vaccine; *SP*, Sanofi Pasteur Ltd; *SOLV*, Solvay; *WA*, Wyeth Canada

Route: IM - intramuscular; SC - subcutaneous

Immunogen:

+ For products in which the immunogens of two different vials or chambers are combined, the contents of the second vial or chamber are noted as + (immunogen)

The following abbreviations are the agreed upon standards for use in Canada:

DTaP-IPV-Hib: diphtheria toxoid, tetanus toxoid, acellular pertussis, polio, *Haemophilus influenzae* type b, pediatric formulation; Tdap: tetanus toxoid, diphtheria toxoid, acellular pertussis, adult formulation; Men — meningococcus; Pneu — pneumococcus; HB: hepatitis B; Chol-Ecol-O: cholera — E.coli

IPV — poliomyelitis vaccine; Inf: influenza; HA: hepatitis A; Rab: rabies; JE: Japanese encephalitis; Typh-I : typhoid — injection; Typh-O: Typhoid — Oral: TBE: tickborne encephalitis

MMR: measles, mumps, rubella; Var: varicella; YF: yellow fever; BCG: Bacilles Calmette-Guérin

Adjuvant: Alum – aluminum-containing adjuvant

Preservative:

P – phenol; PE – 2 phenoxy ethanol; Tm – thimerosal. For the Sanofi Pasteur products, PE is not considered a preservative

The Benefits of Vaccines

Vaccines have improved the lives of every Canadian. For instance, before tetanus immunization was available, the fear of tetanus hovered over every cut and puncture wound. Older adults will easily recall the vigour with which every childhood scrape was disinfected to protect against lockjaw and memories of family or friends paralyzed by polio and summers spent in fear. In the last 50 years, immunization has saved more lives in Canada than any other health intervention. Table 2 and Figures 1 and 2 illustrate the impact of childhood vaccines on infectious diseases in Canada. Please refer to the epidemiology sections in the chapters on *Hepatitis B Vaccine* (page 189) and *Pertussis Vaccine* (page 257) for additional data and charts documenting the recent successes of immunization programs against these two vaccine-preventable diseases.

Many vaccines (and some other public health interventions) result in both a benefit to health and savings in direct medical care costs. For these vaccines, the establishment of publicly funded vaccination programs improves health and results in monetary savings. Therefore, the decision to vaccinate is straightforward. Some newer vaccines result in health benefits but do not save costs. The decision to include these vaccines in vaccination programs then depends on the willingness of society to pay for the health benefits. In general, vaccination programs compare very favourably with other health interventions (Table 3). However, it is important that new vaccination programs be evaluated carefully, and that vaccine researchers and policy makers work together to identify programs that deliver the greatest benefit for the least cost.

Selected references

Centers for Disease Control and Prevention. *An ounce of prevention … what are the returns?* 2nd edition, 1999. URL: <www.cdc.gov/epo/prevent.htm>.

Ess SM, Szucs TD. *Economic evaluation of immunization strategies.* Clinical Infectious Diseases 2002;35:294-7. URL: <http://www.journals.uchicago.edu/CID/journal>.

Tengs TO, Adams ME, Pliskin JS et al. *Five hundred live-saving interventions and their cost-effectiveness.* Risk Analysis 1995;15:369-90.

US National Immunization Program, Centers for Disease Control and Prevention. *Guide to contraindications to vaccinations.* URL: <http://www.cdc.gov/nip/recs/contraindications.htm#micro>.

Table 2. Incidence of Select Vaccine-Preventable Diseases in Canada – Pre-vaccine Era Compared with Five Most Recent Years

Disease	Details	Pre-vaccine era*		2000-2004**	
		5-year average annual incidence per 100,000	Peak annual number of cases	5-year average annual incidence per 100,000	Peak annual number of cases
Diphtheria	Diphtheria toxoid introduced in 1926, routine infant immunization since 1930, national notifiable diseases reporting began in 1924	1925-29 84.2	1925-29 9,010	0.0	1
Invasive *Haemophilus influenzae* type b (Hib) in children < 5 years of age	PRP vaccine introduced in 1986, currently approved Hib PRP-T and PRP-OMP conjugate vaccines introduced in 1991/92, national notifiable diseases reporting of invasive Hib disease began in 1986	1986-90 22.7	1986-90 526	0.9	17
Measles	Live vaccine approved in 1963, MMR universal infant program implemented in 1983, 2 dose MMR introduced 1996/97, no notifiable diseases reporting from 1959-68	1950-54 369.1	1950-54 61,370	0.2	199
Mumps	Vaccine approved in 1969, MMR universal infant program implemented in 1983, 2 dose MMR introduced 1996/97, no notifiable diseases reporting from 1960-85	1950-54 248.9	1950-54 43,671	0.3	202
Pertussis	Whole cell pertussis vaccine approved in 1943, acellular pertussis vaccine replaced whole cell in 1997-98, adolescent/adult acellular formulation approved in 1999	1938-42 156.0	1938-42 19,878	10.4	4,751
Paralytic poliomyelitis	IPV approved in 1955, OPV approved in 1962 and in use in Canada until 1997, IPV used exclusively from 1998-present	1950-54 17.3	1950-54 1,584	0	0

Table 2. Incidence of Select Vaccine-Preventable Diseases in Canada – Pre-vaccine Era Compared with Five Most Recent Years

| Disease | Details | Pre-vaccine era* | | 2000-2004** | |
		5-year average annual incidence per 100,000	Peak annual number of cases	5-year average annual incidence per 100,000	Peak annual number of cases
Rubella	Rubella vaccine introduced 1969, MMR universal infant program implemented in 1983, 2 dose MMR introduced 1996/97	1950-54 105.4	1950-54 37,917	0.1	29
Congenital rubella syndrome (CRS)	See Rubella above. National notifiable diseases reporting of CRS began in 1979	1979-83 2.4†	1979-83 29	0.5†	3

* Five years preceding vaccine introduction

** Provisional numbers from National Disease Reporting System 2002-04

† per 100,000 live births

Table 3. Cost per Life Year Saved for Selected Vaccine Programs and Other Public Health Interventions (adapted from references)

	Cost per life year saved
Vaccines	
Measles, mumps, rubella for children	< 0 ($16 saved per $ spent)
DPT for children	< 0 ($6 saved per $ spent)
Influenza for adults aged ≥ 65 years of age	< 0 ($45 saved per $ spent)
Pneumococcal polysaccharide for adults aged ≥ 65 years	< 0 ($8 saved per $ spent)
Hepatitis B screening in pregnancy and vaccination of children of carriers	$164
Varicella vaccine for children	$16,000
Conjugate pneumococcal vaccine for children	$125,000
Other interventions	
Mandatory seat belt law	$69
Chlorination of drinking water	$3,100
Smoking cessation counseling	$1,000-10,000
Bicycle helmet law	$39,000
Annual screening for cervical cancer	$40,000
Driver and passenger air bags/manual lap belts (vs. airbag for driver only and belts)	$61,000
Smoke detectors in homes	$210,000
Low cholesterol diet for men over age 20 and cholesterol over 4.65 mmol/L (180 mg/dL)	$360,000
Crossing control arm for school buses	$410,000
Radiation emission standard for nuclear power plants	$100,000,000

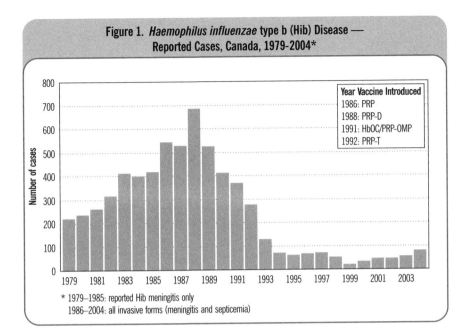

Figure 1. *Haemophilus influenzae* type b (Hib) Disease —
Reported Cases, Canada, 1979-2004*

Year Vaccine Introduced
1986: PRP
1988: PRP-D
1991: HbOC/PRP-OMP
1992: PRP-T

* 1979–1985: reported Hib meningitis only
1986–2004: all invasive forms (meningitis and septicemia)

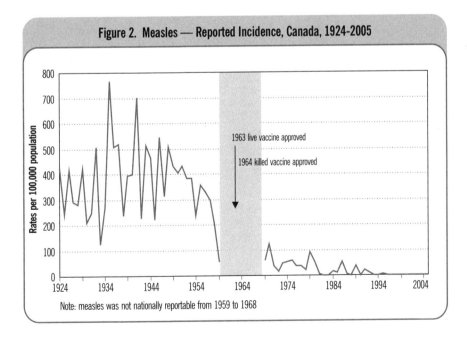

Figure 2. Measles — Reported Incidence, Canada, 1924-2005

1963 live vaccine approved

1964 killed vaccine approved

Note: measles was not nationally reportable from 1959 to 1968

Part 1 — General Guidelines

21

National Guidelines for Immunization Practices

Preamble

The current edition of the *Guide* contains many examples of the effectiveness of provincial/territorial childhood immunization programs in Canada as carried out by both private and public providers. These include elimination of wild-type poliovirus and a decrease of over 95% in the incidence of *Haemophilus influenzae* type b and measles infections. To guarantee continued success it is essential that policy makers, program administrators and providers work together, proactively, to plan, conduct and regularly review immunization programs. Furthermore, several challenges remain, such as continued documented occurrences of "missed opportunities for immunization"; subgroups of Canadians with lower than optimal vaccine coverage; evidence of incorrect handling and storage of vaccine by providers; wide variations in the reporting of adverse events following immunization; and evidence that there is insufficient communication regarding the risks and benefits of vaccines.

Accordingly, the National Advisory Committee on Immunization (NACI) has developed guidelines for immunization practices applicable to both public and private systems of vaccine delivery. The guidelines that follow resulted from extensive consultation with provincial/territorial health authorities; medical, nursing, public health and hospital organizations; and individual providers and child advocacy groups. The original guidelines (*Canadian Immunization Guide*, 6th edition) were officially endorsed by the Canadian Paediatric Society, Advisory Committee on Epidemiology, College of Family Physicians of Canada, Canadian Medical Association, Canadian Nurses Association, Aboriginal Nurses Association of Canada, Society of Obstetricians and Gynaecologists of Canada and the Canadian Public Health Association. They have been slightly modified for this edition.

The guidelines are deliberately broad, far-reaching and rigorous. They define the most desirable immunization practices that health care providers can use to assess their own current practices and identify areas of excellence as well as deficiency. It is recognized that some of the guidelines require involvement of the provinces and territories (e.g., regarding the need to track immunizations and audit coverage levels). Furthermore, some providers/programs may not have the funds necessary to fully implement the guidelines immediately. In such cases the guidelines can act as a tool to clarify immunization needs and to facilitate obtaining additional resources in order to achieve national goals and targets.

The following terms have been used throughout:

- *Provider*: any individual, nurse or physician qualified to give a vaccine

- *Regular provider*: individual usually responsible for a given child's vaccinations
- *Child/children*: the individuals (infancy to adolescence) being considered for immunization
- *Recipient*: the individual being considered for immunization
- *Parent*: the individual(s) legally responsible for the child

These guidelines are recommended for use by all health professionals in the public and private sector who administer vaccines to or manage immunization services for Canadians. Although some guidelines will be more directly applicable to one or other setting, all providers and local health officials should collaborate in their efforts to ensure that there are high coverage rates throughout the community and thus achieve and maintain the highest possible degree of community protection against **vaccine-preventable diseases.**

Guideline 1
Immunization services should be readily available.

Immunization services should be responsive to the needs of vaccine recipients. When feasible, providers should schedule immunization appointments in conjunction with appointments for other health services. Newborn infants should have the first immunization appointment arranged as soon as possible after birth. Immunization services, whether public health clinics or physicians' offices, should be available during the week and at hours that are convenient for working parents. Public sector services should be available on working days, as well as during some other hours (e.g., weekends, evenings, early mornings or lunch hours).

Guideline 2
There should be no barriers or unnecessary prerequisites to the receipt of vaccines.

While appointment systems facilitate clinic planning and avoid unnecessarily long waits, appointment-only systems may act as barriers to the receipt of vaccines. People who appear on an unscheduled basis for vaccination, particularly those in hard-to-reach populations, should be accommodated when possible. Such recipients should be rapidly and efficiently screened without requiring other comprehensive health services.

A reliable decision to vaccinate an adult or a child can be based exclusively on the information elicited from the recipient or from the child's parent, and on the provider's observations and judgment about the health of the potential vaccine recipient at the time. At a minimum, this includes questioning the patient or the child's parent about:

- the recipient's current state of health;
- potential contraindications;
- reactions to previous vaccinations.

Policies and protocols should be developed and implemented so that the administration of vaccine does not depend on individual written orders or on a referral from a primary care provider.

Guideline 3
Providers should use all clinical opportunities to screen for needed vaccines and, when indicated, to vaccinate.

Each encounter with a health care provider, including those encounters that occur during hospitalization, is an opportunity to review the immunization status and, if indicated, administer needed vaccines. Physicians should consider the immunization status at every visit and offer immunization service as a routine part of that care or encourage attendance at the appropriate public health or physician clinic. At each hospital admission the vaccination record should be reviewed and, before discharge from the hospital, patients should receive the vaccines for which they are eligible by age or health status. The patient's current immunization provider should be informed about the vaccines administered in hospital. However, successful implementation requires significant improvements in record-keeping of immunization histories (see Guideline 8).

Home care or public health nurses should use home visits as an opportunity to immunize both adults and children who are home-bound or otherwise unable to access immunization services.

Guideline 4
Providers should educate parents and adult vaccine recipients in general terms about immunization.

Providers should educate people in a culturally sensitive way, preferably in their own language, about the importance of vaccination, the diseases that vaccines prevent, the recommended immunization schedules, the need to receive vaccines at recommended ages and the importance of them bringing their or their child's vaccination record to every health care visit. Parents and adult recipients should be encouraged to take responsibility for ensuring that they or their child complete the full series. Providers should answer all questions recipients may have and provide appropriate educational materials at suitable reading levels, preferably in the patient's preferred language. Providers should familiarize themselves with information on immunization provided by the appropriate health departments as well as by other sources.

Guideline 5
Providers should inform patients and parents in specific terms about the risks and benefits of vaccines that they or their child are to receive.

Information pamphlets about routine vaccines are available from ministries of health in many provinces and territories, and also from the Canadian Paediatric Society. Such pamphlets are helpful in answering many questions that patients and parents may have about immunization, and they facilitate informed consent. Providers should document in the medical record that they have asked the patients and parents if they have any questions and should ensure that satisfactory answers to any questions were given.

Guideline 6
Providers should recommend deferral or withholding of vaccines for true contraindications only.

There are very few true contraindications to vaccination according to current Canadian guidelines, and providers must be aware of them. Accepting conditions that are not true contraindications often results in the needless deferral of indicated vaccines. Minimal acceptable screening procedures for precautions and contraindications include asking questions to elicit a history of possible adverse events following prior vaccinations and determining any existing precautions or contraindications.

Guideline 7
Providers should administer all vaccine doses for which a recipient is eligible at the time of each visit.

Available evidence indicates that most routine vaccines can be administered at the same visit, safely and effectively, including multiple injections. Some vaccines are provided in a combination format whereby more than one is given in a single injection, and others require separate injections. Unless the package insert specifically allows, vaccines should never be mixed in the same syringe.

Guideline 8
Providers should ensure that all vaccinations are accurately and completely recorded.

8.1 Data to be recorded in the patient's record at the time of vaccination

For each vaccine administered the minimum data to be recorded in the patient's record should include the name of the vaccine, the date (day, month and year) and route of administration, the anatomical site, the name of the vaccine manufacturer, the lot number, and the name and title of the person administering the vaccine.

8.2 Updating and maintaining the personal vaccination record

All providers should encourage recipients or parents to maintain a copy of their own or their child's personal vaccination record card and present it at each health care visit so that it can be updated. If a patient or parent fails to bring the card, the provider should ensure that adequate information is given so that the recipient/parent can update the card with the name(s) of the vaccine(s), the date, the provider and the facility.

8.3 Documentation for vaccines given by other providers

Providers should facilitate the transfer of information in the vaccination record to other providers and to appropriate agencies in accordance with requirements. When a provider who does not routinely vaccinate or care for an individual administers a vaccine to that individual, the regular provider should be informed.

8.4 All provinces/territories should develop and maintain electronic immunization registries.

Guideline 9

Providers should maintain easily retrievable summaries of the vaccination records to facilitate age-appropriate vaccination.

Providers should maintain separate or easily retrievable summaries of vaccination records to facilitate assessment of coverage as well as the identification and recall of patients, especially children, who are delayed in the recommended immunization schedule. In addition, immunization files should be sorted periodically and inactive records placed into a separate file. Providers should indicate in their records, or in an appropriately identified place, all primary care services that each patient receives in order to facilitate scheduling with other services.

Guideline 10

Providers should report clinically significant adverse events following vaccination – promptly, accurately and completely.

All individuals who are immunized should be given instructions for post-immunization care. Prompt reporting of adverse events following vaccination is essential to guarantee vaccine safety, allowing for timely corrective action when needed, and to keep information regarding vaccine risk-benefit and contraindications up to date.

Providers should instruct parents to inform them of adverse events following vaccination. Providers should report all clinically significant events to the local public health authority, regardless of whether they believe the events are caused by the vaccine or not. Providers should fully document the adverse event in the medical record at the time of the event or as soon as possible thereafter. At each immunization visit, information should be sought regarding serious adverse events that may have occurred following previous vaccinations.

Guideline 11

Providers should report all cases of vaccine-preventable diseases as required under provincial and territorial legislation.

Providers should know the provincial/territorial requirements for communicable disease reporting. Reporting of vaccine-preventable diseases (VPD) is essential for the ongoing evaluation of the effectiveness of immunization programs, to facilitate public health investigation of vaccine failure and to facilitate appropriate medical investigation of a patient's failure to respond to a vaccine that has been appropriately administered. Provincial data systems for VPD should be linked to electronic immunization registries.

Guideline 12
Providers should adhere to appropriate procedures for vaccine management.

Vaccines must be handled and stored as recommended in manufacturers' package inserts. The temperatures at which vaccines are transported and stored should be monitored according to provincial/territorial guidelines. Vaccines must not be administered after their expiry date, and vaccines that have undergone a breach in the cold chain should not be used without appropriate consultation.

Providers should report usage, wastage, loss and inventory as required by provincial, territorial or local public health authorities.

Providers should be familiar with published national and local guidelines for vaccine storage and handling. Providers must ensure that any office staff designated to handle vaccines are also familiar with the guidelines.

Guideline 13
Providers should maintain up-to-date, easily retrievable protocols at all locations where vaccines are administered.

Providers administering vaccines should maintain a protocol that, at a minimum, discusses the appropriate vaccine dosage, vaccine contraindications, the recommended sites and techniques of vaccine administration, as well as possible adverse events and their emergency management. The *Canadian Immunization Guide* and updates, along with package inserts, can serve as references for the development of protocols. Such protocols should specify the necessary emergency equipment, drugs (including dosage), and personnel to manage safely and competently any medical emergency arising after administration of a vaccine. All providers should be familiar with the content of these protocols, their location, and how to follow them.

Guideline 14
Providers should be properly trained and maintain ongoing education regarding current immunization recommendations.

Vaccines must be administered only by properly trained persons who are recognized as qualified in their specific jurisdiction. Training and ongoing education should be based on current guidelines and the recommendations of NACI and provincial and territorial ministries of health, the National Guidelines for Immunization Practices, and other sources of information on immunization.

Guideline 15
Immunization errors should be reported by providers to their local jurisdiction.

Immunization errors and related incidents should be monitored as a patient safety issue. All immunization errors should be reported by the vaccine provider to the agency or local sector that assumes accountability for the quality of immunization programs. Immunization errors commonly include an error in vaccine type, dose, site, route, person, time or schedule. Immunization-related incidents include a range of events, such as needle injury caused by failed restraint of children, immunization without consent, or fainting with a fall resulting in injury. Methods to detect immunization errors or incidents may include provider self-reporting, direct observation or record audits. Decreasing immunization errors requires an accurate system of error reporting in an open environment that focuses on positive reinforcement rather than punitive action. Activities to prevent immunization error in an agency or organization are a better barometer of quality than the error rate alone. Publishing or sharing information about immunization errors is a first step towards an immunization quality-improvement program that strives to reduce the incidence of errors. Immunization errors can be effectively reduced by systematically identifying, eliminating or minimizing both human and system related factors.

Guideline 16
Providers should operate a tracking system.

A tracking system should generate reminders of upcoming vaccinations as well as recalls for individuals who are overdue for their vaccinations. A system may be manual or automated, and may include mailed or telephone messages. All providers should identify, for additional intensive tracking efforts, patients considered at high risk of failing to complete the immunization series on schedule (e.g., children who start their series late or children who fall behind schedule).

Guideline 17
Audits should be conducted in all immunization clinics to assess the quality of immunization records and assess immunization coverage levels.

In both public and private sectors, an audit of immunization services should include assessment of all or a random sample of immunization records to assess the quality of documentation and to determine the immunization coverage level (e.g., the percentage of 2-year-old children who are up to date). The results of the audit should be discussed by providers as part of their ongoing quality assurance reviews and used to develop solutions to the problems identified.

Communicating Effectively about Immunization

Public concern regarding vaccine safety can reduce vaccine coverage and result in resurgence of vaccine-preventable diseases. As trusted information sources, health care providers have a vital role in the continued success of immunization programs. To be most effective, providers must have skill and expertise, not only in the principles and practices of immunization but also in risk communication. This section outlines the general principles of risk communication and identifies additional resources for providers and the public.

Principles of risk communication

The goal of effective risk communication is the development of an informed decision-making partnership. The process involves both education and advocacy, and is facilitated through advance preparation by all participants, clear messaging, and an open and respectful atmosphere. An individual's perception of risk is influenced by experience as well as personal, religious and cultural contexts. Furthermore, events that are familiar, involve a natural process, seem to be under an individual's control, are of a voluntary nature or involve a decision to forgo something are generally perceived as less risky than those that are unfamiliar, involve a man-made process, involve loss of control, are mandatory or involve a decision to do something rather than avoid something. A decision to become immunized or immunize a child clearly falls into the latter "high risk" category regardless of the true odds. Framing the risks in the right context is very important. Countering an individual's concerns by citing the greater dangers of a familiar event, like driving a car, while true, may be counterproductive.

For effective risk communication, physicians and other health care providers should attempt to do the following:

1. **Communicate current knowledge**, taking into account what an individual already knows and the level of detail requested. The process need not be time-consuming. It is useful to have varied information formats (visual, audio, printed material, Web sites) tailored to a range of educational levels and languages as appropriate to a given practice/clientele. Given the volume, accessibility and variable quality of material available on the Internet, it is also helpful to provide guidance on how to assess Web site reliability. Several excellent resources are listed at the end of this section.

2. **Respect differences of opinion about immunization.** Some individuals will express reluctance or refusal to accept immunization for themselves or their children. It is important to both gauge the strength of this stance as well as discover its underlying reasons.

29

3. **Represent the risks and benefits of vaccines fairly and openly.** Contrast the known and theoretical risks of vaccine with the known risks associated with the vaccine-preventable infection (see at the end of this *Guide* for a table on *Comparison of Effects of Diseases and Vaccines*). It is also important to counter the notion that vaccine-preventable diseases are gone (see box).

4. **Adopt a patient-centred approach.** Effective decision making is best done in a partnership between the provider or vaccinator and the parent or patient. Central to this is the acceptance that individuals have input into the decision to immunize and retain responsibility for their own or their child's health. A decision to do something rather than to avoid something may cause greater concern when it comes to immunizing children. It may be helpful to present the facts and then ask those responsible to consider what the child would choose, were he or she old enough to do so.

5. **Make the most of each opportunity to present clear, evidence-based messages regarding vaccines and immunizations (see box).** Encourage questions, address misinformation, and provide valid and appropriate resources, including authoritative Web sites, for those who want more information.

Conclusion

As long as the diseases that vaccines prevent are rarely seen by the general public today, vaccine safety concerns will continue to have a high profile. Careful and timely counselling can help people to weigh the benefits of vaccines and the risks of the disease that the vaccine will prevent, as well as the small risk posed by the vaccine itself. By providing vaccines in a climate of appropriate informed consent, including discussion of commonly held misconceptions, health care providers can help ensure that immunization will maintain its status as one of the most effective preventive measures in the history of medicine.

Immunization Truths

- Immunization is the best protective strategy against vaccine-preventable diseases.

- The vaccines used in Canada are both effective and safe.

- Health authorities worldwide take vaccine safety very seriously. Expert committees in Canada investigate reports of serious adverse events following immunization.

- Vaccines do not weaken the immune system. Rather, they harness and train it to defend, rapidly, against vaccine-preventable pathogens before illness can occur.

- Vaccine-preventable infections are far more dangerous than vaccines (see the Table on *Comparison of Effects of Diseases and Vaccines* at the end of the Guide).

- The bacteria and viruses that cause vaccine-preventable diseases are not gone.

  - Diphtheria, pertussis, polio, measles, mumps, rubella, varicella, hepatitis A and B are well adapted human pathogens that, to a greater or lesser extent, are contagious and are still occurring in parts of the world.
  - Tetanus is a soil organism – it will never be eliminated.
  - *Haemophilus influenzae* type b, *Streptococcus pneumoniae* and *Neisseria meningitidis* can survive in the nose and throat and will likely never be completely eliminated.

- Unvaccinated individuals have a much greater chance of getting a vaccine-preventable disease than those who have received the vaccine. This is true even in countries where high levels of immunization provide some degree of protection to susceptible individuals (i.e., herd immunity). Three examples:

  - An outbreak of rubella occurred in 2005 among unimmunized individuals in Ontario.
  - Children in the United States who did not receive measles vaccine were 22 to 35 times more likely to get measles than immunized children.
  - Children in the United States who did not receive pertussis vaccine were almost 6 times more likely to get whooping cough than immunized children.

- When vaccine coverage drops, vaccine-preventable diseases return:

  - In Japan, pertussis vaccine coverage dropped from 90% to less than 40% because of public concern over two infant deaths that followed DPT immunization. Prior to the drop in coverage there were 200 to 400 cases of pertussis each year in Japan. From 1976 to 1979, following the marked drop in vaccine coverage, there were 13,000 cases of pertussis, of which over 100 were fatal.
  - In Ireland, measles vaccine coverage dropped to 76% following allegations of a link with autism. The number of measles cases increased from 148 in 1999 to 1200 in 2000, along with several child deaths due to the complications of measles.

References and Web resources for immunization risk communication

A. How to communicate

Spier RE. *Perception of risk of vaccine adverse events: a historical perspective.* Vaccine 2001;20:S78-84.

Stoto MA, Evans G, Bostrom A. *Vaccine risk communication.* American Journal of Preventive Medicine 1998;14(3):237-39.

Summary. Workshop on Vaccine Communication, October 5-6, 2000, Arlington, Virginia. URL: <http://www.dhhs.gov/nvpo/pubs/vcwsummary.pdf>.

Tenrreiro KN. *Time-efficient strategies to ensure vaccine risk/benefit communication.* Journal of Pediatric Nursing 2005;20:469-76.

B. What to communicate

Canadian Coalition for Immunization Awareness and Promotion. *Addressing patient concerns.* URL: <http://www.immunize.cpha.ca/english/links/hlthprv.htm> (English); <http://www.immunize.cpha.ca/francais/hcprovdf/provresf/provparf.htm> (French).

Canadian Paediatric Society. URL: <www.cps.ca>

Children's Hospital of Philadelphia Vaccine Education Center. URL: <http://www.chop.edu/consumer/jsp/microsite/microsite.jsp?id=75918>.

Gold R and Canadian Paediatric Society. *Your child's best shot: a parent's guide to vaccination,* 2nd ed. 2002. URL: <www.cps.ca/english/publications/Bookstore/YourChildsBestShot.htm>.

Immunization Action Coalition. URL: <www.immunize.org>. (Information in several formats, including video.)

National Network for Immunization Information. URL: <www.immunizationinfo.org>. *Communicating with patients about immunization.* URL: <http://www.immunizationinfo.org/healthProfessionals/resource_kit.cfm>.

C. How to evaluate Web site quality and reliability

Centers for Disease Control and Prevention. URL: <http://www.immunizationinfo.org/parents/evaluatingWeb.cfm > (tips on how to assess vaccine Web sites).

World Health Organization. URL: <http://www.who.int/immunization_safety/safety_quality/vaccine_safety_websites/en/>. Vaccine safety net – lists sites with information related to vaccine safety that meet criteria related to credibility, content, accessibility and design.

Principles of Combination Vaccines

Combination vaccine products are already available for many immunizations conducted in Canada. Diphtheria, tetanus and polio vaccines have been available as a combination product for over 30 years. Since 1996, all infants in Canada have been vaccinated against diphtheria, tetanus, pertussis, polio and *Haemophilus influenzae* type b (DTaP-IPV-Hib) with a single, pentavalent vaccine.

Over the past few years, the number of combination vaccine products has grown considerably, and this trend will continue with more vaccines being introduced to the routine immunization schedule for children and adults. As new products are recommended, it is important for the immunization provider to feel comfortable with the principles of combination vaccines. This chapter serves as a general overview of these principles. For details on specific combination vaccines, please refer to the individual chapters in this *Guide*.

What is a combination vaccine?

Combination vaccines are developed to protect against more than one infection. Polyvalent vaccines against multiple strains or serotypes of the same infectious agent are not considered to be combination vaccines. The term "combined vaccines" may also be used to describe the mixture of two separate vaccines in a single vial prior to administration or vaccines that are separately manufactured but combined into one product during the final packaging stages.

General principles of combination vaccines

◆ Combination vaccines are rigorously evaluated before approval for use in Canada. Only those combinations that are known to be safe and efficacious are recommended for routine use. For an overview of vaccine safety, including that of specific combination products, please refer to the chapter on *Vaccine Safety*, page 59.

◆ Ideal combination vaccines are as safe and effective as each of their single component counterparts.

◆ Combination vaccines should fit the currently recommended schedule, be easily stored and easy to administer.

◆ Combination vaccines facilitate adherence to recommended immunization schedules by reducing the number of immunization visits required as well as the number of injections a person receives.

- Combination products can potentially decrease the amount of adjuvants and preservatives when compared with multiple, single-antigen products.

- Health care providers should never combine products that are intended for separate administration.

Efficacy of combination vaccines

- The efficacy of each component in a combination vaccine is compared with established parameters of protection before approval.

- Antibody responses to specific antigens in combination products may be either stronger or weaker than those to separately administered single antigens.

- The impact of any observed changes in antibody titres is assessed against the known human protective levels of antibodies or other indicators of efficacy.

- Combination vaccines approved to date have an efficacy and safety record similar to that of single-component vaccines.

  - The addition of Hib to the combination vaccine with tetanus, diphtheria, acellular pertussis and polio did not result in diminished immune responses to the tetanus, diphtheria, acellular pertussis and polio components. The response to the Hib antigens was somewhat reduced; however, a significant impact on clinical efficacy when the vaccine was administered according to the Canadian immunization schedule was not demonstrated through post-marketing studies.

Safety of combination vaccines

- The currently available combination products in Canada have had excellent safety records.

- Ideal combination vaccines should have fewer adverse reactions or, at the very least, no more than if administering single-antigen products separately.

- The safety of each new combination product is rigorously evaluated prior to approval and compared against the safety of single-antigen products or existing combination vaccines.

- New combination vaccines help to further our knowledge regarding co-administration of antigens as combination vaccines, as they are all well evaluated before approval.

- The vaccine provider may face questions from parents about their feelings that multiple combination vaccines can weaken the immune system.

- With the refinement of vaccine development and production over past decades, children today are exposed to far fewer vaccine antigens than in the past, even though they are immunized against more infections with more combination vaccines.

- Children are naturally exposed to multiple antigens on a routine basis. They respond well to these persistent exposures with no untoward effects on their immune system.

- If multiple antigens posed a problem for the immune system, we would find that infants vaccinated with combination products had less protection against the infection than those vaccinated with single products. This has not been found.

Complexities of combination vaccines

- The efficacy and safety of each component in a combination must be evaluated separately and in its combined form, thereby increasing the complexity of pre-approval clinical trials.

- Clinically important interference between each component of a combination vaccine must be ruled out. Antibody responses to individual antigens in combination products may be diminished. Given that antibody responses are only a surrogate for clinical efficacy, assessing or estimating the clinical relevance of this is complex. In the development of new combination products, acceptable endpoints and immunization goals should be clearly defined.

- The measurement of potency and antigen content of combination products is more complex and difficult.

- Even a single, transient problem in the production of an individual component of a combination product could lead to a significant shortage in vaccine supply for multiple diseases.

- In the context of combination products, the effects of adjuvants can be difficult to assess.

- It can be difficult to determine which component is responsible for an allergic or other adverse event.

- There are usually increased costs associated with combination product procurement.

Principles of Vaccine Interchangeability

This chapter provides the health care provider with an overview of the general principles of vaccine interchangeability for the currently approved vaccines in Canada.

The principles of interchangeability are only applicable to vaccines with the same indication and specified for the same population (i.e., the same age groups). It has now become routine to have similar vaccines from different manufacturers approved for use in Canada. Several factors may necessitate giving different products to the same individual over time. When faced with vaccine shortages, deferring vaccination is not desirable: one study demonstrated that 25% of children whose vaccination had been deferred never returned for the indicated vaccine.

Factors to consider in determining potential candidate vaccines for interchangeability

- The vaccines should be approved with the same indications, specified for the same population and be equally acceptable in terms of safety, reactogenicity, immunogenicity and efficacy.

- A regularly scheduled primary or booster vaccine should not be deferred because of the lack of availability of a particular product.

- Any new regimen should be equally acceptable from a safety, efficacy and scheduling perspective.

- Even when vaccines are approved for the same indications, different manufacturers often use different production methods, antigen concentrations, stabilizers and preservatives. Each of these could affect the immunogenicity, safety or efficacy profile of the product.

Interchangeability following provincial variations in immunization schedules and products

- At present, the immunization schedules as well as the specific products used may vary across the provinces and territories.

- With immigration and migration of people between provinces and territories, issues of vaccine interchangeability have arisen with specific concern regarding measles, mumps, rubella (MMR), varicella and meningococcal conjugate vaccines.

- For DTaP-IPV-Hib, the primary immunization series of three doses given in infancy should, whenever possible, be completed with a single combination product. However, on the basis of expert opinion, if the original vaccine is not known or not available, it is recommended that an alternative combination product be used to complete the primary immunization series. According to expert opinion and the limited data available to date, NACI recommends that the DTaP-IPV-Hib and DTaP-IPV combination vaccine products currently approved for sale in Canada may be used interchangeably for the 18 month and 4-6 year booster, respectively.

◆ On the basis of expert opinion, the MMR products currently available in Canada may be used interchangeably if required.

◆ On the basis of expert opinion, the varicella products currently available in Canada may be used interchangeably if required

Development of evidence for interchangeability

Ideally, as new combination vaccines become available, there should be randomized controlled clinical trials evaluating their interchangeability with existing products. This has only been done in limited instances to date. Most of our knowledge regarding interchangeability has been gathered as a result of situations of vaccine shortages, immigration to areas where different vaccine products are available, and new product purchases with the negotiation of new contracts. Given the importance of this issue and the limited data available regarding the interchangeability of early childhood vaccines, every opportunity should be taken to encourage further research in this area.

Vaccine Administration Practices

Appropriate vaccine administration is a key element to ensuring the optimal safety and efficacy of vaccines. Vaccine administration practices are based on clinical trials that determine the dose, route and schedule for each vaccine. Professional standards for medication and vaccine administration and federal/provincial/territorial policies and procedures, where these exist, also guide vaccination practices. All providers of vaccines should receive education and competency-based training on vaccine administration before providing vaccines to the public. Programs should be in place to monitor the quality of immunization services. The following information provides general guidance for vaccine administration practices.

Pre-vaccination counselling

Prior to vaccination, the vaccine provider should ensure that the vaccine recipient is capable of consenting to the procedure or that, when required, an appropriate guardian or substitute decision maker is present to give consent. Information regarding the risks and benefits of both receiving and not receiving the vaccination should be provided, along with the opportunity to ask questions. Minor side effects that occur frequently and any adverse effects that are severe should be discussed with the individual, guardian or substitute decision maker. This person should be asked about all relevant contraindications and precautions to receiving the vaccine. Care should be taken to determine whether there is a risk of anaphylaxis, such as previous anaphylaxis or severe allergy to any of the vaccine components or latex, if contained in the vaccine products. For more information, please refer to the *General Contraindications and Precautions* chapter, page 73.

Vaccine administration

Vaccines should be administered using the recommended dose, route, site and schedule to optimize vaccine effectiveness and reduce the risk of local reactions or other adverse events.

Vaccine preparation

- ◆ Vaccine inspection: The vaccine identification label and expiry date on the vaccine vial or package should be checked by the vaccine provider before administration. Vaccines should not be used beyond their expiry date. If only the month and year are provided for the expiry date, the vaccine can be used to the end of that month. Multi-dose vials should be labelled with the date of first entry into the vial and, unless otherwise specified by the manufacturer, should be discarded after 30 days of the date of first entry. Before use, vaccine vials should be inspected for any irregularities, e.g., particulate matter, damage or contamination. Vaccines should be mixed with a careful swirling motion until a uniform suspension is achieved prior to administration.

◆ Vaccine reconstitution: Vaccines requiring reconstitution, i.e., a lyophilized product that is mixed with a diluent, should be mixed only with the diluent supplied for the vaccine unless otherwise permitted by the manufacturer.

◆ Pre-loading vaccines in syringes: Ideally, a vaccine should be withdrawn from the vial by the vaccine provider administering the vaccine. Pre-loading syringes with vaccine is discouraged because of the uncertainty of vaccine stability in syringes, risk of contamination, increased potential for vaccine administration errors and vaccine wastage. Pre-loading of syringes in the hospital setting where vaccines are drawn up and labeled in the pharmacy may be considered. In addition, to facilitate timely and efficient administration of a single vaccine to a large number of people in an immunization clinic setting, pre-loading of syringes may be considered. However, if implemented, this practice should be limited to these settings and should include the following: 1) prior agreement on how professional accountability can be ensured if different people pre-load and administer the vaccine, 2) data on stability of pre-loaded product for a specified time period and 3) maintenance of the cold chain.

Syringe and needle selection

◆ Syringe selection: A separate, sterile syringe should be used for each injection, and different vaccines should not be mixed in the same syringe unless specified by the manufacturer as part of the reconstitution and administration procedure. Depending on the dosage, a 3 mL or 1 mL syringe should be selected.

◆ Needle selection: Needle selection should be based on the route of administration, individual's age, size of the muscle mass and viscosity of the vaccine:

  • For intradermal (ID) injections, a 26-27 gauge needle is recommended.

  • For subcutaneous (SC) injections, a 25 gauge, 1.6 cm (5/8") needle is recommended.

  • For intramuscular injections (IM) a 22-25 gauge needle that is long enough to reach muscle is recommended:

    · 2.2 cm (7/8") to 2.5 cm (1") for infants

    · 2.2 cm (7/8") to 2.5 cm (1") for toddlers and older children

    · 2.5 cm (1") to 3.8 cm (1½") for adolescents and adults

The needle should be inserted as far as possible into the muscle. A larger bore needle (e.g., 22 gauge) may be required when administering viscous or larger volume products such as immune globulin.

Restraint

After informed consent, the process of vaccine administration should be shared with the individual, and restraint procedures should be explained. The parent or guardian should hold a child with specific instructions on restraint positioning. Failed restraint can result in inaccurate dose, inappropriate depth of injection or injury to the individual being immunized and/or vaccine provider.

Injection site, route and technique

Vaccines and other biologic products are injected via ID, SC or IM routes.

- ID injections:
  - ID injections are usually administered on the flexor surface of the forearm.
  - The bevel of the needle should be turned upwards and at an angle parallel to the forearm.
  - The needle is inserted so that the bevel penetrates the skin. If done correctly, a small bleb should be observed at the injection site upon injection of the vaccine.
- SC injections: SC injections are usually given at a 45° angle into subcutaneous tissue of the upper triceps area of the arm.
- IM injections:
  - IM injections are administered at a 90° angle into the vastus lateralis muscle (anterolateral thigh) in infants < 1 year of age and the deltoid muscle of anyone ≥ 1 year of age (unless the muscle mass is not adequate). Appropriate site selection is important to avoid inadvertent injection into a blood vessel or injury to a nerve. Some vaccine providers prefer to pull back on the plunger (aspiration) to determine whether the needle has entered a blood vessel. There are no studies that have assessed the need for aspiration prior to IM injection of vaccines in relation to vaccine safety. As well, the syringes provided for immunization may not allow aspiration.
  - The buttock should not be used for active immunization. Immunogenicity is lower to hepatitis B and rabies vaccines if given in the buttock, probably because of injection into adipose tissue where the vaccine is not well mobilized. The buttock is an acceptable site for administration of immune globulin when large volumes are adminis-

tered, but appropriate site selection of the gluteal muscle is necessary to avoid injury to the sciatic nerve.

- Vaccines containing adjuvants are to be injected intramuscularly. If inadvertently injected subcutaneously or intradermally, increased inflammation, induration or granuloma formation may occur.

Please see Table 1, which outlines the route of administration of all vaccines approved for use in Canada, in the *General Considerations* chapter, page 7.

Multiple injections

There are no contraindications to giving multiple vaccines at the same clinic visit, and all opportunities to immunize should be utilized. Giving multiple injections at one visit helps to ensure that children are up to date with the vaccines required for their age. Generally, infants and children have similar immune responses whether vaccines are given at the same time or at different visits. Although children are now receiving more vaccines, they are exposed to fewer antigenic proteins in today's vaccines than in the past because of changes in the vaccine products. Practice considerations for multiple injections include the following:

- Vaccines prepared in separate syringes should be labelled in order to identify which vaccine each syringe contains. The site of administration of each vaccine should be recorded.

- Separate limbs should be used if two IM injections are required. If more than two injections are required, two injections may be administered into the same muscle separated by at least 2.5 cm (1").

- Vaccines that are known to cause more stinging and/or pain should be given last.

Techniques to decrease pain and anxiety

Pain associated with immunizations is generally described as mild and short-lived, and no specific pain reduction strategies are recommended for routine use. However, the following strategies can be considered for individuals who are particularly concerned about immunization pain.

- Swaddling, holding or sucking on a pacifier.

- Breastfeeding infants or offering sweet-tasting solutions such as oral sucrose or glucose.

- Distraction techniques, such as books, video games, cartoons, movies, bubble and party blowers for older children; children can be instructed to "blow away the pain" using party blowers, windmills or bubbles.

- Pharmacologic agents such as EMLA (eutectic mixture of local anesthesia, consisting of 2.5% lidocaine and 2.5% prilocaine), Ametop® gel (4% amethocaine) and vapocoolants (e.g., Fluori-Methane). Studies have demonstrated that EMLA does not affect the immunologic response to MMR, DTaP-IPV-Hib (Pentacel®), hepatitis B (Recombivax®) or Bacille Calmett-Guérin (BCG) vaccinations. EMLA needs to be applied approximately 60 minutes before the injection. Ametop® gel produces anesthesia within 30 to 40 minutes and has been shown not to interfere with the immunologic response to MMR vaccine. Vapocoolants are effective immediately after application.

Techniques to decrease anxiety in adolescents and adults are important to minimize the risk of fainting. These techniques include ensuring that the temperature in the room is comfortable, avoiding long line-ups in mass immunization clinics and administering the vaccine while the person is seated. Patients who appear very anxious should be observed while seated until anxiety has resolved after the immunization.

After the vaccination

After vaccination, vaccine recipients should be counselled on common side effects and the reporting and management of these reactions. Vaccine providers should identify and observe individuals who are particularly anxious about receiving the vaccine. Individuals with presyncopal symptoms such as pallor or sweating should sit or lie down until symptoms resolve. A study using the American Vaccine Adverse Reporting System found that 63% of syncopal events occurred within 5 minutes of vaccination, and 89% occurred within 15 minutes. It is therefore prudent to keep the person in the clinic for 15 minutes after vaccination. This will also facilitate the management of the rare anaphylactic event. All vaccination providers should have the necessary training and equipment to manage anaphylactic events Please refer to the *Anaphylaxis: Initial Management in Non-Hospital Settings* chapter, page 80.

Infection prevention and control (IPC)

Immunization providers should incorporate routine infection control practices into all immunization procedures:

- The vaccine vial should be uncapped, wiped with a suitable disinfectant (e.g., isopropyl alcohol) and allowed to dry prior to withdrawal of vaccine into the syringe.

- Before injection, the skin should be cleansed with a suitable antiseptic and allowed to dry.

- A separate, sterile needle and syringe should be used for each injection.

- Hand hygiene should be performed before vaccine preparation, between vaccine recipients, and whenever the hands are soiled. Alcohol-based hand sanitizers are an alternative to hand washing with soap and water. Glove use during immunization is not routinely recommended, unless the skin on the vaccine provider's hands is not intact. The Health Canada (now the Public Health Agency of Canada) document on Infection Control Guidelines, *Routine Practices and Additional Precautions for Preventing the Transmission of Infection in Health Care,* provides information on IPC precautions.

- Additional practices recommended during immunization include the following:

  - Needles used during immunization should not be recapped after use.

  - Used syringes and needles should be immediately and carefully disposed of in a container designed for this purpose and should never be laid down on the work surface.

  - Used syringes with attached needles and empty or expired vaccine vials should be disposed of according to local waste management legislation or guidelines.

Occupational health

- All vaccine providers should be offered hepatitis B vaccine. Post-immunization serologic testing should be obtained to ensure that there is an adequate antibody response. Please refer to the *Hepatitis B Vaccine* chapter, page 189, for more information.

- Procedures for accidental exposure to blood or body fluids should be in place and understood by vaccine providers.

Vaccine administration check list

- Is the vaccine indicated according to the recommended immunization schedule and the individual's immunization history?
- Has the appropriate consent been obtained?
- Are there any contraindications to vaccination?
- Has the expiry date been checked?
- Has the vaccine provider washed his or her hands or used an alcohol-based hand sanitizer?
- Has the vaccine been appropriately reconstituted and/or mixed?
- Are the dose and route of administration correct?
- Is the appropriate needle gauge and length being used in the correct site?
- Has the appropriate documentation been completed?
- Have post-vaccination instructions been given to the vaccine recipient?

Selected references

Alberta Health and Wellness. *Multiple injections workbook*. 2004. (A participant workbook for use in conjunction with the Multiple Injections video to provide the rationale and evidence-based nursing practice guidelines for administration of multiple injections from an Alberta perspective.)

American Academy of Pediatrics. *Red book 2003: report of the Committee on Infectious Diseases*, 26th edition. Elk Grove Village, Illinois: AAP, 2003.

Atkinson W, Hamborsky J, Wolfe S eds. *Epidemiology and prevention of vaccine-preventable diseases*, 8th edition. Washington DC: Public Health Foundation, 2004;G1-G19.

Braun MM, Patriarca PA, Ellenberg SS. *Syncope after immunization*. Archives of Pediatrics and Adolescent Medicine 1997;151(3):255-59.

Centers for Disease Control and Prevention. *General recommendations on immunization: recommendations of the Advisory Committee on Immunization Practices and the American Academy of Family Physicians*. Morbidity and Mortality Weekly Report 2002;51(RR-2):1-35.

Centers for Disease Control and Prevention. *Suboptimal response to hepatitis B vaccine given by injection into the buttock*. Morbidity and Mortality Weekly Report 1985;34(8):105-108.

Halperin BA, Halperin SA, McGrath P et al. *Use of lidocaine-prilocaine patch to decrease intramuscular injection pain does not adversely affect the antibody response to diphtheria-tetanus-acellular pertussis-inactivated poliovirus-Haemophilus influenzae type b conjugate and hepatitis B vaccines in infants from birth to six months of age*. Pediatric Infectious Disease Journal 2002;21(5):399-405.

Halperin SA, McGrath P, Smith B et al. *Lidocaine-prilocaine patch decreases the pain associated with subcutaneous administration of measles-mumps-rubella vaccine but does not adversely affect the antibody response*. Journal of Pediatrics 2000;136(6):789-94.

Health Canada. *Routine practices and additional precautions for preventing the transmission of infection in health care*. Canada Communicable Disease Report 1999;25(S4). URL: <http://www.phac-aspc.gc.ca/publicat/ccdr-rmtc/99pdf/cdr25s4e.pdf>.

Jacobson RM, Swan A, Adegbenro A et al., Vaccine Research Group. *Making vaccines more acceptable – methods to prevent and minimize pain and other common adverse events associated with vaccines*. Vaccine 2001;19:2418-27.

O'Brien L, Taddio A, Ipp M et al. *Topical 4% amethocaine gel reduces the pain of subcutaneous measles-mumps-rubella vaccination*. Pediatrics 2004;114(6):720-24.

Offit PA, Quarles J, Gerber MA et al. *Addressing parents' concerns: Do multiple vaccines overwhelm or weaken the infant's immune system?* Pediatrics 2002;109(1):124-29.

Reis EC, Holubkov R. *Vapocoolant spray is equally effective as EMLA cream in reducing immunization pain in school-aged children*. Pediatrics 1997;100(6). URL: <http://pediatrics.aappublications.org/cgi/reprint/100/6/e5?maxtoshow=&HITS=10&hits=10&RESULTFORMAT=&author1=Holubkov%2C+R&fulltext=EMLA&searchid=1130332254570_349&stored_search=&FIRSTINDEX=0&sortspec=relevance&journalcode=pediatrics>.

Storage and Handling of Immunizing Agents

Immunizing agents are biologic materials that are subject to gradual loss of potency from deterioration and denaturation. Loss of potency can be accelerated under certain conditions of transport, storage and handling, and may result in failure to stimulate an adequate immunologic response, leading to lower levels of protection against disease. Conditions that result in loss of potency vary among products.

The province or territory should follow Public Health Agency of Canada guidelines to ensure that the manufacturer monitors the cold chain during the shipment of vaccine. Also, the province or territory should have a standard for monitoring shipments to regions, public health units and private offices. Manufacturer and NACI recommendations generally specify that most products should be stored at temperatures from +2° to +8° C. Exceptions exist (e.g., yellow fever) for which the recommended storage conditions are −30° to +5° C, as outlined in the manufacturer's product leaflets.

The term "cold chain" as used in this statement refers to all equipment and procedures used to ensure that vaccines are protected from inappropriate temperatures and light, from the time of transport from the manufacturer to the time of administration.

The effects of exposure to adverse environmental conditions, such as freezing, heat and light, are cumulative. Data are available to indicate that certain products remain stable at temperatures outside of +2° to +8° C for specified periods of time, but mechanisms rarely exist for monitoring the effect of cumulative exposures. Additionally, different products are often transported and stored in the same container. Therefore, it is recommended that all biologics for immunization be maintained at +2° to +8° C at all times, unless otherwise specified in the product leaflet. Management of products that have been exposed to adverse conditions should be guided by specific instructions pertaining to the conditions from the vaccine supplier.

Monitoring of the vaccine cold chain is required to ensure that biologics are being stored and transported at recommended temperatures. Testing of product potency or seroconversion rates as indicators of cold chain integrity are rarely feasible.

Refer to the product leaflet of each immunizing agent for specific instructions related to storage and handling. The following general principles apply.

Multidose vials

Multidose vials should be removed from the refrigerator only to draw up the dose required and should be replaced immediately. Although the practice of drawing vaccines and leaving them in the refrigerator in advance of administration is strongly discouraged (see page 39 in the *Vaccine Administration Practices* chapter), two exceptions are noted:

- Pre-loading of syringes in the hospital setting where vaccines are drawn up and labeled in the pharmacy. Strict adherence to cold chain procedure for transport of the vaccine to the ward and patient bedside is required.

- Pre-loading of syringes in an immunization clinic setting. This may be considered in order to facilitate the flow of the clinic. Proper labeling and adherence to cold chain is required

Vaccine providers should observe strict aseptic technique when using multidose vials. Multidose vials should be dated once entered and used only for the period of time specified in the manufacturer's product leaflet. If no directions are given the vaccine should not be used beyond 30 days after initial entry into the vial.

Lyophilized (freeze-dried) vaccines

For optimal potency, freeze-dried vaccines (e.g., measles, mumps rubella [MMR], varicella, Bacille Calmette-Guérin [BCG], *Haemophilus influenzae* type b) should be reconstituted immediately before use with the diluent provided for that purpose. Reconstituted vaccines, including yellow fever vaccine, should be used within 1 hour of reconstitution; if unused, they should be discarded. There are slight variations in the time intervals recommended by specific manufacturers, and users should refer to the product leaflet to guide timing of reconstitution.

Light exposure

MMR, varicella and BCG vaccines should be protected from light at all times by storage of the vials in the cartons provided. After reconstitution, if vaccines are not used immediately, they **must** be kept at +2° to +8° C, protected from light and used within the time frame recommended in the product leaflet.

Freezing

Vaccine providers are reminded that the maintenance of cold chain also requires that vaccines not be exposed to temperatures lower than those recommended. Liquid inactivated and adsorbed vaccines should not be used if they have been frozen. These include Tdap, DTaP, DT, DTaP-Polio, DT-Polio, Td, Td-Polio, hepatitis A and B vaccines, influenza, pneumococcal and meningococcal vaccines. Before use, liquid vaccines should be inspected and should not be used if the usual appearance is altered or a temperature recording device shows that the vaccine was exposed to temperatures below zero.

Expiry

Vaccines should not be used beyond their expiry date. For expiry dates specified as month/year, products are deemed to expire on the last day of the specified month. The error of administration of expired vaccine should be reported to the local public health authority.

Disposal of spoiled or expired vaccines

All vaccines that cannot be used because of expiry or adverse environmental exposure should be returned to the source for appropriate recording of returns and disposal or should be appropriately disposed of according to local or regional standards.

Refrigerators

The temperature in frost-free refrigerators may cycle widely and should be monitored to ensure that cycling is within the acceptable range. Special maximum-minimum thermometers are commercially available for purchase and are useful for most office storage. Vaccine providers should record daily current maximum and minimum refrigerator temperatures and contact the local public health unit if vaccines are exposed to temperatures outside the recommended range. More expensive, constant chart-recording thermometers with alarms are appropriate for larger vaccine storage depots. Non-frost-free refrigerators should be defrosted regularly and immunizing agents stored in a functioning refrigerator during the defrosting process. Refrigerators older than 10 years are more likely to malfunction and to have breaks in the seal around the door, leading to temperature instability. Half-size/under the counter/bar refrigerators are less reliable than full-size kitchen refrigerators. Vaccine providers in private practice will discover that the cost of replacing ageing bar refrigerators with newer and full-size equipment is offset by the savings in hydroelectric power and staff time dealing with reporting and fixing cold chain breaks.

Placement of full, plastic water bottles in the lower compartment and door shelves of the refrigerator and ice packs in the freezer compartment will help stabilize temperatures, especially in the event of a power failure.

Recommended office procedures

The following office procedures should be implemented to ensure that storage of vaccines is optimized:

♦ Designate and train a specific staff person to be responsible for managing vaccines.

♦ Post storage and handling guidelines on the refrigerator.

♦ Use insulated storage containers with ice packs for transport of vaccines; to avoid freezing, do not place vaccine packages in direct contact with ice packs. Practitioners transporting vaccines out of the office (e.g., to housebound seniors) should observe these cold chain precautions as well.

♦ When transporting vaccines, keep a log of pre- and post-transport vaccine temperatures and the specific batches transported.

♦ Place newly delivered vaccines into the refrigerator immediately upon delivery to the office.

♦ Store vaccines in the middle of the refrigerator to avoid the coldest and warmest parts of the refrigerator; do not store vaccines on the door shelves.

♦ Place a maximum-minimum thermometer on the middle shelf of the fridge.

♦ Read, record and re-set the thermometer at least once daily.

♦ Secure the electrical cord from the fridge to the wall outlet to prevent accidental power interruptions.

♦ Ensure that the fridge door does not accidentally swing open by installing a fail-safe (e.g., Velcro™) closing mechanism.

♦ Do not store food or biologic specimens in the same fridge as vaccines.

♦ Rotate stock so that vaccines with the earliest expiry date are at the front of the shelf. Place expired vaccine into a marked box in the refrigerator for appropriate disposal, based on consultation with local public health authorities.

♦ Vaccine should only be removed from the refrigerator immediately prior to administration.

♦ If refrigerator malfunction is suspected on the basis of temperature readings, obtain servicing immediately and store the vaccine in an alternative refrigerator in the meantime.

♦ In the event of an identified cold chain break, seek advice from your local public health authority about whether the vaccine(s) may continue to be used; while awaiting advice, keep the vaccines stored in appropriate cold chain conditions and ensure that they are not administered until a determination has been made by the public health authority.

- When a cold chain break is identified after vaccine has been administered, consult with the local health department about management of the situation. Information required to assess the circumstances will include the name of the vaccine(s), and the duration and temperatures of exposure. People immunized with vaccines whose potency is likely to have been jeopardized may need to be tested for serologic evidence of immunity or be re-vaccinated.

Ongoing cold chain monitoring should be integrated into immunization practice. Periodic cold chain surveys are worthwhile to evaluate awareness, equipment and practices as well as the frequency of breaks in the cold chain during transport from depots and storage in peripheral offices. These should be undertaken by provincial/territorial and local immunization programs.

Selected references

Carrasco P, Herrera C, Rancruel D et al. *Protecting vaccines from freezing in extremely cold environments.* Canada Communicable Disease Report 1995;21(11):97-101.

Cheyne J. *Vaccine delivery management.* Reviews of Infectious Diseases 1989;11(S3): S617-S622.

Deasy T, Deshpande R, Jaiyeola A et al. *Evaluating the cold chain in Ontario: results of a province-wide study.* Public Health Epidemiological Report, Ontario 1997;8(3):44-52.

Dimayuga RC, Scheifele DW, Bell A. *Survey of vaccine storage practices: Is your office refrigerator satisfactory?* British Columbia Medical Journal 1996;38(2):74-7.

Gold MS, Martin L, Nayda CL et al. *Electronic temperature monitoring and feedback to correct adverse vaccine storage in general practice.* Medical Journal of Australia 1999;171(2):83-4.

Guthridge SL, Miller NC. *Cold chain in a hot climate.* Australian and New Zealand Journal of Public Health 1996;20(6):657-60.

Health Canada. *Guidelines for temperature control of drug products during storage and transportation.* Ottawa: Health Canada, 2005. URL: <http://www.hc-sc.gc.ca/dhp-mps/compli-conform/gmp-bpf/docs/gui-0069_tc-tm_e.html>. Accessed November 17, 2005.

Health Canada. *National guidelines for vaccine storage and transportation.* Canada Communicable Disease Report 1995;21(11):93-7.

Jeremijenko A, Kelly H, Sibthorpe B et al. *Improving vaccine storage in general practice refrigerators.* British Medical Journal 1996;312(7047):1651-52.

Kendal AP, Snyder R, Garrison PJ. *Validation of cold chain procedures suitable for distribution of vaccines by public health programs in the USA.* Vaccine 1997;15(12-13):1459-65.

Krugman RD, Meyer BC, Enterline JC et al. *Impotency of live-virus vaccines as a result of improper handling in clinical practice.* Journal of Pediatrics 1974;85(4):512-14.

Lerman SJ, Gold E. *Measles in children previously vaccinated against measles.* Journal of the American Medical Association 1971;216(8):1311-14.

Milhomme P. *Cold chain study: danger of freezing vaccines.* Canada Communicable Disease Report 1993;19(5):33-8.

Steinmetz N, Furesz J, Reinhold C et al. *Storage conditions of live measles, mumps and rubella virus vaccines in Montreal.* Canadian Medical Association Journal 1983;128(2):162-63.

Woodyard E, Woodyard L, Alto WA. *Vaccine storage in the physician's office: a community study.* Journal of the American Board of Family Practice 1995;8(2):91-4.

World Health Organization. *Expanded programme on immunization: stability of vaccines.* Weekly Epidemiological Record 1990;65(30):233-35.

World Health Organization. *Report of the Technical Review Group Meeting, 7-8 June 1998: achievements and plan of activities, July 1998-June 1999.* Geneva: World Health Organization, 1998 (Technical Report Series, No. 98.02).

Yuan L, Daniels S, Naus M et al. *Vaccine storage and handling: knowledge and practice in primary care physicians' offices.* Canadian Family Physician 1995;41:1169-76.

Timing of Vaccine Administration

For most products that require more than one dose or booster doses for full immunization, intervals longer than those recommended between doses do not lead to a reduction in final antibody concentrations. Therefore, as a general rule, *interruption of a series of vaccinations for any reason does not require starting the series over again, regardless of the interval elapsed.* By contrast, doses given at less than the recommended interval may result in less than optimal antibody response and should not be counted as part of a primary series.

There are obvious practical advantages to giving more than one vaccine at the same visit, especially for infant immunization schedules, for travel immunization or when there is doubt that an individual will return for further doses of vaccine. No increase in the frequency or severity of clinically significant side effects has been observed. The immune response to each antigen is generally adequate and comparable to that found in persons receiving these vaccines at separate times.

Simultaneous administration of childhood vaccines (diphtheria, tetanus, acellular pertussis [DTaP]; inactivated poliovirus [IPV]; *Haemophilus influenzae* type b [Hib]; measles, mumps, and rubella [MMR]; varicella; pneumococcal conjugate and hepatitis B vaccine) is encouraged for children who are the recommended age to receive these vaccines and for whom no contraindications exist. If not given during the same visit as other live virus vaccines, administration of two live vaccines should generally be separated by at least 4 weeks. A number of vaccines that deliver protection against more than one disease (i.e., combination vaccines) are available and approved for use in Canada.

Simultaneously administering pneumococcal polysaccharide vaccine and inactivated influenza vaccine elicits a satisfactory antibody response without increasing the incidence or severity of adverse reactions. Therefore, simultaneous administration is strongly recommended for all persons for whom both vaccines are indicated.

Different formulations of vaccine against the same disease (e.g., pneumococcal conjugate and pneumococcal polysaccharide vaccine or meningococcal conjugate and meningococcal polysaccharide vaccine) cannot be given simultaneously, and a minimum time interval should elapse between the administration of the two formulations.

Vaccines administered simultaneously should be given using separate syringes at separate sites unless otherwise specified by the manufacturer, with consideration being given to the precautions that apply to each individual vaccine.

Part 1 — General Guidelines

51

MMR vaccine can decrease the immunologic response to tuberculin skin testing, resulting in false-negative results. Therefore, tuberculin skin tests should be given either on the same day as MMR immunization or at least 4-6 weeks later. The effect of other live virus vaccines such as varicella and yellow fever vaccines on tuberculin reactivity is currently unknown, and no recommendations for postponement of tuberculin skin testing can be made at this time.

Please refer to the specific vaccine chapters in this *Guide* for further information.

Selected references

Centers for Disease Control and Prevention. *General recommendations on immunization: recommendations of the Advisory Committee on Immunization Practices (ACIP) and the American Academy of Family Physicians (AAFP)*. Morbidity and Mortality Weekly Report 2002;51(RR-2):1-35.

Centers for Disease Control and Prevention. *Travelers' health: yellow book. Health information for international travel, 2005-2006*. URL: <http://www.cdc.gov/travel/>.

Centers for Disease Control and Prevention. *Typhoid immunization: recommendations of the Advisory Committee on Immunization Practices (ACIP)*. Morbidity and Mortality Weekly Report 1994;43(RR-14):1-7.

Centers for Disease Control and Prevention. *Yellow fever vaccine: recommendations of the Advisory Committee on Immunization Practices (ACIP), 2002*. Morbidity and Mortality Weekly Report 2002;51(RR-17):1-10 .

DeStefano F, Goodman RA, Noble GR et al. *Simultaneous administration of influenza and pneumococcal vaccines*. Journal of the American Medical Association 1982;247(18):2551-54.

Halperin S, McDonald J, Samson L et al. *Simultaneous administration of meningococcal C conjugate vaccine and diphtheria-tetanus-acellular pertussis-inactivated poliovirus-Haemophilus influenzae type b conjugate vaccine in children: a randomized double-blind study*. Clinical and Investigative Medicine 2002;25(6):243-51.

King GE, Hadler SC. *Simultaneous administration of childhood vaccines: an important public health policy that is safe and efficacious*. Pediatric Infectious Disease Journal 1994;13(5):394-407.

Yvonnet B, Coursaget P, Deubel V et al. *Simultaneous administration of hepatitis B and yellow fever vaccines*. Journal of Medical Virology 1986;19(4):307-11.

Recent Administration of Human Immune Globulin Products

Passive immunization with products of human origin can interfere with the immune response to live viral vaccines. For measles vaccine and varicella vaccine, the recommended interval between immune globulin (Ig) or other blood products and subsequent immunization varies from 3 to 11 months, depending on the specific product and dose given, as shown in Table 4 (page 54).

For an optimum response to rubella or mumps vaccine given as individual components, there should be an interval of at least 3 months between administration of Ig or blood products and immunization. If given as combined measles, mumps and rubella (MMR) vaccine, as is the usual circumstance in Canada, longer intervals, as recommended in Table 4, should be followed to ensure that there is an adequate response to the measles component.

For women susceptible to rubella who are given Rh Ig in the peripartum period, MMR should be administered as soon as possible following delivery to increase the likelihood that these susceptible women get vaccinated. Serologic testing should be done 2 months later and non-immune women should be re-vaccinated. After receipt of an Rh Ig product, an interval of 2 months should elapse before varicella vaccine is administered to varicella-susceptible women.

If administration of an Ig preparation becomes necessary after varicella or MMR or any of the individual MMR component vaccines have been given, interference can also occur. If the interval between administration of any of these vaccines and subsequent administration of an Ig preparation is < 14 days, immunization should be repeated at the interval indicated in Table 4, unless a serologic test conducted after this recommended interval (given in the Table) indicates immunity. If the Ig product is given > 14 days after the vaccine, immunization does not have to be repeated.

Studies have found no evidence that Ig administration interferes with the response to inactivated vaccines, toxoids or the live vaccines for yellow fever or polio. Orally administered polio vaccine is no longer used in Canada. Yellow fever vaccine is not affected by either the simultaneous or previous use of Ig preparations. The background antibody level for typhoid is low in Canada, and therefore an Ig preparation produced in Canada is unlikely to interfere with typhoid immunization. Because there is little interaction between Ig preparations and inactivated vaccines or the live vaccines specified above, these vaccines can be given before, concurrently or after an Ig preparation has been used. The vaccine and Ig preparation should be given at different sites. Dukoral™ (oral, inactivated travellers' diarrhea and cholera vaccine) is the only vaccine currently marketed in Canada for protection against cholera and, as noted previously for other inactivated vaccines, no interference should be expected when Ig is administered.

A humanized, monoclonal anti-respiratory syncytial virus (RSV) antibody (palivizumab) is available for prevention of respiratory syncytial virus infection in high-risk infants and young children. This product contains only antibody to RSV and therefore will not interfere with the immune response to vaccines; it can be administered at the same time at a separate site.

Table 4. Guidelines for the Interval Between Administration of Immune Globulin Preparation or Blood Products and MMR or Varicella Vaccines*

Product	Dose	Interval (months)
General products†		
Immune globulin (Ig)	0.02-0.06 mL/kg	3
	0.25 mL/kg	5
	0.50 mL/kg	6
Intravenous immune globulin (IVIg)	160 mg/kg	7
	320 mg/kg	8
	640 mg/kg	9
	> 640-1280 mg/kg	10
	> 1280-2000 mg/kg	11
Plasma and platelet products	10 mg/kg	7
Reconstituted RBCs	10 mg/kg	3
Washed RBCs	10 mg/kg	0
Agent-specific products		
Hepatitis B immune globulin (HBIg)	0.06 mL/kg	3
Rabies immune globulin (RabIg)	20 IU/kg	4
RSV Ig (palivizumab)	15 mg/kg/month	0
Rh immune globulin (RhIg)	300 µg	2**
Tetanus immune globulin(TIg)	250 units	3
Varicella immune globulin (VarIg)	12.5 units/kg	5

* This table was originally developed for guidance related to the use of measles vaccines. It has been generalized to include recommendations related to the use of varicella vaccine.

† RBC = red blood cells

** Based on expert opinion: for women susceptible to rubella who are given Rh Ig in the peripartum period, MMR should be administered as soon as possible following delivery and serologic testing done 2 months later to assess the immune response.

Immunization Records

Vaccines administered to an individual should be recorded in three locations:

- the personal immunization record held by the person or his or her parent/guardian;
- the record maintained by the health care provider who gave the immunization; and
- the local or provincial registry.

Each method of recording should include the following:

- trade name of the product;
- disease(s) against which it protects;
- date given (day, month and year);
- dose;
- site and route of administration;
- manufacturer;
- lot number;
- name and title of person administering the vaccine.

Pre-printed, peel-off labels and bar coding of products will facilitate such recording. Manufacturers are encouraged to produce these labels and to bar code products. Immunization registries should have mechanisms that will allow bar coded information about the products to be read into the database.

Personal immunization records: Each person who is immunized should be given a permanent personal immunization record. Individuals should be instructed to keep the record in a safe place and bring it to immunization visits. Parents should maintain these records on behalf of their children and pass them on to their children at the appropriate time, such as when they are leaving home. Immunization records may be required for children to attend school or child-care centres. Adults may be required to produce these records in order to work in certain professions, such as health care, teaching or occupations requiring foreign travel. Relevant information, such as rubella and hepatitis B serology or tuberculin skin test results, can also be recorded in the personal immunization record.

Health care provider records: Health care providers must also maintain a record of all vaccinations provided. In addition to information about vaccinations given, the health care provider's record should include all relevant serologic data (e.g., rubella serologic results, hepatitis B surface antibody titres) and should document adverse events following immunization as well as contraindications, exemptions or reasons for deferring vaccination. It is recommended that a summary of immunizations, serologic results and any significant adverse vaccine reactions be stored in an easily retrievable manner that permits regular checking and updating of the individual's immunization status (i.e., immunization information should not be archived in a medical record). Electronic medical records used by health care providers should have the capacity to collect and easily retrieve all required vaccination information. Vaccine providers should forward the immunization information to other providers and/or to agencies, such as public health, as appropriate or required by legislation.

Immunization registries: There are several advantages to maintaining immunization records in a registry. On an individual level, immunization registries prevent immunizations already given by another health care provider from being duplicated.

A comprehensive immunization registry system will serve the following functions:

- facilitate the timely, accurate recording of all relevant immunization information regardless of where and by whom the vaccines were administered;
- identify children and adults who are overdue for immunizations and generate reminders and recalls for these individuals;
- allow health care providers to review immunization status at each encounter in a confidential, secure manner and produce immunization records for their patients;
- provide data for public health professionals to assess immunization rates, and plan and evaluate targeted interventions for populations with less than optimal immunization rates.

Where immunization registries exist, immunization providers should be aware of legislative or other requirements to report immunization information to these registries. Incomplete information can significantly decrease the benefits derived from an immunization registry. Strategies should be employed to maximize participation by health care providers.

Refer to the *National Guidelines for Immunization Practices,* page 22, for additional information about the use and maintenance of immunization records.

Selected references

Canadian Immunization Registry Network (CIRN). URL: <http://www.phac-aspc.gc.ca/im/cirn-rcri/index.html>.

Feikema SM, Klevens RM, Washington ML et al. *Extraimmunization among US children.* Journal of the American Medical Association 2000;283(10):1311-17.

Health Canada. *Functional standards and minimum (core) data sets for a National Immunization Registry Network and Vaccine Associated Adverse Event Surveillance System.* Canada Communicable Disease Report 2002;28(S6):1-38.

Part 2

Vaccine Safety and Adverse Events Following Immunization

Vaccine Safety

Introduction

Vaccine safety is of the highest importance and concern for all vaccine stakeholders. As vaccine-preventable infections have decreased, the spotlight of public and mass media concern has shifted to vaccine safety. Since vaccines are usually given to healthy people, especially children, tolerance for adverse events is low. Perceived vaccine safety risks get as much attention as real ones and can be difficult to dispel despite credible scientific evidence. Loss of confidence threatens the continued success of immunization programs.

Health care providers have essential and pivotal roles to play in gaining and maintaining public confidence in the safety of vaccines These include providing evidence-based information on the benefits and risks of vaccines; helping clients and patients to interpret media and Internet vaccine safety messages; and identifying and reporting adverse events following immunization. Any single occurrence of an unusual event following immunization may be coincidental or caused by the vaccine. An accumulation of reports, sometimes as few as four or five, may signal a risk due to the vaccine. Thus, each and every report submitted by vaccine providers is important.

This new chapter has been added to the *Canadian Immunization Guide* for the following reasons:

- to highlight the critical importance of ongoing post-marketing vaccine safety surveillance by describing how vaccines are evaluated and regulated, and the scientific limitations of pre-marketing assessments;

- to provide an overview of Canada's vaccine safety surveillance system with specific information not only on how to report adverse events but also on how such information is used to ensure that immunization programs, in Canada and internationally, remain as safe as possible;

- to provide an overview of the type and quality of evidence available to inform vaccine safety;

- to summarize the current status of key vaccine safety issues;

- to provide a list of key resources and references on vaccine safety.

Vaccine evaluation and regulation

The development of a new vaccine starts with pre-clinical laboratory testing to ensure that vaccine candidates produce the immune response needed to prevent disease and have no toxicities that would prevent their use in people. Human studies then proceed through several phases involving progressively more subjects. Table 1 describes the phases of vaccine evaluation in terms of how many subjects are studied and what is learned.

Depending on the specific vaccine, it may take years to decades to gather the scientific immunogenicity, safety and efficacy data needed to obtain authorization for marketing. However, pre-marketing vaccine studies do not have sufficient numbers of subjects to detect rare or very rare adverse events, the frequency of which is shown in Table 2. Furthermore, all potential target populations have not been fully studied prior to marketing approval. Thus, ongoing post-marketing studies of vaccine safety and effectiveness are essential, not only to gather data on new vaccines but also to monitor existing vaccines for any change in the frequency of known events that might occur if newly released vaccine lots do not perform as expected. Post-marketing data help to refine the benefit-risk assessment of a given vaccine as well as add to key information regarding contraindications, warnings and concomitant use with other vaccines.

The Biologics and Genetic Therapies Directorate (BGTD) of Health Canada is the regulatory authority responsible for establishing the safety, efficacy and quality of all biologics for human use, including vaccines (http://www. hc-sc.gc.ca/dhp-mps/brgtherap/index_e.html). BGTD reviews the clinical and chemistry/manufacturing information of vaccine submissions, and conducts on-site evaluations of manufacturing facilities and laboratory analysis of vaccines. The clinical information includes data from clinical trials, and post-marketing safety and efficacy information. BGTD will

Table 1. Stages of Clinical Vaccine Assessment and Detectable Adverse Events

Phase	Number of subjects	Key study objectives
I	10-<100	• Immunogenicity • Local/systemic reactions
II	50-500	• Optimal dose/schedule in target population(s) • Ongoing safety assessment
III	300-30,000	• Immunogenicity/efficacy in target population(s) • Ongoing safety assessment
Regulatory authorization for vaccine marketing		
IV	Varies with study objectives (100 to many thousands)	• Immunogenicity/efficacy in not yet studied populations • Possible interactions with other vaccines • Expanded safety assessment
Post-marketing passive or active surveillance	General population	• "Real world" effectiveness • Rare or unexpected adverse events ("signals")

grant a marketing authorization for the vaccine if the evidence to support the safety, efficacy and quality of the vaccine is considered adequate and sufficient.

Subsequently, if there are any changes in chemistry/manufacturing procedures or new clinical information pertaining to approved products, vaccine manufacturers must submit information for BGTD approval. The nature, extent and importance of the changes affecting the approved vaccine will determine whether additional clinical testing is required and whether the changes must be communicated to vaccine users through updated labeling and revisions of the product monograph.

A product monograph is the official labeling document for a vaccine and must be approved by Health Canada when the vaccine is first authorized for marketing and each time the information is updated. It is a factual, scientific document that, devoid of promotional material, describes the properties, claims, indications, conditions and any other information required for optimal, safe and effective use of the vaccine. It must accurately reflect important information and results from clinical trials and other relevant information submitted to Health Canada for evaluation. The product monograph consists of three parts:

◆ **Health professional information:** contains prescribing information, including indications, contraindications, warnings and precautions, adverse reactions, interactions, dosage, administration and storage instructions.

◆ **Scientific information:** contains a summary description of the preclinical, toxicological and clinical testing of the vaccine and any other pertinent scientific information with relevant references.

◆ **Consumer information:** contains an abbreviated summary, written in simplified language, to communicate essential information to the vaccine or product recipient/user.

Table 2. Description of Terms Used for the Frequency of Adverse Events Following Immunization

Related adjective	Detectable range*
Very common	> 1/10
Common	> 1/100 and < 1/10
Uncommon	> 1/1000 and < 1/100
Rare	> 1/10,000 and < 1/1,000
Very rare	< 1/10,000

* The units for the detectable range may vary depending on how the data were derived and may be doses of vaccine administered, number of subjects immunized or doses of vaccine distributed.

Product monographs may contain proprietary information and thus are not generally made available in their entirety, although many manufacturers now publish them on their Web sites. The package insert in marketed vaccines is an abbreviated form of the product monograph and usually contains the same prescribing information as is found in part 1 of the full monograph. Information on a specific vaccine found in other publications, including the *Compendium of Pharmaceuticals and Specialties* (CPS), is not controlled by Health Canada. The vaccine manufacturer may choose to include all, selected or modified parts of the information from the product monograph.

To further establish ongoing quality, safety and efficacy, all vaccines are released on a lot-by-lot basis. For each lot, BGTD reviews production protocols submitted by the manufacturer and performs selective confirmatory testing as appropriate to each vaccine.

Vaccine safety surveillance and assessment in Canada

In 2005 the name of Canada's vaccine safety surveillance system was changed from the Vaccine Associated Adverse Event Surveillance System (VAAESS) to the Canadian Adverse Event Following Immunization Surveillance System (CAEFISS). This change harmonizes Canadian terminology with what is used by the World Health Organization (WHO) and many other countries. Furthermore, it describes the nature of such events more accurately, in that adverse events do indeed follow immunization, but the temporal association is not proof that the event was caused by the vaccine.

In Canada a standard report form is available on the Internet (http://www.phac-aspc.gc.ca/im/aefi-form_e.html), through public health units and in the CPS. This form includes check boxes to facilitate the reporting of selected adverse events of special interest (e.g., anaphylaxis, injection site reactions, neurologic events) but also should be used to report all other severe, unusual or unexpected adverse events that are of concern to the vaccine provider, health care provider, vaccine recipient or his/her parent(s)/caregiver(s). Vaccinees and/or their parents/caregivers should therefore be advised to notify their health care provider about any adverse event of concern. Information on the report form facilitates monitoring and follow-up of adverse events at the local/provincial level, and causality assessment and signal detection at the national level. Confidentiality and privacy of health information are maintained throughout.

Surveillance

Monitoring vaccine safety in Canada involves passive and active surveillance and, as necessary, focused ad hoc studies.

◆ **Passive surveillance:** this encompasses all spontaneous adverse event reporting. Health care providers complete reports and submit them to their local health unit or Medical Officer of Health. From there, reports are sent to the central provincial/territorial health department, which in turn forwards them to the Immunization and Respiratory Infections Division within the Centre for Infectious Disease Prevention and Control at the Public Health Agency of Canada (PHAC). This federal office is responsible for maintaining a national database of all reported adverse events. The database also includes reports from vaccine manufacturers, which are required by law to submit all adverse event reports to PHAC and, if serious, to do so within 15 calendar days of receipt (http://www.phac-aspc.gc.ca/publicat/ccdr-rmtc/00vol26/26s1/26s1e_e.html). In some jurisdictions, reports related to vaccines that are not publicly funded are submitted by vaccine providers directly to PHAC. If in doubt it is best to check with the provincial/territorial public health department as to where the report should be sent.

♦ **Active surveillance:** for severe adverse events following childhood immunizations this type of surveillance has been conducted in Canada since 1991 by the Immunization Monitoring Program ACTive (IMPACT). This is a pediatric, hospital-based network funded by PHAC and administered by the Canadian Paediatric Society. The 12 IMPACT hospitals encompass approximately 90% of tertiary care pediatric beds in Canada. Details on the network and lists of relevant publications can be found at http://www.cps.ca/english/proadv/IMPACT/IMPACT.htm. All serious adverse events detected by IMPACT are to be reported to the vaccinee's home provincial/territorial public health authorities, as well as to PHAC.

♦ **Ad hoc studies:** additional surveillance, as well as epidemiologic or clinical studies, may be undertaken by public health or academic investigators to further characterize adverse events of concern, assess whether or not there is a causal link between the vaccine and a given adverse event or learn about risk factors that increase the likelihood that an adverse event will occur. Examples of such studies include those done following the recognition of oculorespiratory syndrome (ORS) following influenza vaccination.

Causality assessment

Special review of serious and unusual adverse events (life-threatening, such as anaphylaxis or those associated with 3 or more days of hospitalization, congenital abnormality, residual damage or death) is conducted by the Advisory Committee on Causality Assessment (ACCA), which comprises pediatricians, immunologists, epidemiologists and other experts. In addition, any unusual events or cluster of events may be reviewed by ACCA. The primary mandate of ACCA is to evaluate the degree to which such events are linked to the implicated vaccine (for more information see http://www.phac-aspc.gc.ca/im/vs-sv/acca_e.html). The process of causality assessment requires sufficient case detail to be sure the adverse event diagnosis is accurate and to judge the potential contribution of underlying disease, intercurrent illness or concomitant medication(s). Since details are often missing in the submitted report it is usually necessary to contact the original reporter for additional information before ACCA can review a case. Plausible biologic mechanisms, as well as the availability and strength of existing scientific evidence to support or reject a causal association between the vaccine and a given adverse event, are all taken into consideration. The findings of ACCA are communicated back to the provinces/territories from which the report originated.

Global partners in vaccine safety

Canada actively participates in several international endeavours to monitor and improve vaccine safety on a global scale. Adverse event reports are forwarded to the WHO Uppsala Monitoring Centre for entry into a global pharmacovigilance database (http://www.who-umc.org/DynPage. aspx?id=13140&mn=1514). These data are regularly scanned to identify any safety signals of potential concern. Canada is an active participant in the Brighton collaboration (http://www.brightoncollaboration.org), which seeks to standardize and harmonize adverse event definitions for use in all phases of vaccine testing, as outlined in Table 1. Canada is represented on the WHO Global Advisory Committee on Vaccine Safety (http://www.who. int/vaccine_safety/en/) and also participates in ad hoc consultations and committees set up by the WHO to review specific issues in vaccine safety. Canada also cooperates with the Council for International Organizations of Medical Sciences (CIOMS, http://www.cioms.ch/), which is an international, non-governmental, non-profit organization established jointly by WHO and UNESCO in 1949 to facilitate and promote international activities in the field of biomedical sciences, including making recommendations on the assessment and monitoring of adverse reactions.

Evidence pertaining to vaccine safety: where to find it, how to interpret it

Temporal associations

Since vaccines are usually given to healthy people, any event that follows soon after immunization may be perceived as being due to the vaccine. This is particularly true for events with no proven cause, such as autism, most encephalopathies and multiple sclerosis. Multiple immunizations are given during early childhood because that is the period of greatest human vulnerability to vaccine-preventable morbidity and mortality. However, it is also a critical period of growth and development during which damage due to genetic, in utero and/or other post-natal influences may first become apparent. Consideration should always be given to the possibility of an association between the vaccine and an adverse event. However, other possibilities must also be considered. These include infections and concomitant medications, as well as diseases due to genetic, environmental or other factors. Adverse events due to these other causes may simply occur by chance after the administration of a vaccine.

Chance associations illustrate the greatest vulnerability of universal immunization programs. If a vaccine truly causes a given event, even if rare, the association can be proven by a well-designed study with sufficient subjects. In contrast, the absence of association or "zero risk" cannot be proven by epidemiologic methods. Even if no association is repeatedly shown in a number of studies, it is always possible to theorize that an association might be found in another group of individuals who have not been studied. It is not possible to demonstrate that there is a 100% certainty that no person has ever had the adverse event of interest. An element of doubt will always remain, although it can be stated that the risk is very close to zero.

Clinical trials have repeatedly shown that placebo recipients experience adverse events, which clearly cannot be due to the vaccine. In a randomized placebo-controlled trial of varicella vaccine among healthy children aged 1 to 14 years, the vaccinees ($n = 491$) and placebo recipients ($n = 465$) had a similar frequency of irritability (24% and 20%, respectively), tiredness (20%, 22%), headache (15%, 16%), cough (45%, 48%), common cold (63%, 65%), poor sleep (12%, 13%) and loss of appetite (11%, 13%) during the 8-week period after immunization. Rigorous trials such as this are very helpful because they allow the assessment of the degree to which adverse events are attributable to the vaccine as opposed to other factors.

Vaccine attributable risk

This is defined as the difference between the frequency of adverse events in otherwise comparable vaccinated and unvaccinated individuals. Figure 1 illustrates that not all health problems noted after immunization are caused by vaccine. In a population of immunized children, the number of illnesses or clinical symptoms compatible with an adverse event increased in the week after hepatitis B immunization but returned to pre-vaccination levels thereafter. The vaccine can be implicated only for this "excess" of illness (or attributable risk [AR]).

As another example, in a Finnish study of cross-over design, each twin of 581 pairs was given either measles, mumps and rubella (MMR) vaccine or placebo in a blinded fashion, and 3 weeks later was administered the other substance. Adverse events were monitored for 21 days after immunization. Table 3 clearly shows that some children in the placebo group experienced fever throughout the follow-up period, but the only significant differences (AR) between placebo and MMR groups occurred from days 7 to 12.

Randomized, placebo-controlled trials

These trials provide the most reliable and valid evidence pertaining to vaccine safety. Unfortunately such trials are not done for all vaccines nor are they usually large enough to detect rare adverse events.

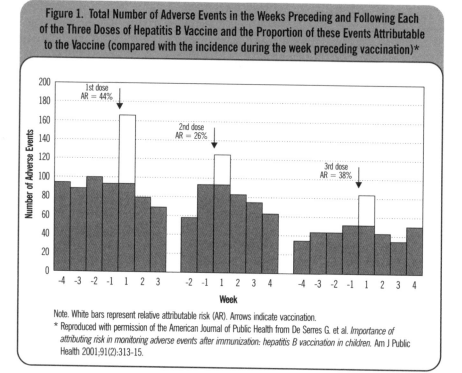

Figure 1. Total Number of Adverse Events in the Weeks Preceding and Following Each of the Three Doses of Hepatitis B Vaccine and the Proportion of these Events Attributable to the Vaccine (compared with the incidence during the week preceding vaccination)*

Note. White bars represent relative attributable risk (AR). Arrows indicate vaccination.

* Reproduced with permission of the American Journal of Public Health from De Serres G. et al. *Importance of attributing risk in monitoring adverse events after immunization: hepatitis B vaccination in children.* Am J Public Health 2001;91(2):313-15.

Table 3. Percentage of Children with Fever after MMR Immunization or Placebo Injection in 581 Twin Pairs*

	Days after injection				
	1-6	7-8	9-10	11-12	13-21
MMR	17.2%	20.3%	24.0%	19.9%	16.2%
Placebo	17.0%	18.0%	17.9%	17.5%	16.5%
Difference or attributable risk	0.2%	2.3%	6.1%	2.4%	−0.3%

* Calculated from data presented in Table II in Peltola H, Heinonen OP. *Frequency of true adverse reactions to measles, mumps, rubella vaccine.* Reprinted with permission from Elsevier Science. Lancet 1986;1(8487):939-42

Population-based epidemiologic studies

Such studies use **cohort** (i.e., they compare the adverse event rate in immunized versus non-immunized populations) or **case-control** methodologies (i.e., they compare the proportion of cases with an adverse event and controls without an adverse event who were exposed to vaccine) to test hypotheses regarding a causal association between a given vaccine and an adverse event. However, the validity, generalizability and utility of data from such studies are highly dependent on study design. Since exposure to vaccine is not random in the study populations, several sources of bias exist that may confound the results.

Ecologic studies

Ecologic studies take advantage of "natural experiments" to test hypotheses regarding vaccines and adverse events. For example, the occurrence of autism might be compared during two separate periods of time in a country that switched from thimerosal-containing to thimerosal-free vaccines. As another example, the prevalence of multiple sclerosis might be compared in a country that has never introduced hepatitis B vaccine to one that has been using the vaccine for decades. A major methodologic problem with such studies is the inability to control for multiple confounding factors that may not be equally distributed or applicable to the time periods or geographic areas being compared. For example, differences in diagnostic criteria, standards of health practice and/or health-seeking behaviour could confound the results in favour of or against the hypothesis.

Reports of single or multiple cases

These reports often represent the first evidence of a possible link between a vaccine and an adverse event. As discussed earlier, chance temporal associations between vaccine(s) and subsequent adverse events are relatively common occurrences given the frequency of disease that occurs in any given population. In certain rare instances, a well-documented case report can establish a causal relation such as death due to disseminated BCG or unrelenting measles infection following administration of BCG vaccine or measles vaccine, respectively, to a severely immunocompromised host. The vaccine strains are distinguishable from naturally circulating disease strains (commonly referred to as "wild type"). Thus recovery of the vaccine types from body tissue(s) in conjunction with histopathological changes consistent with severe infection is usually considered proof of causality. However, the vast majority of case reports represent unproven temporal associations that require confirmation using scientifically sound methodologies.

Spontaneously submitted reports to passive surveillance systems

Reports sent to CAEFISS or the Vaccine Adverse Event Reporting System (VAERS) in the United States provide the weakest evidence of a causal association between a vaccine and the reported adverse event. It is essential to understand that proving causality is not the intent of passive surveillance. Rather, such systems are put in place to identify signals of concern as early as possible. Subsequently, specific studies must be designed to test the hypothesis that the adverse event is truly caused by vaccine. Illustrative of this process is the recent US experience with rotavirus vaccine. Regular analysis of VAERS data revealed an increased frequency of reports of intussusception (the "signal") in infants following the introduction of live attenuated rotavirus vaccine. Subsequently, several case-control studies confirmed the hypothesis of a link between rotavirus vaccine and intussusception, and the vaccine was withdrawn from the market. In Canada oculorespiratory syndrome (ORS) following immunization with influenza vaccines used in 2000 was recognized through an increased frequency of reports to the passive surveillance system. Following those observations several studies were done to characterize the causes and determinants of ORS, and modifications were made to one of the implicated vaccines before the 2001 influenza vaccine campaign.

There is currently public access to data from VAERS. Public access to CAEFISS data is planned, with announcements to be posted at the PHAC vaccine safety web site, http://www.phac-aspc.gc.ca/im/vs-sv/index.html, as soon as it is initiated. This is essential, given the need for transparency and openness regarding reported adverse events in order to maintain public confidence in immunization programs. However, the data are frequently misinterpreted and used to draw inappropriate conclusions regarding risks associated with immunization. Since many of the allegations presented on the Internet and in mass media result from inappropriate use of such data, health care professionals need to clearly understand both the purpose (as described above) and the limitations of passive surveillance systems:

- lack of an appropriate control group

- reporting bias. This stems from several factors that increase the rate of reporting other than a true increased frequency of a given adverse event. Examples include the following:
  - major media focus on allegations such as a link between autism and MMR vaccine
  - markedly increased frequency of immunization such as occurs during mass vaccine campaigns for outbreaks of infection due to *Neisseria meningitidis*
  - enhanced awareness following recognition of clusters of specific adverse events such as ORS

- lack of use of and/or adherence to standard case definitions

- incomplete detail to support a given diagnosis and/or to consider other possible causes, such as intercurrent infection or concomitant medication

- underreporting

- inability to determine the frequency of association since the total number of persons immunized is unknown:
  - the Internet often contains allegations of "hot lots" based on data from VAERS, which publishes the lot numbers associated with adverse event reports. However, the number of actual vaccine doses distributed for a given lot can vary from thousands to millions. If the lot size is unknown it is impossible to determine the lot-specific incidence of a given adverse event.

Expert-based reviews of vaccine safety issues

Vaccine safety is an issue of global concern. Although there are variations in vaccine products used in different countries, the similarities in terms of immunogen are such that much can be learned from expert reviews of specific issues, including examination of published and unpublished data. Currently, there are three sources of such reviews: the WHO, the Institute of Medicine and the Cochrane Collaboration.

World Health Organization: Details of the many WHO initiatives involving vaccine safety are available on the Internet (http://www.who.int/immunization_safety/en/). Two initiatives deserve further mention here as sources of reliable information on vaccine safety issues. In 1999 the Global Advisory Committee on Vaccine Safety (GACVS) was established to provide prompt, scientific evidence-based responses to safety issues of global concern. The expert committee meets every June and December, and soon afterwards posts reports of its deliberations on the WHO Web site (http://www.who.int/vaccine_safety/en/) and publishes these in the Weekly Epidemiological Record (http://www.who.int/wer/en/). The Web site also has a "topics" page that not only summarizes committee conclusions and recommendations but also provides links to other key publications or information on the specific issue. The other initiative, Vaccine Safety Net (http://www.who.int/immunization_safety/safety_quality/vaccine_safety_websites/en/), has been developed by GACVS to promote and identify Web sites on vaccine safety that adhere to good information practices.

Institute of Medicine (IOM): Formed in 1970 by the U.S. National Academy of Sciences (NAS), the IOM functions as an independent, expert professional body that examines issues of relevance to the health of the public (http://www.iom.edu). From 1977 through 1994 the IOM committees reviewed childhood vaccines and other vaccine safety issues. In 2001 a new IOM Immunization Safety Review Committee was assembled and included 13 individuals with broad expertise. To avoid real or perceived conflict of interest, an absolute criterion for membership was lack of any association with vaccine manufacturers or their parent organizations and no prior function as a legal expert witness. From 2001 through 2004 the committee reviewed and published its findings on eight specific vaccine safety issues (http://www.iom.edu/; a search on <immunization safety> will lead to all activities since 2001). For each issue studied, the Committee reviewed all pertinent theoretical, experimental, clinical and epidemiologic evidence and heard presentations from the public and health professionals. The Committee started from a neutral position, with no prior assumption regarding a positive or negative connection between the vaccine and the issue at hand. The scientific evidence was then reviewed, and biologic mechanisms for a possible causal association were carefully considered. Prior to publication, each report was reviewed by an independent expert panel, chosen by the NAS and IOM but anonymous to the committee. Reviewer's comments are given due consideration, but ultimately the final published report represents the consensus of the IOM safety panel alone. To view reports online and/or purchase copies see the National Academies Press site, http://lab.nap.edu, and search on vaccine or immunization safety.

The **Cochrane Collaboration** (www.cochrane.org) also conducts systematic reviews of vaccines, which may include information on vaccine safety. Since reviews are limited to randomized controlled trials, information regarding rare adverse events is unlikely to be covered.

Vaccine safety data in the Canadian Immunization Guide

In each chapter of this *Guide*, pre-licensure and post-marketing evidence-based safety data are presented for specific vaccines, as appropriate. At the time of publication of the *Guide* post-marketing surveillance of reports submitted to the CAEFISS has demonstrated continued vaccine safety and no unexpected serious adverse events. Detailed summaries of Canadian safety surveillance data for all reports by year, as well as for subgroups by vaccine and specific adverse event, will be published periodically on the Internet, in the *Canada Communicable Disease Report* and in peer reviewed publications as appropriate to the content. An updated list of published materials can be found at the PHAC Vaccine Safety Web site (http://www.phac-aspc.gc.ca/im/vs-sv/index.html, see "Safety data and publications").

Vaccine safety controversies

Space does not permit a detailed discussion of past or current controversies. Table 4 summarizes the conclusions of the IOM safety panel on several recent vaccine safety issues. Topical information on new, as well as past, controversies can be found at the PHAC's Vaccine Safety Web site. Additionally, in the suggested reading and resources given later, Web addresses are provided for the IOM's detailed reports as well as for meeting reports from the GACVS. Also, see the WHO Vaccine Safety Net Web site for a list of sites whose content on vaccine safety has been judged to meet the necessary criteria for credibility, content, accessibility and design.

Suggested reading and resources

Final report: National Immunization Strategy, 2003: http://www.phac-aspc.gc.ca/publicat/nat_immunization_03/index.html

WHO Global Advisory Committee on Vaccine Safety

Folb PI, Bernatowska E, Chen R et al. *A global perspective on vaccine safety and public health: the Global Advisory Committee on Vaccine Safety.* American Journal of Public Health 2004;94(11):1926-1931. This is an overview of the committee's role and activities. Downloadable pdf file at http://www.who.int/vaccine safety/about/en/vaccine.pdf.

GACVS. Bi-annual meeting reports, including summary lists of the topics discussed and full text details, can be found at http://www.who.int/vaccine_safety/reports/en/

Table 4. Events Judged Not To Be Linked to Vaccines*

Exposure	Events judged not to be causally linked with exposure	Year reviewed and National Academies Press site address for specific citation
Multiple immunizations	• Increased susceptibility to infection • Type 1 diabetes mellitus • Sudden infant death syndrome	2002 http://fermat.nap.edu/catalog/10306.html 2003 http://fermat.nap.edu/catalog/10649.html
• MMR vaccine • Thimerosal-containing vaccines	• Autism	2004 http://fermat.nap.edu/catalog/10997.html
Haemophilus influenzae type b conjugate vaccines	• *H. influenzae* infection shortly after immunization	1994 http://fermat.nap.edu/catalog/2138.html
Hepatitis B vaccine	• Incident cases/relapses of multiple sclerosis in adults	2002 http://fermat.nap.edu/catalog/10393.html
Influenza vaccine	• Relapses of multiple sclerosis	2004 http://fermat.nap.edu/catalog/10822.html
Diphtheria and/or tetanus toxoid containing vaccines	• Acute/chronic encephalopathy • Sudden infant death syndrome • Infantile spasms (hypsarrythmia)	2003 http://fermat.nap.edu/catalog/10649.html 1994 http://fermat.nap.edu/catalog/2138.html
Whole cell pertussis vaccines	• Sudden infant death syndrome	2003 http://fermat.nap.edu/catalog/10649.html

* Based on review of scientific evidence by an expert safety review panel of the IOM (see www.iom.edu or specific citation in Table)

WHO Vaccine Safety Net

http://www.who.int/immunization_safety/safety_quality/vaccine_safety_websites/en/

Institute of Medicine

To read and/or purchase reports on vaccine and immunization safety issues, see the National Academies Press site, http://lab.nap.edu, and search on vaccine or immunization safety.

Guidelines for preparing core clinical safety information on drugs – report of the Council for International Organizations of Medical Sciences (CIOMS) Working Group III. Geneva: World Health Organization (WHO), 1995. (Chapter 5, Good Safety Information Practice).

Canadian Coalition for Immunization Awareness and Promotion

Tips for assessing Web sites (usually for health professionals and the public) can be found at the Canadian Coalition for Immunization Awareness and Promotion

English version: http://www.immunize.cpha.ca/english/poster/intip_e.htm
French version: http://www.immunize.cpha.ca/francais/posterf/intip_f.htm

---

BOX 1. The W5 of AEFI (Adverse Event Following Immunization) Reporting in Canada

- WHY to report:
  - to ensure that the vaccines used in Canada are safe
  - to maintain public confidence in Canada's immunization programs
  - it is a health care professional responsibility
  - it is a legal requirement in many Canadian jurisdictions

- WHO should report:
  - all vaccine providers
  - all health care professionals caring for patients who may have had an AEFI
  - all vaccine manufacturers to whom an AEFI report is submitted

- WHEN to report:
  - when an AEFI is
    - severe (death, hospitalization for > 3 days, congenital abnormality, residual abnormality, life threatening)
    - unexpected (in terms of type or frequency)
    - of concern (to the vaccinee, his/her caregiver(s) or AEFI reporter)
  - when an AEFI occurs within a timeframe that is generally consistent with one or more of the following:
    - immunizing agent: 30 days after live vaccine/7 days after killed or subunit vaccine
    - plausible biologic mechanism: up to 8 weeks for immune-mediated events
    - reporter suspects the AEFI may be linked to immunization

- WHAT to report: details regarding
  - vaccinee – unique identifier, date of birth and sex;
  - immunization event(s) – province/territory where given, date, all vaccines given including name, manufacturer, lot number, administration site and route, as well as the number in series of vaccine doses if relevant;
  - adverse event(s) – description, including time of first onset following immunization, duration, health care utilization, treatment and outcome;
  - relevant medical history – underlying disease, known allergies, prior AEFI;
  - concomitant event(s) – acute illness, current medication, injury, exposure to environmental toxins.

- WHERE to find the AEFI report form:
  - Web (http://www.phac-aspc.gc.ca/im/aefi-form_e.html)
  - Local public health units
  - *Compendium of Pharmaceuticals and Specialties*

General Contraindications and Precautions

Contraindications

A **contraindication** is a condition that significantly increases the chance that a serious adverse event will occur if the vaccine is given. In general, vaccines should not be given when a contraindication exists.

The only three contraindications to vaccines approved in Canada that may exist are the following:

- anaphylaxis to a component of the vaccine (can occur with any vaccine)
  - A patient who has had an anaphylactic reaction to a vaccine or who has a history of anaphylaxis to a component of a vaccine should not receive the same vaccine again. Such patients should be referred to an allergist to determine the specific cause of the allergic reaction and to assess which vaccines should be avoided and for how long. Anaphylactic reactions to vaccines are rare (approximately 2 per million doses administered) but can be life threatening. All vaccine providers should be prepared to respond to anaphylactic reactions to vaccines. For more information see the *Anaphylaxis: Initial Management in Non-Hospital Settings* chapter, page 80.

- significant immunosuppression (live vaccines only)
  - In patients significantly immunocompromised, live viral or bacterial vaccines may cause serious adverse events because of uncontrolled replication of the virus or bacteria. For more information see the chapter on *Immunization of Immunocompromised Persons*, page 117.

- pregnancy (live vaccines only) (see Table 5)
  - If a pregnant woman receives a live vaccine, the infection with the vaccine-strain virus or bacteria might affect the fetus. Although this has been confirmed to occur only for smallpox vaccine, safety data for other live virus vaccines in pregnant women are very limited. Thus women should not receive live vaccines during pregnancy unless their risk from the illness is clearly greater than the potential risk from the vaccine. For more information, see *Immunization in Pregnancy and Breast-Feeding* chapter, page 107.

Precautions

A precaution is a condition that may increase the chance of an adverse reaction following immunization or that may compromise the ability of the vaccine to produce immunity. In general, vaccines are deferred when a precaution is present. However, there may be circumstances when the benefits of giving the vaccine outweigh the potential harm, or when reduced vaccine immunogenicity still results in significant benefit to a susceptible, immunocompromised host.

The precautions associated with each vaccine are discussed in detail in the chapters about specific vaccines. See also Table 6 regarding concerns associated with multiple vaccines.

Two precautions deserve further comment:

◆ Persons who have chronic underlying illness or who are immunocompromised, in whom there may be a reduced response to vaccines.

  • Even a less than optimal response may provide important benefit to such patients, who are also at high risk of morbidity and mortality due to vaccine-preventable infection. For more information please refer to the *Immunization of Immunocompromised Persons* chapter, page 117.

◆ Persons with a history of Guillain-Barré syndrome (GBS) with onset within 8 weeks of a previous immunization.

  • Subsequent doses of the same vaccine should only be given if the benefit of vaccination outweighs the potential risk of recurrence of the GBS if vaccine is given.

As noted in Table 6, children and adults with neurologic conditions other than GBS are not at increased risk of adverse events after vaccination and may be at greater risk of morbidity and mortality from vaccine-preventable diseases than healthy individuals. Recommended vaccines should not be avoided in children or adults with neurologic conditions. For more information, please refer to the *Immunization of Persons with Neurological Disorders* chapter, page 131.

Table 5. Contraindications and Selected Precautions for Vaccine Administration

Issue of concern (see indicated page for more detailed discussion)	Type of vaccine	
	Inactivated/ subunit	Live
Allergy to vaccine component (page 80)	Contraindication if the specific vaccine contains that particular component	
Severely immunocompromised (page 117)	Precaution	Contraindication
Pregnancy (page 107)	None	Contraindication
Recent administration of blood product containing antibodies (page 53)	None	Precaution
Recent administration of live virus vaccine (page 51)	None	Precaution
Severe bleeding disorder (page 134)	Precaution	Precaution

Not contraindications

There are a number of conditions or circumstances that some health care providers inappropriately consider to be contraindications to vaccination. This may result in missed opportunities for needed vaccination. Information about some of these conditions is provided in Table 6.

In particular, mild common illnesses (e.g., upper respiratory tract infections, otitis media, colds, diarrhea) or concurrent antibiotic therapy do NOT interfere with the immune response and are NOT a contraindication to vaccination. Almost no acute illness, however severe, interferes significantly with the immune response to vaccine. Some people argue that the occurrence of systemic adverse events may complicate the medical management of the other acute illness or that events associated with the acute illness may mistakenly be thought to be vaccine-related adverse events. These are both theoretical concerns. Almost invariably, this potential risk is much less important than the risk associated with missing an opportunity to give a recommended vaccine.

Table 6. Conditions that are NOT Contraindications to Immunization

Conditions	Comments
Concurrent condition in vaccinee	
Premature birth	• Premature infants • respond adequately to vaccines used in infancy • are not at significantly increased risk of adverse events. • Immunize on schedule, according to child's chronological age. • **EXCEPTION:** Hepatitis B vaccine for infants weighing < 2000 g • Mother HBV negative: defer vaccine until infant weighs > 2000 g or is 1 month of age. • Mother HBV positive: give infant hepatitis B immune globulin and first dose of hepatitis B vaccine immediately after birth. Will need 4th dose of HBV (see chapter *Immunization of Infants Born Prematurely*, page 113).
Breast-feeding	• After immunization of either a mother or her infant, during breast-feeding there is • no reduction in maternal or infant response to vaccines • no increase in the risk of adverse events for either mother or breast-feeding infant, following immunization of either.
Pregnancy (inactivated vaccines)	• All **inactivated vaccines** are safe in pregnancy and should be administered if indicated.

Table 6. Conditions that are NOT Contraindications to Immunization

Conditions	Comments
Concurrent condition in vaccinee	
Neurologic disorder	• No evidence of increased risk of any adverse event following immunization. • Such persons may be at increased risk of complications from vaccine-preventable diseases such as influenza and should be immunized appropriately. • **EXCEPTION:** precaution for repeat doses of any vaccine that was temporally associated with an episode of Guillain-Barré syndrome (onset within 8 weeks after immunization).
Cancer (inactivated vaccines)	• No increased incidence of adverse reactions to inactivated vaccines • No interference between treatment of cancer and inactivated vaccine • The immune response may be less than that of healthy adults and children, but any protection following immunization is important because of the increased risk of infection and associated complications
Minor acute illness (with or without fever of ≥ 39.5° C)	• No interference with response to vaccine. • No increase in risk of adverse event(s) following immunization.

Antibiotic therapy	• No effect on response to most inactivated or live vaccines used in Canada.
	• **EXCEPTIONS**
	  · **Live oral typhoid** vaccine should be delayed until 48 hrs after receipt of the last dose of antibiotics active against *Salmonella typhi* (penicillins, cephalosporins, trimethoprim-sulfamethoxazole, fluoroquinolones, azithromycin, tetracyclines).
	  · **Live attenuated varicella** vaccine may have reduced effectiveness if given concurrently with antivirals active against herpesviruses. If possible discontinue antivirals active against herpesvirus ≥ 24 hours before immunization and do not re-start until 4 weeks after vaccination.

Convalescence from or exposure to an infection	• No interference with response to vaccine. • No increase in risk of adverse event(s) following immunization.
Tuberculin skin testing	• Any vaccine can be given at the same time as, or at any time after, a tuberculin skin test. • Tuberculin skin tests can be given at the same time as, or any time after, any vaccine. However, MMR vaccine may suppress the tuberculin reaction and cause false-negative skin test results if skin tests are administered in the 4-6 weeks after vaccination. The effect of other live virus vaccines such as varicella and yellow fever vaccines on tuberculin reactivity is currently unknown, and no recommendations for postponement of tuberculin skin testing can be made at this time.

Table 6. Conditions that are NOT Contraindications to Immunization

Conditions	Comments
Concurrent condition in household contact of vaccinee	
Pregnant or immunosuppressed individuals living in household with vaccinee	• No risk from any vaccine marketed in Canada to household contacts of vaccinees. • Immunization of household contacts of immunosuppressed patients and neonates provides important protection against transmission of disease in the household. Vaccination opportunities in such persons should not be missed.
Concern regarding possible allergy in vaccinee	
Gastrointestinal intolerance to eggs	The inability to eat eggs for reasons other than allergy is not associated with an increase of adverse events to any vaccine.
Child, not yet exposed to egg protein	There is no reason to avoid any recommended vaccine. It is very unlikely that such children would have an egg allergy severe enough to cause them to react to the minute quantity of egg protein contained in some vaccines.

History of allergy that does not involve vaccine or component of vaccine	• It is safe to immunize people with any of the following:
	  • non-specific allergies
	  • environmental allergies
	  • family histories of allergies
	  • administration of allergy shots (desensitization therapy for allergy)
	  • allergies to commonly used antibiotics
	• **EXCEPTION:** vaccines containing neomycin +/or polymyxin (see Table 1, General Considerations chapter, page 7 are contraindicated in individuals with IgE-mediated allergies to these antibiotics.

Concern regarding past adverse reaction	
History of large local reaction following immunization	• A large local reaction to one vaccine is not associated with an increased risk of local reactions to other vaccines. • A large local reaction to the fourth dose of DTaP-IPV-Hib does not predict a large reaction to the fifth dose booster (DTaP-IPV), which should be given on schedule. • In other circumstances, repeating a dose of a vaccine that previously gave a large local reaction may result in another large local reaction. However, there is no increased risk of systemic adverse events.
Febrile seizures	Childhood vaccines prevent serious diseases that pose a much greater risk to most children's health than seizures that might be associated with a febrile reaction after vaccination.

Part 2 — Vaccine Safety and Adverse Events Following Immunization

Table 6. Conditions that are NOT Contraindications to Immunization

Conditions	Comments
Concern regarding past adverse reaction	
Family history of adverse reactions to vaccines	• Adverse reactions to vaccines are not known to be inherited. • **EXCEPTION:** a family history of an overwhelming infection or fatality after administration of a live vaccine may suggest inheritable severe immunodeficiency, which should be ruled out before administering live vaccines.
Concern regarding capacity to respond to vaccine	
Concern about exposure to too many antigens	This concern is not substantiated given the following facts: • The vaccines used today are much more highly purified than those in the past, so that even though infants and children now receive more vaccines than they did 30 years ago, the total number of vaccine antigens to which they are exposed is much lower today than it used to be. • The human immune system has an enormous capacity to respond to antigens. • Infants can respond to about 10,000 different antigens at any one time. Immunization does not add, significantly, to the daily load of foreign antigens even for a 2-month-old baby. • The vaccines given at 2, 4 and 6 months of age in Canada engage less than 0.01% of an infant's immune response capacity.

Concern about too many needles	• A Canadian study has shown that
	  · immunization providers are more concerned about multiple injections than are parents
	  · most parents accept multiple injections if it means getting a vaccine with fewer side effects.

Pre-immunization screening for contraindications and precautions

Every patient should be screened for contraindications and precautions before receiving any vaccine dose. Checklists and routine screening questions are useful ways to ensure that this takes place. Effective screening requires only a few questions: sample questions for two circumstances are shown in the box. (Please refer to the *Vaccine Administration Practices* chapter, page 38.)

Selected references

Centers for Disease Control and Prevention. *An ounce of prevention ... what are the returns?* 2nd edition, 1999. URL: <www.cdc.gov/epo/prevent.htm>.

Ess SM, Szucs TD. *Economic evaluation of immunization strategies.* Clinical Infectious Diseases 2002;35:294-97. URL: <http://www.journals.uchicago.edu/CID/journal/issues/v35n3/011581/011581.html>.

Halperin BA, Eastwood BJ, Halperin SA. *Comparison of parental and health care professional preferences for the acellular or whole cell pertussis vaccine.* Pediatric Infectious Disease Journal 1998;17(2):103-9.

Tengs TO, Adams ME, Pliskin JS. *Five hundred live-saving interventions and their cost-effectiveness.* Risk Analysis 1995;15(3):369-90.

US National Immunization Program. *Guide to contraindications to vaccinations.* URL: <http://www.cdc.gov/nip/recs/contraindications.htm#micro>.

Sample screening questions for the parents of children about to receive a dose of any vaccine:

- How is your child today?
- Does your child have any allergies to food or medication?
- Did your child have any problems after his or her previous vaccines/shots?

If the vaccine to be given is a live viral or live bacterial vaccine, add

- Does your child have any problems with his or her immune system?
- Has your child received any transfusions or blood products in the last year?

Sample screening questions for adults being offered influenza vaccine:

- Have you had influenza vaccine before? If yes, did you have any problems after the vaccine?
- Have you had any reactions to vaccines in the past?
- Have you ever fainted after a needle or vaccine?
- Do you have any allergies to food or medications?

Part 2 — Vaccine Safety and Adverse Events Following Immunization

Anaphylaxis: Initial Management in Non-Hospital Settings

This section is intended as a guide for the initial management of patients in a public health clinic, medical office or similar non-hospital setting. For a patient with severe, life-threatening anaphylaxis, establishment of intravenous access for drug and fluid administration will be necessary, and endotracheal intubation and other manoeuvres may be required. These interventions are ordinarily best performed in a hospital's emergency department.

Since the publication of the 2002 *Canadian Immunization Guide*, the following changes have been made: 1) the management of an urticarial rash at the injection site has been outlined; 2) the use of self-injectors (Epipen® or Twinject™) has been reviewed; 3) and the use of diphenhydramine hydrochloride (Benadryl®) has been expanded and the dose reduced for some age groups.

Anaphylaxis is a potentially life-threatening allergic reaction to foreign protein antigens such as food and bee stings. It is a rare complication of immunization but, even so, it should be anticipated in every vaccinee. Prevention is the best approach. Pre-vaccination screening should include questions about possible allergy to any component of the product(s) being considered in order to identify this contraindication. As avoidance is not always possible, every vaccine provider should be familiar with the symptoms of anaphylaxis and be ready to initiate management and administer appropriate medications. Most instances begin within 30 minutes after an injection of vaccine; shorter intervals to onset foretell more severe reactions. Thus vaccine recipients should be kept under supervision for at least 15 minutes after immunization; 30 minutes is a safer interval when there is a specific concern about possible vaccine allergy. In low-risk situations, supervision can include having vaccinees remain within a short distance of the vaccinator (e.g., within a school being used for immunization) and return immediately for assessment if they feel unwell.

Anaphylaxis is one of the rarer events reported in the post-marketing surveillance system for vaccine adverse events. According to the latest analysis of complete national data collected through passive surveillance, the estimated annual reported rate of anaphylaxis ranges from 0.4 to 1.8 reports per 1,000,000 doses of vaccines distributed in Canada.

Anaphylaxis must be distinguished from fainting (vasovagal syncope), anxiety and breath-holding spells, which are more common and benign reactions. During fainting, the individual suddenly becomes pale, loses consciousness and collapses to the ground. Fainting is sometimes accompanied by brief clonic seizure activity (i.e., rhythmic jerking of the limbs), but this generally requires no specific treatment or investigation. Fainting is managed simply by placing the patient in a recumbent position. Recovery of consciousness occurs within a minute or two, but patients may remain pale, diaphoretic and mildly hypotensive for several more minutes. The likelihood of fainting is reduced by measures that lower stress in those awaiting immunization, such as short waiting times, comfortable room temperature, preparation of vaccines out of view of recipients and privacy during the procedure. To reduce injuries during fainting spells those at risk are best immunized while seated.

People experiencing an anxiety spell may appear fearful, pale and diaphoretic and complain of lightheadedness, dizziness and numbness, as well as tingling of the face and extremities. Hyperventilation is usually evident. Treatment consists of reassurance and rebreathing using a paper bag until symptoms subside.

Breath-holding spells occur in some young children when they are upset and crying hard. The child is suddenly silent but obviously agitated. Facial flushing and perioral cyanosis deepens as breath-holding continues. Some spells end with resumption of crying, but others end with a brief period of unconsciousness during which breathing resumes. Similar spells may have been observed in other circumstances. No treatment is required beyond reassurance of the child and parents.

In the case of anaphylaxis, changes develop over several minutes and usually involve at least two body systems (affecting the skin, respiration, circulation). Unconsciousness is rarely the sole manifestation of anaphylaxis. It occurs only as a late event in severe cases.

The cardinal features of anaphylaxis are

♦ itchy, urticarial rash (in over 90% of cases);

♦ progressive, painless swelling (angioedema) about the face and mouth, which may be preceded by itchiness, tearing, nasal congestion or facial flushing;

♦ respiratory symptoms, including sneezing, coughing, wheezing, labored breathing and upper airway swelling (indicated by hoarseness and/or difficulty swallowing) possibly causing airway obstruction;

♦ hypotension, which generally develops later in the reaction and can progress to cause shock and collapse.

Gastrointestinal symptoms like nausea, vomiting and diarrhea may occur with anaphylaxis.

Swelling and urticarial rash at the injection site can occur but are not always caused by an allergic reaction. This reaction can be managed by observation. Ice can be put at the site of reaction for comfort. It can also be treated with diphenhydramine hydrochloride (Benadryl®, see step 7 in the next section) alone. If diphenhydramine is given to treat such a reaction, the patient should be kept under close supervision for 1 hour after the dose. If the hives or swelling disappear without additional treatment, the patient does not need to be kept under further observation. However, if any other symptoms arise, even if considered mild (e.g., sneezing, nasal congestion, tearing, coughing, facial flushing) or if the hives progress despite the use of diphenhydramine, epinephrine should be given (see below). There is little risk to the unnecessary use of epinephrine, whereas delay in its administration when required may result in difficulty to treat anaphylaxis and in death.

Features of severe disease include obstructive swelling of the upper airway, marked bronchospasm and hypotension.

Management of anaphylaxis

The following steps describe the management of anaphylaxis. Steps 1 to 4 are meant to be done rapidly or simultaneously. **The priority is prompt administration of epinephrine (step 1)**, which should not be delayed if earlier steps cannot quickly be completed.

1. **Promptly administer 0.01 mL/kg (maximum 0.5 mL) of aqueous epinephrine 1:1000 by subcutaneous or intramuscular injection in the opposite limb to that in which the vaccination was given.** Speedy intervention is of paramount importance: failure to use epinephrine promptly is more dangerous than using it improperly (see text below for discussion of epinephrine).

2. Call for assistance, including an ambulance.

3. Place the patient in a recumbent position, elevating the feet if possible.

4. Establish an oral airway if necessary.

5. If oxygen is available, it should be given to patients with cyanosis, dyspnea or any other severe reaction. Monitor with pulse oximetry if available.

6. If the vaccine was injected subcutaneously, an additional dose of 0.005 mL/kg (maximum 0.3 mL) of aqueous epinephrine 1:1000 can be injected into the vaccination site to slow absorption. This should be given shortly after the initial dose of epinephrine (Table 7) in moderate to severe cases. It is generally not repeated. Local injection of epinephrine into an intramuscular vaccination site is contraindicated because it dilates vessels and speeds absorption of the vaccine.

7. As an adjunct to epinephrine, a dose of diphenhydramine hydrochloride (Benadryl®) can be given. Oral treatment (oral dose: 1-2 mg/kg to a maximum single dose of 50 mg) is preferred for conscious patients who are not seriously ill, because Benadryl® is painful when given intramuscularly. This drug has a high safety margin, making precise dosing less important. The approximate doses for injection (50 mg/mL solution) are shown in Table 8.

8. If available, consider inhaled β-agonist if there is a bronchospasm resistant to an adequate dose of epinephrine (e.g., nebulized salbuta-

mol 2.5-5.0 mg in 3 mL of saline or 1 puff per 3 kg to a maximum of 10 puffs by metered dose inhalers).

9. Monitor vital signs and reassess the situation frequently, to guide medication use.

10. Arrange for rapid transport to an emergency department. Since 20% of anaphylaxis episodes follow a biphasic course with recurrence of the reaction after a 2-9 hour asymptomatic period, hospitalization or a long period of observation is recommended for monitoring. For all but the mildest cases of anaphylaxis, patients should be hospitalized overnight or monitored for at least 12 hours.

The subcutaneous or intramuscular route for epinephrine injection is appropriate. Epinephrine dosing can be repeated twice at 5-minute intervals if necessary, for a total of three doses, again avoiding the limb in which the vaccination was given. A different limb is preferred for each dose to maximize drug absorption.

The epinephrine dose should be carefully determined. Calculations based on body weight are preferred when weight is known. Recording the weight of children before routine immunization is recommended when feasible. Excessive doses of epinephrine can add to patients' distress by causing palpitations, tachycardia, flushing and headache. Although unpleasant, such side effects pose little danger. Cardiac dysrhythmias may occur in older adults but are rare in otherwise healthy children.

When body weight is not known the dose of aqueous epinephrine 1:1000 can be approximated from the subject's age (Table 7).

Table 7. Appropriate Dose of Epinephrine (1:1000) According to Age

Age	Dose	
2 to 6 months*	0.07 mL	(0.07 mg)
12 months	0.10 mL	(0.10mg)
18 months to 4 years*	0.15 mL	(0.15 mg)
5 years	0.20 mL	(0.20 mg)
6-9 years	0.30 mL	(0.30 mg)
10-13 years	0.40 mL†	(0.40 mg)
≥ 14 years	0.50 mL†	(0.50 mg)

*   Dose for children between the ages shown should be approximated, the volume being intermediate between the values shown or increased to the next larger dose, depending on practicability.

†   For a mild reaction a dose of 0.3 mL can be considered.

Table 8. Appropriate Dose of Diphenhydramine Hydrochloride

Age	Dose	
	Injected (50 mg/mL)	Oral or injected
< 2 years	0.25 mL	(12.5 mg)
2-4 years	0.50 mL	(25.0 mg)
5-11 years	0.50-1.00 mL	(25-50 mg)
≥ 12 years	1.00 mL	(50 mg)

An epinephrine self-injector (Epipen® or Twinject™) can also be used if the person who administers it is knowledgeable about proper use. The junior preparations contain 0.15 mL of epinephrine 1:1000, which is ideal for children weighing 15 kg. The regular preparations contain 0.3 mL of epinephrine 1:1000 and should be used for people weighing ≥ 30 kg. For those weighing below 15 kg or between 15 and 30 kg, judgement should be used to decide which, if any, self-injector should be used.

The anaphylactic state in patients receiving β-adrenergic antagonist therapy (for elevated blood pressure) will be more resistant to epinephrine therapy.

Epinephrine vials and other emergency supplies should be checked on a regular basis and replaced if outdated.

Recommended epinephrine kit contents

- Copy of the anaphylaxis procedures and doses recommended of epinephrine and diphenhydramine for weight and age
- 2–1 cc syringes with attached needles (1–25 gauge, 5/8" needle; 1–25 gauge, 1" needle)
- 2 vials of epinephrine 1:1000 (check expiry date monthly and replace once expired)
- 1 vial of diphenhydramine (pills or oral solutions optional, check expiry date monthly and replace once expired)
- 1 – 25 gauge, 5/8" needle (extra)
- 1 – 25 gauge, 1" needle (extra)
- 2 alcohol swabs (optional)

Selected references

Ellis AK, Day JH. *Anaphylaxis: diagnosis and treatment.* Allergy Asthma 2000;13(3): 22-35.

Joint Task Force on Practice Parameters; American Academy of Allergy, Asthma and Immunology; American College of Allergy, Asthma and Immunology; Joint Council of Allergy, Asthma and Immunology. *The diagnosis and management of anaphylaxis: an updated practice parameter.* Journal of Allergy and Clinical Immunology 2005;115: S483-523.

Thibodeau JL. *Office management of childhood vaccine-related anaphylaxis.* Canadian Family Physician 1994;40:1602-10.

Anaphylactic Hypersensitivity to Egg and Egg-Related Antigens

Changes since the publication of the 2002 *Canadian Immunization Guide* include the following: 1) no special precaution when administering measles, mumps, and rubella (MMR) vaccine to egg-allergic individuals; 2) information on the new rabies vaccine (RabAvert®), which is derived from virus grown in chick embryo cell culture; and 3) chicken allergy as a contraindication to vaccination with the yellow fever vaccine.

General considerations

In this chapter, egg or chicken allergy is defined as an IgE-mediated hypersensitivity causing symptoms like, but not limited to, urticaria, swelling of the mouth and throat, difficulty breathing or hypotension. Chicken allergy refers to allergy to chicken meat as opposed to allergy to feathers.

Egg allergy is one of the most common food allergies of childhood, with a prevalence of 1%-3% in children under 3 years of age. As most children outgrow their egg allergy, the prevalence in adulthood is much lower. Isolated chicken allergy is a very rare condition.

Vaccines that contain small quantities of egg protein can cause hypersensitivity reactions in some people with allergies to eggs. The likelihood of such reactions occurring varies considerably among vaccines. The yellow fever vaccines are prepared from virus grown in chick embryos and are the most likely to cause allergic reaction in egg- or chicken-allergic individuals. Allergic reactions can also occur to vaccines against influenza, which are prepared from viruses grown in embryonated eggs. In contrast, the MMR vaccine viruses most widely used in Canada and one of the rabies vaccines (RabAvert®) are grown in chick embryo cell culture. The final vaccine products *may* contain trace quantities of egg proteins, but the amount is not felt to be enough to cause an allergic reaction, especially for MMR. Some extra precautions are still recommended for RabAvert®. Egg proteins are not involved in the manufacturing process of the other rabies vaccine (Imovax® Rabies).

MMR vaccine

Anaphylaxis after measles vaccination is rare. It has been reported both in people with anaphylactic hypersensitivity to eggs and in those with no history of egg allergy. In some of these instances it is hypersensitivity to gelatin that is responsible for the anaphylactic reaction. As well, allergy to other components of the vaccine, such as neomycin, has been hypothesized but not proven. The minute quantity of egg proteins contained in the MMR vaccine seems to be insufficient to cause an allergic reaction in egg-allergic people.

Several studies have reported uneventful routine MMR immunization in egg-allergic people and in those with positive MMR skin tests, whereas others have reported occasional adverse reactions despite the use of MMR skin testing and graded challenge vaccination. Therefore the use of skin testing with MMR vaccines in egg-allergic individuals is no longer recommended.

The largest published review of the literature provides data on 1227 egg-allergic patients who received the MMR vaccine as a usual single dose. Only two had any symptoms suggesting an allergic reaction, and they were from the same case report, whereas in better studies no patient reacted. These combined data indicate that 99% of children who are allergic to egg can safely receive the vaccine (95% confidence interval (CI) 99.41%-99.98%). Four of the best studies from this review of the literature are summarized below.

♦ Fasano et al (1992) studied 140 children whose double-blind placebo-controlled food challenges to egg were positive or who had a convincing history of recent anaphylaxis to egg ingestion and a positive skin test to eggs. Seventy-one children were immunized prospectively and 69 children had already received the MMR vaccine. None had any reaction to the vaccine.

♦ James et al (1995) prospectively evaluated the administration of MMR vaccine to 54 children with positive skin test to eggs and either a positive food challenge to egg or convincing history of severe or recent anaphylactic reaction to egg. None had any reaction to the vaccine.

♦ Aickin et al (1994) described 242 children with documented allergic reaction after the ingestion of egg and positive skin test to egg. None had any reaction to the vaccine.

♦ Freigang et al (1994) described 500 children with convincing history of egg allergy and positive skin test to egg. None had any reaction to the vaccine.

In view of the cumulative data indicating the safety of MMR immunization in people with a history of anaphylactic hypersensitivity to hens' eggs and the lack of evidence of the predictive value of MMR skin testing, the National Advisory Committee on Immunization (NACI) does not recommend routine MMR skin testing or any special precaution in these individuals. As for all vaccines, NACI recommends immunization by personnel with the capability and facilities to manage adverse events following immunization such as anaphylaxis.

Rabies vaccine

Immunization with rabies vaccine obtained by viruses grown in chick embryo cell culture (RabAvert®) is probably safe in egg-allergic individuals because the vaccine contains only a minute quantity of egg proteins; however, no safety data exist. An alternative vaccine, if available, should be used in egg-allergic individuals. If an alternative vaccine is not available, post-exposure prophylaxis should be administered with strict medical monitoring in facilities where emergency treatment of anaphylaxis is available. For pre-exposure vaccination when no alternative vaccine is available referral to an allergy specialist prior to vaccination is recommended, as vaccination might be possible after careful evaluation, skin testing and graded challenge or desensitization.

Influenza vaccine

Allergic reactions have been reported in patients with egg allergy receiving the influenza vaccine. In the few studies evaluating immunization with influenza vaccine in egg-allergic children, allergic reactions ranged from 0%-40%.

Most influenza vaccines probably contain only a very small amount of egg proteins, but manufacturers do not report the egg content of their influenza vaccine. In some studies in which investigators have determined the egg content of some influenza vaccines, it was found that the egg protein content varied by several logarithmic factors from manufacturer to manufacturer and from year to year.

Egg-allergic individuals should not be routinely vaccinated with the influenza vaccine. Of these individuals, those who are at risk of the complications of influenza should be evaluated by an allergy specialist, as vaccination might be possible after careful evaluation, skin testing and graded challenge or desensitization. If such an evaluation is not possible, the risk of an allergic reaction to the vaccine must be weighed against the risk of influenza disease.

Yellow fever vaccine

The yellow fever vaccine has the greatest likelihood of containing sufficient amounts of egg or chicken proteins to cause an allergic reaction in egg- or chicken-allergic individuals. There have been several reports of anaphylactic reactions to the yellow fever vaccine in egg- or chicken-allergic individuals but no studies have been done in which the vaccine was administered to such individuals in order to monitor for the reaction. The yellow fever vaccine should not be routinely administered to egg- or chicken-allergic individuals. Referral to an allergy specialist is recommended, as vaccination might be possible after careful evaluation, skin testing and graded challenge or desensitization.

Summary of guidelines for vaccination of egg- or chicken-allergic individuals

- ◆ Individuals should be asked about allergy to egg prior to vaccination with influenza vaccine, yellow fever vaccine and the rabies vaccine RabAvert®.

- Individuals should be asked about allergy to chicken prior to vaccination with yellow fever vaccine.

- Prior egg ingestion should not be a prerequisite for immunization with egg-containing vaccine.

- Atopic diseases are not a contraindication to immunization with egg-containing vaccine.

- Egg allergy is not a contraindication to immunization with MMR. People with these allergies may be immunized in the routine manner without prior testing.

- Influenza vaccines that are prepared from viruses grown in embryonated eggs should not be given to egg-allergic individuals unless the risk of the disease outweighs the small risk of a systemic hypersensitivity reaction. Referral to an allergy specialist is recommended, as vaccination might be possible after careful evaluation, skin testing and graded challenge or desensitization.

- Yellow fever vaccines should not be given to egg- or chicken-allergic individuals unless the risk of the disease outweighs the small risk of a systemic hypersensitivity reaction. Referral to an allergy specialist is recommended, as vaccination might be possible after careful evaluation, skin testing and graded challenge or desensitization.

- When no alternative vaccines are available for egg-allergic individuals, post-exposure vaccination with RabAvert® should be performed in facilities where treatment for anaphylaxis is available. For pre-exposure vaccination when no alternative vaccine is available, referral to an allergy specialist is recommended as vaccination might be possible after careful evaluation, skin testing and graded challenge or desensitization.

- Re-immunization with MMR, yellow fever, influenza or rabies vaccine is contraindicated in an individual with a previous anaphylactic reaction to that vaccine. Referral to an allergy specialist is recommended to find out which component of the vaccine was responsible for the allergic reaction

Selected references

Aickin R, Hill D, Kemp A. *Measles immunisation in children with allergy to egg*. British Medical Journal 1994;309:223-25.

Fasano MB, Wood RA, Cooke SK et al. *Egg hypersensitivity and adverse reactions to measles, mumps and rubella vaccine*. Journal of Pediatrics 1992;120(6):878-81.

Freigang B, Jadavji TP, Freigang DW. *Lack of adverse reactions to measles, mumps and rubella vaccine in egg-allergic children*. Annals of Allergy 1994;73:486-88.

Herman JJ, Radin R, Schneiderman R. *Allergic reactions to measles (rubeola) vaccine in patients hypersensitive to egg protein*. Journal of Pediatrics 1983;102(2):196-99.

James JM, Burks AW, Roberson PK et al. *Safe administration of the measles vaccine to children allergic to eggs.* New England Journal of Medicine 1995;332(19):1262-66.

Kelso JM, Yunginger JW. *Immunization of egg-allergic individuals with egg- or chicken-derived vaccines.* Immunology and Allergy Clinics of North America 2003;23(4):635-48.

Zeiger RS. *Current issues with influenza vaccination in egg allergy.* Journal of Allergy and Clinical Immunology 2002;110(6):834-40.

Part 3

Recommended Immunization

Recommended Immunization Schedules

Few measures in preventive medicine are of such proven value and as easy to implement as routine immunization against infectious diseases. Immunization carried out as recommended in the following schedules will provide good basic protection for most children against the diseases shown.

Following a standard schedule ensures that the maximal achievable protection is achieved. However, modifications of the recommended schedule may be necessary because of missed appointments or intercurrent illness. Interruption of a recommended series does not require starting the series over again, regardless of the interval elapsed. Children, youth and adults with interruptions to their vaccines should be vaccinated to complete the appropriate schedule for their *current* age.

Similar vaccines are now available from different manufacturers but may not be identical. It is therefore essential for the user to read the appropriate chapter in this *Guide* as well as the manufacturer's package insert.

Table 1. Routine Immunization Schedule for Infants and Children

Age at vaccination	DTaP-IPV	Hib	MMR	Var	HB	Pneu-C-7	Men-C	Tdap	Inf
Birth					Infancy 3 doses				
2 months	●	✦				◼	◉		
4 months	●	✦			★	◼	(◉)		
6 months	●	✦				◼	◉ or		6-23 months
12 months			◼	●		◼ 12-15 months	◉ if not yet given		◎ 1-2 doses
18 months	●	✦	◼		or				
4-6 years	●		or ◼						
14-16 years					Pre-teen/ teen 2-3 doses		◉ if not yet given	▲	

Table 2. Routine Immunization Schedule for Children < 7 Years of Age Not Immunized in Early Infancy

Timing	DTaP-IPV	Hib	MMR	Var	HB	Pneu-C-7	Men-C	Tdap
First visit	◉ ✓	✦ ✓	■	●	★ ✓	✓ ⊠	◉	
2 months later	◉	(✦)	■		★	(⊠)	(◉)	
2 months later	◉					(⊠)		
6-12 months later	◉	(✦)			★			
4-6 years of age	(◉)							
14-16 years of age								▲

Table 3. Routine Immunization Schedule for Children ≥ 7 Years of Age up to 17 Years of Age Not Immunized in Early Infancy

Timing	Tdap	IPV	MMR	Var	HB	Men-C
First visit	▲	◆	■	●	★	◉
2 months later	▲	◆	■	(●)	(★)	
6-12 months later	▲	◆			★	
10 years later	▲					

Table 4. Routine Immunization Schedule for Adults (≥ 18 Years of Age) Not Immunized in Childhood

Timing	Tdap	Td	MMR	Var	Men-C	Pneu-C-23	Inf
First visit	▲		■	●	(◉)		
2 months later		◫	(■)	●		(▪)	(⊖)
6-12 months later		◫					
10 years later		◫					

Notes

( )   Symbols with brackets around them imply that these doses may not be required, depending upon the age of the child or adult. Refer to the relevant chapter for that vaccine for further details.

◉   **Diphtheria, tetanus, acellular pertussis and inactivated polio virus vaccine (DTaP-IPV):** DTaP-IPV(± Hib) vaccine is the preferred vaccine for all doses in the vaccination series, including completion of the series in children who have received one or more doses of DPT (whole cell) vaccine (e.g., recent immigrants). In Tables 1 and 2, the 4-6 year dose can be omitted if the fourth dose was given after the fourth birthday.

- ✦ **_Haemophilus influenzae_ type b conjugate vaccine (Hib):** the Hib schedule shown is for the _Haemophilus_ b capsular polysaccharide — polyribosylribitol phosphate (PRP) conjugated to tetanus toxoid (PRP-T). For catch up, the number of doses depends on the age at which the schedule is begun (see _Haemophilus Vaccine_ chapter). Not usually required past age 5 years

- ■ **Measles, mumps and rubella vaccine (MMR):** a second dose of MMR is recommended for children at least 1 month after the first dose for the purpose of better measles protection. For convenience, options include giving it with the next scheduled vaccination at 18 months of age or at school entry (4-6 years) (depending on the provincial/territorial policy) or at any intervening age that is practical. In the catch-up schedule (Table 2), the first dose should not be given until the child is ≥ 12 months old. MMR should be given to all susceptible adolescents and adults.

- ● **Varicella vaccine (Var):** children aged 12 months to 12 years should receive one dose of varicella vaccine. Susceptible individuals ≥ 13 years of age should receive two doses at least 28 days apart.

- ★ **Hepatitis B vaccine (HB):** hepatitis B vaccine can be routinely given to infants or pre-adolescents, depending on the provincial/territorial policy. For infants born to chronic carrier mothers, the first dose should be given at birth (with hepatitis B immunoglobulin), otherwise the first dose can be given at 2 months of age to fit more conveniently with other routine infant immunization visits. The second dose should be administered at least 1 month after the first dose, and the third at least 2 months after the second dose, but these may fit more conveniently into the 4 and 6 month immunization visits. A two-dose schedule for adolescents is an option (see _Hepatitis B Vaccine_ chapter).

- ▣ **Pneumococcal conjugate vaccine – 7-valent (Pneu-C-7):** recommended for all children under 2 years of age. The recommended schedule depends on the age of the child when vaccination is begun (see _Pneumococcal Vaccine_ chapter).

- ▢ **Pneumococcal polysaccharide – 23-valent (Pneu-P-23):** recommended for all adults ≥ 65 years of age (see _Pneumococcal Vaccine_ chapter).

- ◉ **Meningococcal C conjugate vaccine (Men-C):** recommended for children under 5 years of age, adolescents and young adults. The recommended schedule depends on the age of the individual (see _Meningococcal Vaccine_ chapter) and the conjugate vaccine used. At least one dose in the pimary infant series should be given after 5 months of age. If the provincial/territorial policy is to give Men-C to persons ≥ 12 months of age, one dose is sufficient.

- ▲ **Diphtheria, tetanus, acellular pertussis vaccine – adult/adolescent formulation (Tdap):** a combined adsorbed "adult type" preparation for use in people ≥ 7 years of age, contains less diphtheria toxoid and pertussis antigens than preparations given to younger children and is less likely to cause reactions in older people.

- ▥ **Diphtheria, tetanus vaccine (Td):** a combined adsorbed "adult type" preparation for use in people ≥ 7 years of age, contains less diphtheria toxoid antigen than preparations given to younger children and is less likely to cause reactions in older people. It is given to adults not immunized in childhood as the second and third doses of their primary series and subsequent booster doses; Tdap is given only once under these circumstances as it is assumed that previously unimmunized adults will have encountered _Bordetella pertussis_ and have some pre-existing immunity.

- ◔ **Influenza vaccine (Inf):** recommended for all children 6-23 months of age and all persons ≥ 65 years of age. Previously unvaccinated children < 9 years of age require two doses of the current season's vaccine with an interval of at least 4 weeks. The second dose within the same season is not required if the child received one or more doses of influenza vaccine during the previous influenza season (see _Influenza Vaccine_ chapter).

- ◆ **IPV Inactivated polio virus**

Immunization of Adults

Prevention of infection by immunization is a lifelong process. There are a number of vaccines that all adults (≥ 18 years) require. There are also other vaccines that need to be tailored to meet individual variations in risk resulting from occupation, foreign travel, underlying illness, lifestyle and age.

Immunization does not stop at childhood!

Childhood immunization programs have significantly reduced vaccine-preventable diseases among children, but Canada's population has an increasing number of adults who remain vulnerable to these diseases. For example, a random digit dialing telephone survey conducted in 2002 among Canadians aged ≥ 18 found that only 54% of respondents had adequate coverage for tetanus, and this rate was lowest in those aged ≥ 60. Furthermore, although overall rates of vaccination are rising as compared with previous years, only two-thirds of Canadians aged ≥ 65 surveyed in 2000/2001 reported receiving influenza vaccination, and only 47% of those aged ≥ 20 with at least one chronic complication placing them at increased risk of influenza had been vaccinated.

Reasons for adults not being immunized

The following are common reasons for incomplete immunization in the adult years:

- lack of recommendation from their physician
- misrepresentation/misunderstanding of the risks of vaccine and benefits of disease prevention in adults
- lack of understanding of vaccine safety and efficacy
- missed opportunities for receiving the vaccine at health care encounters in physicians' offices, hospitals and nursing homes
- lack of publicly funded vaccine and reimbursement to health care providers
- lack of coordinated immunization programs for all adults
- lack of regulatory or legal requirements
- fear of injections
- lack of availability of up-to-date records and recording systems.

Health care provider as health advocate

Health professionals have the responsibility to prevent vaccine-preventable diseases in those under their care. Failure to maintain adult immunization results in significant individual risk, increased mortality and community risk for preventable diseases. Society not only expects health practitioners to promote newly approved interventions that maintain health and prevent disease but also to ensure that the population under their care has continuing and updated protection through appropriate immunization. Health care providers are recognized as leaders in their community, and their behaviours and attitudes can be a positive force for health promotion. They must present factual information concerning immunization and vaccines and also be able to review the benefits and risks of these interventions. This must be done in a manner that promotes the well-being of the individual, the family and the community.

Strategies to improve vaccine uptake in adults

Four categories of effective intervention that increase vaccine uptake have been described by Shefer et al. Interventions that increase the demand include community education, patient reminders, incentives and patient-held records. Educational programs for health care providers are also effective. However, the two interventions that had the greatest success in enhancing access to immunization were programs that decrease costs and those that include legal or regulatory interventions. Stone et al. in their meta-analysis of controlled clinical trials concluded that organizational changes, such as the introduction of specific clinics and the participation of non-physician staff to execute the specific prevention strategies, were the most effective ways to enhance uptake. Johnston and Conly have conducted an excellent review of these issues.

All adults should be counselled concerning their personal immunization status. Health care providers should regularly review the patients under their care to ensure not only that their immunization status is up to date but also that they have been made aware of new vaccines. Practitioners should regularly audit their patients' immunization records during clinical encounters that coincide with a mid-decade birthday (i.e., 15, 25, 35, 45, 55 years etc.).

There are a number of patient encounters/situations that provide opportunities for general vaccine counselling in adults:

◆ "new" patient/client encounter as part of the "history";
◆ patient hospitalization, especially when the diagnosis is a chronic disease;
◆ patients requesting specific vaccination(s), e.g., pneumococcal vaccine or influenza vaccine;
◆ patients with evidence of "risk taking" behaviour, such as illicit drug use or a sexually transmitted disease;
◆ individuals requesting advice concerning international travel;
◆ periodic health examinations;
◆ visits for chronic disease management;
◆ management protocols on admission to nursing and long-term care institutions;

- pregnancy and the immediate post-partum period;
- assessment of new immigrants to Canada;
- new employee assessments in health care and health care-related facilities;
- parents attending their children's vaccination visits.

Immunizations recommended for adults – routine

All adults should be immunized against diphtheria, tetanus, pertussis, measles, mumps, rubella and varicella. The schedule for adults who have no record or an unclear history of prior immunization as well as for booster dosing of those who have completed a prior primary series is shown in Table 5.

All Canadian adults require maintenance of immunity to tetanus and diphtheria, preferably with combined (Td) toxoid and a single dose of acellular pertussis vaccine. The first priority is to ensure that children receive the recommended series of doses, including the school leaving dose at 14 to 16 years of age, and that adults have completed primary immunization with Td. Currently, only a single dose of acellular pertussis (given as Tdap) is recommended in adulthood because the duration of protection from Tdap has yet to be determined. For adults not previously immunized against pertussis only one dose of Tdap is required as it is assumed that most adults will have some degree of immunity due to prior pertussis infection.

Combined measles, mumps, rubella vaccine (MMR) is preferred for vaccination of individuals not previously immunized against one or more of these viruses. Adults born before 1970 may be considered immune to measles. Adults born in 1970 or later who do not have documentation of adequate measles immunization or who are known to be seronegative should receive MMR vaccine. One additional dose of vaccine should be offered only to adults born in 1970 or later who are at greatest risk of exposure and who have not already received two doses or demonstrated immunity to measles. These people include travellers to a measles-endemic area, health care workers, students in post-secondary educational settings and military recruits. MMR is recommended for all adults without a history of mumps or mumps immunization. MMR vaccine should also be given to all adults without a history of rubella vaccination. Female adolescents and women of childbearing age should be vaccinated before pregnancy or post-partum, unless they have documented evidence of detectable antibody or prior vaccination. In addition, it is also important that health care workers of either sex be actively immunized against rubella because they may, through frequent face-to-face contact, expose pregnant women to rubella.

A history of chickenpox infection is adequate evidence of varicella immunity. Serologic testing should be performed in adults without a history of disease, as the majority of such adults will be immune and do not require the varicella vaccine. It is particularly important to promote varicella immunization with immigrants and refugees from tropical countries, women of

Table 5. Adult Immunization Schedule – Routinely for All

Vaccine	Dosing schedule (no record or unclear history of immunization)	Booster schedule (primary series completed)
Tetanus and diphtheria (page 312) given as Td; and pertussis given as Tdap	Doses 1 and 2, 4-8 weeks apart and dose 3 at 6-12 months later; one of the doses should be given as Tdap for pertussis protection	Td every 10 years; 1 dose should be given as Tdap if not previously given in adulthood
Measles, mumps and rubella (page 231) given as MMR	1 dose for adults born in or after 1970 without a history of measles or those individuals without evidence of immunity to rubella or mumps; second dose for selected groups (page 231)	Not routinely required
Varicella (page 335)	Doses 1 and 2, at least 4 weeks apart for susceptible adults (no history of natural disease or seronegativity)	Not currently recommended

childbearing age, those who are at occupational risk of exposure, including health care and child care workers, household contacts of immunocompromised persons, those with cystic fibrosis, and those susceptible adults exposed to a case of varicella. There are no data at present to guide recommendations for varicella booster dosing in adults following the primary vaccination series.

Immunizations for adults – specific risk groups

There are several specific groups of adults for whom certain vaccines are recommended because of the presence of risk factors for disease, and these are summarized in Table 6. In many cases, individual factors, and in particular the presence of underlying co-morbid illnesses, define groups that specifically benefit from certain vaccines. However, there are two commonly encountered groups of healthy adults who require assessment for a series of vaccines: health care workers and international travelers. In both of these groups, the priority should be to ensure that routinely recommended immunizations are completed and booster doses provided as indicated.

Health care workers, including hospital employees, other staff who work or study in hospitals (e.g., students in health care disciplines and contract workers), other health care personnel (e.g., those working in clinical laboratories, nursing homes and home care agencies) and child care workers, are at risk of exposure to communicable diseases because of their contact with patients or material from individuals with infections, both diagnosed and undiagnosed.

Hepatitis B is the most important vaccine-preventable infectious occupational disease for health care workers. The risk of being infected is a consequence of the prevalence of virus carriers in the population receiving care, the frequency of exposure to blood and other body fluids and the contagiousness of hepatitis B virus. Hepatitis B vaccine is recommended for health care workers and others who may be exposed to blood or blood products, or who may be at increased risk of sharps injury, bites or penetrating injuries (for example, clients and staff of institutions for the developmentally challenged). Annual influenza immunization is recommended for all health care personnel who have contact with individuals in high-risk groups. Such personnel include physicians, nurses and others in both hospital and outpatient settings; employees of chronic care facilities; and providers of home care, visiting nurses and volunteers. Influenza immunization of health care workers has been shown to reduce the mortality and morbidity of patients under their care in long-term settings and to reduce worker illness and absenteeism during the influenza season. Other vaccines may be indicated for certain workers at particularly high risk of exposure, such as laboratory workers in specialized reference or research facilities. These include but are not limited to typhoid, meningococcal, BCG, rabies, and smallpox vaccines. An individualized risk-benefit assessment is required.

International travelers represent another defined group requiring specific vaccine consideration. Ensuring that traveling adults have completed a primary series of routine vaccinations is the first priority (Table 6). This is particularly important because many vaccine-preventable diseases remain endemic in developing countries. Although completion of primary polio vaccination is adequate in most adults, a one-time polio booster (> 10 years since primary vaccination) is recommended for adults who have not had a previous booster and are traveling to polio-endemic countries. It is also important that travelers who are in specific risk groups for routine vaccines (such as pneumococcal and influenza vaccines in those ≥ 65) receive the ones indicated. With travel-specific vaccines, an individualized approach is required that considers a patient's health status, risk of exposure and complications from vaccine-preventable illness, as well as location and duration of travel. Most commonly these include consideration for immunization against yellow fever, Japanese encephalitis, typhoid, cholera, meningococcal disease, rabies, and hepatitis A and B, as listed in Table 6.

Adults ≥ 65 years of age and those with conditions that increase their chances of complications should receive one dose of pneumococcal vaccine and yearly influenza vaccine. Opportunities to increase influenza vaccination should be taken; it is estimated that less than one-half of high-risk Canadians receive influenza vaccine annually. Increasing the rate of influenza vaccination of health care workers and household contacts of individuals with increased risk of influenza complications will not only affect the vaccinated individuals but may also result in substantial secondary benefit to others.

Hepatitis A vaccination is recommended for those at increased risk of exposure (see *Hepatitis A Vaccine* chapter). Universal immunization against hepatitis B is recommended in childhood in Canada, and opportunities should be provided for adults to receive hepatitis B vaccine. Adults who are at increased risk of exposure to hepatitis B by virtue of their occupation, lifestyle or environment should receive the vaccine at the earliest possible clinical encounter. Patients may be vaccinated simultaneously for hepatitis A and B using a combined vaccine. Because of their increased risk for complications, all non-immune patients with chronic liver disease should be vaccinated against hepatitis A and B.

Cholera vaccine should be considered for high-risk travelers to cholera-endemic countries (please refer to the *Immunization of Travellers* chapter).

Meningococcal C conjugate vaccines are recommended for immunization of young adults to prevent the increased risk of serogroup C meningococcal disease in these age groups. Meningococcal vaccine is recommended for certain groups with increased risk of meningococcal disease (please refer to the *Meningococcal Vaccine* chapter). Such individuals include those with functional or anatomic asplenia; persons with complement, properdin or factor D deficiency; military recruits; research, industrial and clinical laboratory personnel who are routinely exposed to *Neisseria meningitidis* cultures; and travelers to high-risk areas. In cases in which risk is restricted to group C disease, monovalent serogroup C meningococcal conjugate vaccine may be preferred. Meningococcal vaccine is also used for outbreak management.

Although oral poliovirus vaccine is no longer used in Canada, individuals who have received a primary vaccination series with this vaccine are considered immune. Immunization of adults against poliovirus should be considered for those at increased risk (see *Poliomyelitis Vaccine* chapter).

Rabies vaccine should be offered, before exposure, to those individuals at high risk as a result of occupational or travel exposure to rabid animals. These may include veterinarians, laboratory workers, animal control and wildlife workers, spelunkers, trappers and hunters, and travelers to endemic countries where there may be limited access to safe and effective post-exposure prophylaxis.

Typhoid vaccine is recommended for high-risk international travelers, including those with prolonged (> 4 weeks) exposure in an endemic region or those with shorter duration of stay in particularly high-risk situations (please refer to the *Typhoid Vaccine* chapter). Although routine vaccination of health care workers is not required, laboratory workers who frequently handle live cultures of *Salmonella typhi* should be vaccinated.

Part 3 — Recommended Immunization

Table 6. Adult Immunization Schedule – Specific Risk Situations

Vaccine or toxoid	Indication	Schedule
Influenza (page 209)	Adults ≥ 65 years; Adults < 65 years at high risk of influenza-related complications, their household contacts, health care workers, and all those wishing to be protected against influenza.	Every autumn using current recommended vaccine formulation
Pneumococcal polysaccharide (page 267)	Adults ≥ 65 years; Adults < 65 who have conditions putting them at increased risk of pneumococcal disease	1 dose
Hepatitis A (page 179)	Occupational risk, life-style, travel and living in areas lacking adequate sanitation. Outbreak control, post-exposure immunoprophylaxis. Patients with chronic liver disease.	2 doses 6-12 months apart
Hepatitis B (page 189)	Occupational risk, life-style, post-exposure immunoprophylaxis. Patients with chronic liver disease.	3 doses at 0, 1 and 6 months
Bacille Calmette-Guérin (BCG) (page 149)	Rarely used. Consider for high-risk exposure in selected cases.	1 dose
Cholera (page 158)	High-risk exposure in travelers to endemic area(s)	1 oral dose of live attenuated vaccine; 2 doses at least 1 week apart but not greater than 6 weeks of oral inactivated vaccine
Japanese encephalitis (page 221)	Travel to endemic area(s) or other exposure risk	3 doses at days 0, 7 and 30
Poliomyelitis (page 277)	Travel to endemic area(s) or other risk group	Primary series doses 1 and 2, 4-8 weeks apart and dose 3 at 6-12 months later; 1 booster dose if > 10 years since primary series
Meningococcal conjugate	Young adults	1 dose
Meningococcal polysaccharide (page 239)	High-risk exposure groups	1 dose
Rabies, pre-exposure use (page 285)	Occupational or high-risk travelers	3 doses at days 0, 7 and 21
Typhoid (page 317)	High-risk travelers to endemic area(s) or other high-risk exposure	Parenteral capsular polysaccharide 1 dose; live attenuated 3-4 oral doses depending on preparation

Table 6. Adult Immunization Schedule – Specific Risk Situations

Vaccine or toxoid	Indication	Schedule
Yellow fever (page 343)	Travel to endemic area(s) or if required for foreign travel	1 dose with booster every 10 years if required
Smallpox	Laboratory staff working with vaccinia or other orthopoxviruses	1 dose

Naturally occurring smallpox has been eradicated worldwide, and as a result vaccination is highly restricted. Laboratory workers who handle vaccinia or other orthopoxviruses should be considered for vaccination.

Selected references

Canadian Association for the Study of the Liver. *Canadian Consensus Conference on the Management of Viral Hepatitis.* Canadian Journal of Gastroenterology 2000;14(Suppl B):5B-20B.

Committee to Advise on Tropical Medicine and Travel (CATMAT). *Statement on poliomyelitis vaccination for international travellers (evidence-based medicine recommendations).* Canada Communicable Disease Report 1995;21(16):145-48.

Committee to Advise on Tropical Medicine and Travel (CATMAT); National Advisory Committee on Immunization (NACI). *Statement on new oral cholera and travellers' diarrhea vaccination.* Canada Communicable Disease Report 2005;31(ACS-7):1-11.

Coulibaly N, De Serres G. *Coverage of anti-tetanus vaccinations in adults in Canada – year 2002.* Canadian Journal of Public Health 2004;95(6):456-59.

Health Canada. *Smallpox vaccination of laboratory workers.* Canada Communicable Disease Report 2004;30(19):167-9.

Johansen H, Nguyen K, Mao L et al. *Influenza vaccination.* Health Reports 2004;15(2):33-43.

Johnston BL, Conly JM. *Routine adult immunization in Canada: recommendations and performance.* Canadian Journal of Infectious Diseases 2002;13(4):226-31.

Lau DT, Hewlett AT. *Screening for hepatitis A and B antibodies in patients with chronic liver disease.* American Journal of Medicine 2005;118(Suppl 10A):28S-33S.

National Advisory Committee on Immunization (NACI). *Statement on recommended use of meningococcal vaccines.* Canada Communicable Disease Report 2001;27(ACS-6):2-36.

National Advisory Committee on Immunization (NACI). *Statement on smallpox vaccination.* Canada Communicable Disease Report 2002;28(ACS-1):1-12.

National Advisory Committee on Immunization (NACI). *Prevention of pertussis in adolescents and adults.* Canada Communicable Disease Report 2003;29(ACS-5):1-9.

National Advisory Committee on Immunization (NACI). *Update on varicella.* Canada Communicable Disease Report 2004;30(ACS-1):1-26.

Shefer A, Briss P, Rodewald L et al. *Improving immunization coverage rates: an evidence-based review of the literature.* Epidemiologic Reviews 1999;21(1):96-142.

Part 3 — Recommended Immunization

Spira AM. *Preparing the traveller.* Lancet 2003;361(9366):1368-81.

Statement on travellers and rabies vaccine. Canadian Medical Association Journal 1995;152(8):1241-45.

Stone EG, Morton SC, Hulscher ME et al. *Interventions that increase use of adult immunization and cancer screening services: a meta-analysis.* Annals of Internal Medicine 2002;136(9):641-51.

Immunization of Children and Adults with Inadequate Immunization Records

Many people present to health care providers and public health officials with inadequate immunization records. In the absence of a standardized approach to their management, they may be under- or over-immunized. The concern with over-immunization relates to vaccination against diphtheria, pertussis or tetanus because of the potential for a higher incidence of local adverse reactions. Local reactions increase with the number of doses administered. These local reactions can include large swelling at the injection site, but pain is generally limited, and such reactions are not a contraindication to continuing the recommended schedule. Recent studies have indicated that tetanus and diphtheria booster doses given in a combination product with acellular pertussis and administered at intervals of less than 5 years do not result in increased local reactions in adolescents.

In every instance, an attempt should be made to obtain the person's immunization records from his or her previous health care provider. Written documentation of immunization is preferred for both children and adults. In some instances, information obtained by telephone from the health care provider with the exact dates of immunization may be accepted. For children, parental recall of prior immunization, in the absence of documentation provided by the administrator of the vaccine, correlates poorly with immunizations received and should not be accepted as evidence of immunization. Adults without immunization records should also be considered unimmunized. Additional information on the immunization of people who have newly arrived in Canada can be found in the chapter entitled *Immunization of Persons New to Canada*, page 144.

Routine serologic testing to determine immunity of children and adults without records is generally not practical. Instead, the following approach is recommended:

- All children and adults lacking written documentation of immunization should be started on a primary immunization schedule as appropriate for their age. For more information, please refer to the *Recommended Immunization Schedules* chapter, page 93.

- Measles, mumps, and rubella (MMR), polio, *Haemophilus influenzae* type b conjugate, pneumococcal conjugate, meningococcal conjugate, hepatitis B and A, varicella and influenza vaccines can be given, if indicated, on the basis of age and/or risk factors without concern about prior receipt of these vaccines. This is acceptable because adverse effects of repeated immunization with these vaccines have not been demonstrated.

- Persons who develop a serious adverse local reaction after administration of vaccines containing tetanus, diphtheria and pertussis should be individually assessed before they receive additional doses of these vaccines. The benefit of continuing the series needs to be weighed against the risk of further adverse reactions. Serologic testing for diphtheria and tetanus antitoxin levels may demonstrate immune status and guide the need for continued immunization. There are no established serologic correlates for protection against pertussis.

◆ Pneumococcal polysaccharide vaccine should be given, if indicated when a record cannot be found, since in most studies local reaction rates after revaccination have been similar to rates following initial vaccination. For more information, please refer to the *Pneumococcal Vaccine* chapter, page 267.

Immunization in Pregnancy and Breast-Feeding

Introduction

Pregnancy provides a situation in which engagement in medical care may be greater than at any time in an otherwise healthy adult woman's life. It allows for evaluation of the woman's vaccine status as well as consideration of vaccines that may be beneficial to the neonate, if given to the woman, in order to decrease the risk of neonatal vaccine-preventable illness.

This chapter will review general issues regarding immunization in pregnancy, but particular issues will be addressed in vaccine-specific chapters. It is important that the obstetric care provider be familiar with both the potential risks of vaccination in pregnancy and the potential benefits in preventing disease at that time and providing neonatal protection. Ideally, this planning should occur before conception. If a woman of reproductive age presents with the intent to become pregnant, the adult immunization schedule should be reviewed and vaccines updated as indicated. For more information, please refer to the *Recommended Immunization Schedules* chapter, page 93.

Maternal benefits

Although pregnancy is an immunologically altered state, there are no data to support an inadequate response to vaccines. This is supported by data from trials of tetanus toxoid and polio vaccine in which normal adult immunologic responses were observed in pregnant women. There are a number of indications for immunization of pregnant women for the benefit of their own health. Recommendations include hepatitis B vaccine in a person with ongoing exposure risks, hepatitis A vaccine in a traveler or close contact of a person with hepatitis A, tetanus toxoid, meningococcal vaccine in an outbreak setting, and pneumococcal and influenza vaccines for all adult indications.

Maternal safety issues

There does not appear to be any evidence of increased risk of adverse reactions to vaccines administered in pregnancy. Reactions to vaccines in pregnancy are usually limited to local reactions, and no increase in anaphylactic reactions or events that might induce pre-term labour has been observed.

Safety and benefit of immunization in pregnancy for the fetus/infant

A major issue to consider regarding immunization in pregnancy is the risk or benefit of the vaccine for the fetus or neonate. There are no published data showing that any of the currently approved vaccines are teratogenic or embryotoxic, or have resulted in specific adverse pregnancy outcomes. In contrast, there are a good deal of data supporting the beneficial effects of antenatal vaccines on the prevention of disease in the neonate. In order for a vaccine to be beneficial to a neonate, a protective concentration of maternal antibody needs to be transferred to the infant transplacentally. It is known that all subclasses of IgG are transported from mother to infant across the placenta, but the majority of transfer occurs during the third trimester. Active placental transfer of IgG is specific and has variable efficacy. The mechanism is not well understood but can result in a range of cord blood levels that can be 20% to 200% of maternal levels. Maternal IgG typically has a half-life of 3-4 weeks in the newborn, waning during the first 6-12 months of life. Current pediatric vaccine schedules take into consideration the potential effect that maternally transferred antibodies may have on infant vaccinations and incorporate this into the vaccine schedules and dosing.

Risks associated with vaccines in pregnancy are primarily theoretical risks associated with the administration of live virus vaccines. There are circumstances in which vaccination with a live-attenuated product may be considered (e.g., yellow fever vaccine). If live vaccine is inadvertently given to a pregnant woman, termination of the pregnancy is not recommended (see specific chapters for details).

Immunization in pregnancy: review of specific vaccine categories

1. Live-attenuated vaccines

In general, live-attenuated virus vaccines (such as measles, mumps and rubella (MMR) or varicella) are contraindicated in pregnancy as there is a theoretical risk to the fetus. However, it is important to mention that to date, there is no evidence to demonstrate a teratogenic risk from such vaccines.

◆ **Rubella vaccine: please see the *Rubella Vaccine* chapter, page 298**

Rubella vaccine is available in combination with measles and mumps (MMR). It is a live attenuated vaccine and therefore contraindicated during pregnancy. The vaccine is indicated post-partum or pre-conception in susceptible women. It is advised that women should delay pregnancy by 1 month following such immunization.

Inadvertent rubella vaccinations in pregnancy were reportable to the U.S. Centers for Disease Control and Prevention between 1971 and 1989. Analysis of the accumulated data revealed that subclinical infection was detected in 1%-2% of fetuses but that there was no evidence of congenital rubella syndrome in any of the offspring of 226 inadvertently vaccinated women. In addition, in a prospective study by Motherisk in Toronto, infants of 94 women immunized 3 months before conception or during pregnancy did not have an increased rate of malformation compared with an unexposed cohort. Termination of pregnancy should not be recommended following inadvertent rubella immunization on the basis of fetal risks. However, given the small theoretical fetal risk, immunization with the rubella vaccine is best delayed until after delivery. Breast-feeding and Rh immune globulin administration are not contraindications to immunization. Nevertheless, because of possible decreased immunogenicity of the vaccine in the presence of Rh immune globulin, it is recommended that rubella antibody status be checked at 2 months post-partum.

◆ **Varicella vaccination: please see the *Varicella Vaccine* chapter, page 327**

Immunity to varicella should be reviewed in women of reproductive age, and vaccination should be recommended to non-pregnant women. Since the varicella vaccine is a live attenuated virus vaccine, its use should be avoided in pregnancy. A program to ensure that varicella vaccine is administered to the susceptible post-partum woman should be developed, with two doses given at least 4 weeks apart. In women receiving Rh immune globulin postpartum, an interval of 2 months should elapse before varicella vaccine is given. This is because of a theoretical risk of interference with immunogenicity.

Breast-feeding is not a contraindication to vaccination nor is household contact with a newborn.

In a study of 362 women, no cases of congenital varicella occurred as a result of inadvertent exposure to the vaccine in pregnancy. Inadvertent exposure to the vaccine, therefore, does not constitute a reason to recommend pregnancy termination. However, it is recommended that non-pregnant women who are vaccinated should delay conception by 1 month.

Following exposure of a pregnant woman to varicella, a history of previous vaccination or of chickenpox illness should be sought, as it has been shown to correlate well with seropositive immune status. In the absence of such a history, the mother's immunity should be verified by testing for varicella IgG. Exposed susceptible women should be offered varicella immunoglobulin (VarIg) within 96 hours of exposure in an attempt to prevent the disease or reduce the severity of their infection. The recommended dosage is 125 IU for each 10 kg body weight up to a maximum of 625 IU. Although a study has shown that congenital varicella syndrome did not occur in the fetuses of 97 pregnant women given VarIg, this study is too small to conclude that VarIg will prevent or alter disease in the fetus (please refer to the *Passive Immunizing Agents* chapter, page 353, for more specific recommendations). Susceptible pregnant women should be given varicella vaccine after delivery as long as 5 months have passed since VarIg administration.

◆ **Other live attenuated vaccines:**

Other live attenuated vaccines must be evaluated on an individual risk/benefit ratio. For instance, if a pregnant woman **must** travel to an area endemic for yellow fever, the vaccine may be administered when the risk of exposure is high and the travel cannot be postponed.

2. Inactivated viral and bacterial vaccines, toxoids

There is no evidence to suggest a risk to the fetus or to the pregnancy from maternal immunization with these vaccines.

◆ **Influenza vaccination:**

All pregnant women who are at high risk of influenza-related complications should be particularly targeted for influenza vaccination (see *Influenza Vaccine* chapter, page 209). Recent trends have indicated an increase in maternal age and higher rates of multiple gestation, both of which may present an increased risk of medical complications, including cardiorespiratory diseases, that would warrant influenza vaccination as per the adult indications. There is some evidence, although limited, suggesting that healthy pregnant women are at increased risk of complications from influenza. Mortality rates among pregnant women in the 1918 and 1957 pandemics were reported to be as high as 45%. This is presumably because pregnancy is associated with significant cardiovascular and respiratory demands, with increased stroke volume, heart rate and oxygen consumption. A more recent report demonstrated that the need for hospitalization was 4 times greater in pregnant than non-pregnant women with influenza. The risks were, in fact, calculated to be equivalent to those of non-pregnant women with high-risk conditions for whom immunization has traditionally been recommended.

However, given these limited data, more research is needed to clarify the feto-maternal advantages of influenza vaccine. The data regarding safety of the vaccine appear to be reassuring. A study of 252 pregnant women vaccinated during pregnancy at a mean gestational age of 26.1 weeks (range 14-39 weeks) had no adverse events and no difference in perinatal outcomes compared with a non-vaccinated group.

Immunization and breast-feeding

Breast-feeding is considered safe following immunization of the mother and has not been shown to adversely influence the maternal immune response. Therefore, breast-feeding does not represent a contraindication to any maternal immunization, and breast-feeding women who have not received all recommended adult immunizations may be safely immunized. Infants who are breast-fed should receive all recommended vaccines at the usual times.

Passive immunization

There is no known risk to the fetus and/or mother from administration of immune globulin for passive immunization during pregnancy. Therefore, these products should be administered as required.

Table 7. Indication for Use in Pregnancy

Vaccine	Indication for use in pregnancy	Comment
Measles, mumps, and rubella (MMR)	Contraindicated Immunize susceptible women post-partum.	No known fetal effects but live vaccine – theoretical risk. Not reason for termination of pregnancy.
Varicella	Contraindicated Immunize susceptible women post-partum.	No known fetal effects but live vaccine – theoretical risk. Not reason for termination of pregnancy.
Poliomyelitis Salk (IPV)	Not contraindicated	To be considered if pregnant woman needs immediate protection (high-risk situation/travel). No known fetal effects.
Yellow fever	Generally contraindicated unless travel to high-risk endemic area is unavoidable.	No data on fetal safety although fetuses exposed have not demonstrated complications. Not a reason for pregnancy termination.
Influenza	Safe	No adverse effects.
Rabies	Not contraindicated for post-exposure prophylaxis.	Prudent to delay pre-exposure immunization unless substantial risk of exposure.
Hepatitis A	No apparent risk	To be considered in high-risk situations in which benefits outweigh risks.
Hepatitis B	No apparent risk	Vaccine recommended for pregnant women at risk.
Pneumococcal polysaccharide	No apparent risk	Vaccine recommended for pregnant women in high-risk categories.
Meningococcal	Polysaccharide vaccine safe and effective in pregnancy. Conjugate vaccine: no data available.	Polysaccharide vaccine to be administered as per general guidelines for non-pregnant women. Conjugate – considered in situations in which benefit outweighs risk.

Table 7. Indication for Use in Pregnancy

Vaccine	Indication for use in pregnancy	Comment
Cholera	No data on safety.	To be used in high-risk situation only (e.g., outbreak).
Typhoid	No data on safety. Some preparations are live.	To be considered only in high-risk cases (e.g., travel to endemic areas).
Diphtheria/tetanus	No evidence of teratogenicity.	Susceptible women to be vaccinated as per general guidelines for non-pregnant women.
Pertussis	Lack of data confirming the safety and immunogenicity of acellular pertussis vaccine in pregnant women	Warranted when the risk of disease outweighs the risk of vaccine both for the mother and the fetus
Japanese encephalitis Live	No data on safety.	To be considered only in high-risk cases (e.g., travel to endemic areas if benefit outweighs risk).
Vaccinia (smallpox) Live	Contraindicated	Has been reported to cause fetal infection.

Selected references

Bar-Oz B, Levichek Z, Moretti ME et al. *Pregnancy outcome following rubella vaccination: a prospective controlled study.* American Journal of Medical Genetics 2004;130(1):52-4.

Centers for Disease Control and Prevention. *Measles, mumps and rubella vaccine use and strategies for elimination of measles, rubella, and congenital rubella syndrome and control of mumps: recommendations of the Advisory Committee on Immunization Practices (ACIP).* Morbidity and Mortality Weekly Report 1998;32(RR-8):32.

Freeman DW, Barno A. *Deaths from Asian influenza associated with pregnancy.* American Journal of Obstetrics and Gynecology 1959;78:1172-75.

Harris JW. *Influenza occurring in pregnant women: a statistical study of thirteen hundred and fifty cases.* Journal of the American Medical Association 1919;72(978):980.

Kanariou M, Petridou E, Liatsis M et al. *Age patterns of immunoglobulins G, A and M in healthy children and the influence of breast feeding and vaccination status.* Pediatric Allergy and Immunology 1995;6(1):24-9.

Munoz FM, Greisinger AJ, Wehmanen OA et al. *Safety of influenza vaccination during pregnancy.* American Journal of Obstetrics and Gynecology 2005;192(4):1098-1106.

Neuzil KM, Reed GW, Mitchel EF et al. *Impact of influenza on acute cardiopulmonary hospitalizations in pregnant women.* American Journal of Epidemiology 1998;148(11):1094-1102.

Pabst HF, Godel J, Grace M et al. *Effect of breast-feeding on immune response to BCG vaccination.* Lancet 1989;1(8633):295-97.

Pabst HF, Spady DW. *Effect of breast-feeding on antibody response to conjugate vaccine.* Lancet 1990;336(8710):269-70.

Shields KE, Galil K, Seward J et al. *Varicella vaccine exposure during pregnancy: data from the first 5 years of the pregnancy registry.* Obstetrics and Gynecology 2001;98(1):14-9.

Immunization of Infants Born Prematurely

Premature infants whose clinical condition is satisfactory should be immunized with age-appropriate doses of vaccine at the same chronological age and according to the same schedule as full-term infants, regardless of birth weight. In premature infants, maternally derived antibody is present at lower titres and for a shorter duration than in mature infants. As well, the severity of vaccine-preventable illnesses may be greater in this population. Therefore, immunization of premature infants should not be delayed.

Antibody response to immunization is generally a function of chronologic age and not of maturity. Although studies demonstrate conflicting results, premature infants may have lower antibody responses than full-term controls to several vaccinations. Despite this, vaccine efficacy remains high. Several recent studies have demonstrated that healthy premature infants generally tolerate immunizations well, with low rates of adverse events that are similar to those of full-term infants. These studies have evaluated the pentavalent combination vaccine products, hepatitis B vaccine and the newer conjugated pneumococcal and meningococcal vaccines.

Premature and very low birthweight infants (i.e., 1500 g) still hospitalized at the time of immunization, however, may experience a transient increase or recurrence of apnea and bradycardia following vaccination. This subsides within 48 hours and does not alter the overall clinical progress of the child. The risk of these events is greater among infants with ongoing cardiorespiratory issues at the time of vaccination, but such events can also occur in those who are clinically stable. Given these findings, it is recommended that hospitalized premature infants have continuous cardiac and respiratory monitoring for 48 hours after their first immunization.

Hepatitis B

The response to hepatitis B vaccine may be diminished in infants with birth weights < 2000 g. Routine immunization of infants of mothers known to be negative for hepatitis B surface antigen (HBsAg) should be delayed until the infant reaches 2000 g or 1 month of age. Premature infants born to women who are HBsAg positive should, however, still receive hepatitis B immune globulin (HBIg) within 12 hours of birth and the appropriate dose of vaccine starting at birth. These infants require a fourth dose of hepatitis B vaccine (please refer to the *Hepatitis B Vaccine* chapter, page 189, for more information).

If the mother's status is unknown, the vaccine should be given in accordance with the recommendations for the infant of an HBsAg-positive mother. The maternal status should be determined within 12 hours, and if the mother is HBsAg positive the infant should also receive HBIg.

Part 3 — Recommended Immunization

113

Influenza

All children < 2 years of age are now considered to be at high risk of significant morbidity and mortality from influenza and should be immunized starting at 6 months of age. This includes infants born prematurely. Household contacts of all infants < 23 months of age, including those < 6 months of age, who are too young to receive influenza immunization themselves, should also be immunized to prevent household transmission to the infant (please refer to the *Influenza Vaccine* chapter, page 209, for more information).

Respiratory syncytial virus (RSV)

Infants born at 32 weeks and 0 days' gestation or earlier who are ≤ 6 months of age (with or without bronchopulmonary dysplasia [BPD]) at the start of the RSV season, infants born between 32 and 35 weeks' gestation in isolated communities where hospital care is not readily accessible, as well as children ≤ 24 months of age with BPD who required oxygen and/or medical therapy for that illness within the 6 months preceding the RSV season and children < 2 years of age with hemodynamically significant cyanotic or acyanotic congenital heart disease should be considered for monoclonal anti-RSV antibody, palivizumab, to decrease the likelihood of serious RSV infection requiring hospitalization, and supplemental oxygen therapy (please refer to the *Passive Immunizing Agents* chapter, page 353 for more information).

Immunization of Patients in Health Care Institutions

Taking an immunization history from those admitted to hospital or attending outpatient clinics and vaccinating them before discharge provides an important opportunity to maintain up-to-date immunization for all patients. For patients without regular sources of care or those followed in specialized clinics, the only opportunities for immunization may be during clinic visits or hospitalization. There is good evidence that using provider reminders and standing orders, and evaluating vaccine coverage with feedback to providers improves vaccine uptake. Immunization status should also be verified during emergency department visits and vaccine offered as appropriate.

The admission of elderly patients and others at high risk of influenza complications or pneumococcal disease is an opportunity to ensure that these people are immunized. Effective programs to immunize such patients before discharge will guarantee that they do not miss immunization in the community during the limited influenza vaccination period.

All pregnant women should be screened for chronic hepatitis B virus (HBV) infection, and newborns of HBV-infected women should receive hepatitis B immune globulin and start a course of vaccine within 12 hours of birth. As well, administering the first dose of hepatitis B vaccine, before discharge, to other newborns at high risk of exposure to hepatitis B virus may be considered. Please refer to the *Hepatitis B Vaccine* chapter, page 189, for more information on the timing of vaccination and on other recommended recipients.

Women susceptible to rubella or varicella should receive vaccine post-partum before discharge. Please refer to the *Recent Administration of Human Immune Globulin Products* chapter, page 53, for specific recommendations for women who have received Rh immune globulin post-partum. Arrangements should also be made for the parents, other adolescent or adult family members, and other caretakers of the newborn to receive, as soon as possible, one dose of pertussis-containing vaccine formulated for adolescents and adults if they have not already received one.

Residents of long-term care institutions, like members of the general population, should receive all routine immunizations appropriate for their age and individual risk status. Annual immunization against influenza is essential for residents of long-term care institutions, and robust programs to ensure that this occurs should be put in place. As well as the proven strategies of provider reminders, standing orders, and evaluation of vaccine coverage with feedback to providers, it is advisable to inform patients or their surrogate decision makers of the facility's immunization policy on admission and every effort made to obtain informed consent before the influenza season.

Part 3 — Recommended Immunization

In both acute-care and long-term care settings, it is most important that immunization efforts be part of organized care plans within each department, with clear accountability for program planning, implementation and evaluation.

Selected references

Centers for Disease Control and Prevention. *Recommendations of the Advisory Committee on Immunization Practices: programmatic strategies to increase vaccination rates – assessment and feedback of provider-based vaccination coverage information.* Morbidity and Mortality Weekly Report 1996;45(10):219-20.

Task Force on Community Preventive Services. *The guide to community preventive services.* URL: <www.thecommunityguide.org/vaccine/default.htm>. Accessed February 5, 2006.

Immunization of Immunocompromised Persons

The number of immunocompromised people in Canadian society is steadily increasing for a variety of reasons. These include our increased understanding of "normal" and altered immunity; recognition of the subtle immunodeficiencies associated with chronic illnesses (e.g., liver disease, renal disease); increased numbers of individuals with absent or dysfunctional spleens; the expanding range of illnesses treated with immuno-modulatory agents (e.g., autoimmune diseases, inflammatory conditions); the HIV pandemic; increased numbers of long-term survivors after organ transplantation; and the increased use of ablative therapy for cancer and other conditions.

The number of immunizations to which immunocompromised people are likely to be exposed is also increasing. There is an ever-enlarging spectrum of vaccines available, and an increasing number of vaccines are included in routine programs. Efforts are under way to fully immunize adolescents, adults and the elderly. As well, individuals with significant illness can now travel with relative ease, for example, people infected with HIV. For more information, please visit http://www.phac-aspc.gc.ca/tmp-pmv/catmat-ccmtmv/index.html.

Therefore, the frequency and complexity of questions dealing with immunization in immunocompromised hosts will only increase with time. Still further complexity is added by the fact that the relative degree of immunodeficiency varies over time in many people. The decision to recommend for or against any particular vaccine will depend upon a careful, case-by-case analysis of the risks and benefits. Consultation with a specialist with expertise in vaccination should be considered when immunizing immunocompromised persons.

There is potential for serious illness and death in the underimmunization of immunocompromised people, and every effort should be made to ensure adequate protection through immunization. However, the inappropriate use of live vaccines can cause serious adverse events in some immunocompromised hosts as a result of uncontrolled replication of the virus or bacterium. Children with a known or suspected family history of congenital or hereditary immunodeficiency that is a contraindication to vaccination with live virus should not receive live vaccines unless their immune competence has been established. As many congenital immunodeficiencies are autosomal recessive, the history of immunodeficiency may not be present in first-degree relatives. Vaccine providers should also be alert to such clues as multiple neonatal or infant deaths in a family. Although questioning about personal or family history of immunodeficiency is recommended before any live vaccine is administered, the family history is of paramount importance if such vaccines are to be given before 1 year of age, as signs or symptoms of congenital immunodeficiency may not be present in younger

117

children. Immunization of those with significant immunodeficiency should be performed only in consultation with experts.

General principles

Several general principles apply to the immunization of immunocompromised individuals:

- ◆ maximize benefit while minimizing harm;
- ◆ make no assumptions about susceptibility or protection
  - a history of childhood infection or previous immunization may be irrelevant;
- ◆ immunize at the time when maximum immune response can be anticipated
  - immunize early, before immunodeficiency begins, if possible
  - delay immunization if the immunodeficiency is transient (if this can be done safely)
  - stop or reduce immunosuppression to permit better vaccine response, if appropriate;
- ◆ consider the immunization environment broadly
  - vaccinate household contacts when appropriate (see below for specific recommendations)
  - consider the immunization status of both the donor and/or recipient in the setting of hematopoietic stem cell transplantation;
- ◆ avoid live vaccines, unless
  - data are available to support their use
  - the risk of natural infection is greater than the risk of immunization;
- ◆ monitor vaccinees carefully and boost aggressively
  - the magnitude and duration of vaccine-induced immunity are often reduced in immunocompromised individuals.

Approach to vaccination of immunodeficient individuals

Chronic liver disease

Hepatitis A and B immunizations are recommended in people with chronic liver disease, since they are at risk of fulminant hepatitis. Vaccination should be done early in the course of the disease, as the immune response to vaccine is suboptimal in advanced liver disease. For more information, please refer to the hepatitis A and B chapters, pages 205.

Chronic renal disease and patients undergoing dialysis

Bacterial and viral infections are a major cause of morbidity and mortality in patients who have renal disease or who are undergoing chronic dialysis. Many of these infections are vaccine preventable. All the standard immunizations are required (see *Recommended Immunization Schedules*, page 93).

Particular attention should be paid to ensuring that there is optimal protection against varicella, hepatitis B, influenza and pneumococcal diseases. Influenza immunization is recommended yearly; household members should also be vaccinated. The schedule proposed for immunization against pneumococcal disease in patients with splenic disorders (see below) should be followed for people with chronic renal disease and for dialysis patients. Some data suggest that there is a poor response to hepatitis B vaccine in the dialysis population and that hepatitis B surface antibody levels might decline rapidly. In adults, immunization with a higher dosage is recommended (see the *Hepatitis B Vaccine* chapter for details). Data on alternative vaccination schedules for children undergoing hemodialysis are limited. The antibody level to hepatitis B surface antigen should be measured yearly and booster doses should be given if the level decreases to less than 10 IU/L (see the *Hepatitis B Vaccine* chapter for details). Varicella vaccine should be given to susceptible transplant candidates before transplantation because varicella is a significant cause of morbidity and mortality, but the vaccine is contraindicated in immunosuppressed patients after transplantation (see below). See section on solid organ transplantation for renal transplant recipients.

Splenic disorders

Asplenia or hyposplenism may be congenital, surgical or functional. A number of conditions can lead to functional hyposplenism. These include sickle cell anemia, thalassemia major, essential thrombocytopenia, celiac disease and inflammatory bowel disease. There are no contraindications to the use of any vaccine for patients known to be functionally or anatomically hyposplenic. Particular attention should be paid to providing optimal protection against encapsulated bacteria (*Streptococcus pneumoniae*, *Haemophilus influenzae* type b [Hib], *Neisseria meningitidis*), to which these individuals are highly susceptible. They should also receive all routine immunizations and yearly influenza vaccination. Careful attention should be paid to immunization status when "elective" surgical splenectomy is planned so that all of the necessary vaccines can be delivered at least 2 weeks before removal of the spleen. In the case of an emergency splenectomy, vaccines should be given 2 weeks after the splenectomy. If the patient is discharged earlier and there is a concern that he/she might not return, vaccination should be given before discharge.

The following immunization schedule is recommended for hyposplenic and asplenic individuals.

Part 3 — Recommended Immunization

- ◆ **Meningococcal disease:**

  - Children < 2 years of age with asplenia or hyposplenia should be vaccinated with Men-C-C as described in the routine infant schedule (please refer to the *Recommended Immunization Schedules* chapter, page 93 and then receive quadrivalent Men-P-ACYW at 2 years of age and at least 2 weeks after the Men-C-C.

  - Children > 2 years of age and adults should receive both the Men-C-C and the Men-P-ACYW. The Men-C-C should be given first and the Men-P-ACYW at least 2 weeks later. If the Men-P-ACYW vaccine is given first, an adequate response to Men-C-C has been observed after a delay of 6 months in adults, and this remains the recommended interval until further data are available.

  - A booster dose of Men-P-ACYW is recommended every 2 to 5 years depending on the age at immunization. Please refer to the meningococcal chapter, page 237, for more information on recommended usage.

- ◆ **Pneumococcal disease:**

  - Children ≤ 23 months of age: Pneu-C-7 is recommended as described in the routine infant schedule (please refer to the *Recommended Immunization Schedules* chapter, page 93). They should receive the Pneu-P-23 at 2 years of age and ≥ 8 weeks after the last dose of Pneu-C-7.

  - Children 24 to 59 months not previously vaccinated: two doses of Pneu-C-7, administered 2 months apart, followed by one dose of Pneu-P-23 administered ≥ 8 weeks after the second dose of Pneu-C-7.

  - Children 24 to 59 months who have completed the Pneu-C-7 vaccination series before age 2: one dose of Pneu-P-23 (≥ 8 weeks after the last dose of Pneu-C-7).

  - Children aged 24 to 59 months who have already received Pneu-P-23 but not Pneu-C-7: two doses of Pneu-C-7 administered 2 months apart. Vaccination with Pneu-C-7 should be initiated ≥ 8 weeks after vaccination with Pneu-P-23.

  - Children ≥ 5 years of age and adults who have not previously received pneumococcal vaccines should be vaccinated with Pneu-P-23. Pneu-C-7 is not contraindicated in children ≥ 5 years of age with high-risk conditions. When circumstances permit, some experts suggest that the conjugate vaccine may be given as the initial dose followed by the polysaccharide vaccine, as this may theoretically improve antibody response and immunologic memory. However, the polysaccharide vaccine is the vaccine of choice for these individuals, and if only one vaccine can be provided it should be the polysaccharide vaccine.

- A single booster with Pneu-P-23 is recommended after 5 years in those aged > 10 years at the time of initial immunization and after 3 years for those who received their initial vaccine when they were ≤ 10 years.

♦ **Haemophilus influenzae type b:**

Vaccination with the age-appropriate primary series of Hib conjugate vaccine should be completed (if not already complete) for all children < 5 years of age with asplenia. Despite limited efficacy data and the low overall risk of Hib sepsis in individuals > 5 years of age, especially in the era of high Hib immunization coverage in the population, some experts recommend that all asplenic individuals > 5 years of age receive a single dose of conjugate Hib vaccine, regardless of previous Hib immunization.

Congenital immunodeficiency states

This is a varied group of conditions that includes defects in antibody production (e.g., agammaglobulinemia, isotype and IgG subclass deficiencies, common variable immunodeficiency), complement deficiencies, defects in one or more aspects of cell-mediated immunity and mixed deficits. Individuals with defects in antibody and complement have unusual susceptibility to the encapsulated bacteria and members of the Enteroviridae family (e.g., polio, coxsackie and echoviruses), and individuals with mixed and T cell defects are particularly susceptible to intracellular pathogens (virtually all viruses and some bacteria, fungi and parasites). Although the defects and susceptibility patterns are very different, the approach to immunization is quite similar for these individuals. Component and inactivated vaccines can and should be administered in all of these conditions, despite the fact that many vaccinees will respond poorly, if at all. Live vaccines are generally not recommended for these patients, although some exceptions exist (see below).

♦ **Antibody defects:**

Immune response to a vaccine might be decreased and antibody levels might decrease more quickly in people with congenital B cell deficiency. As a general rule, people with antibody defects can be protected from many of the vaccine-preventable infections with the use of intravenous immunoglobulin (IVIg) or pathogen-specific Ig preparations. However vaccination is recommended in these people to increase the level of protection.

Particular attention should be given to ensuring that individuals with these conditions are immunized against pneumococcal, meningococcal and Hib diseases. Yearly influenza vaccine is also recommended. Although oral poliovirus vaccine (OPV) is no longer used in Canada, it remains an approved product and is used in many other countries. OPV should not be used in the affected individual or any of his or her family members. Measles (available as MMR) and varicella vaccines should be considered if the patient is not receiving regular Ig replacement therapy (which may affect the efficacy of the vaccines); but all other live vaccines are contraindicated (except in isolated IgA deficiency).

◆ **T cell, natural killer and mixed cell-mediated antibody defects:**

All live vaccines are contraindicated. Inadvertent live vaccine administration and exposure to natural infections can be dealt with by rapid administration of serum Ig or pathogen-specific Ig with or without appropriate antiviral or antibacterial treatment. Yearly influenza vaccine is recommended.

◆ **Phagocytic defects:**

Live bacterial vaccines (BCG [Bacille Calmette-Guérin] and oral typhoid vaccine) are contraindicated. Yearly influenza vaccine is recommended.

◆ **Complement deficiency:**

There are no contraindications to the use of any vaccine. However, immunity can decrease over time. Measurement of antibody titres and re-immunization, if needed, should be considered. Individuals with complement deficiency should receive meningococcal vaccine because of increased susceptibility to this pathogen (see the section on high-risk groups in the meningococcal chapter for details). Immunizations against common bacterial pathogens such as pneumococcus and Hib are also recommended.

◆ **Household contact:**

Even if contraindicated for the patients, household contacts can receive MMR vaccine if indicated. Varicella vaccine is recommended for susceptible contacts of immunocompromised individuals. No precautions need to be taken after vaccination unless the recipient develops a rash. In such circumstances, the rash should be covered and the vaccine recipient should avoid direct contact with the immuncompromised person for the duration of the rash. Yearly influenza vaccination and up-to-date routine immunizations are also recommended for household contacts of immunocompromised individuals

Immunosuppressive therapy

Long-term immunosuppressive therapy (e.g., long-term steroids [discussed below], cancer chemotherapy, radiation therapy/azathioprine, cyclosporine, cyclophosphamide/infliximab) is used for organ transplantation and an increasing range of chronic infectious and inflammatory conditions (e.g., inflammatory bowel disease, psoriasis, systemic lupus erythematosis). These therapies have their greatest impact on cell-mediated immunity, although T cell-dependent antibody production can also be adversely affected.

There is no contraindication to the use of any inactivated vaccine in these people, and particular attention should be paid to the completion of childhood immunizations, annual influenza immunization and pneumococcal immunization (with a booster after 3-5 years). Ideally, all appropriate vaccines or boosters should be administered to these individuals at least 14 days before the initiation of therapy. If this cannot be done safely, a period of at least 3 months should elapse after immunosuppressive drugs have been stopped before administration of both inactivated and component vaccines (to establish immunogenicity, although inactivated vaccines can be administered if required for post-exposure or outbreak management) and live vaccines (to reduce the risk of dissemination). However, the interval may vary with the intensity of the immunosuppressive therapy, underlying disease and other factors. If immunosuppressive therapy cannot be stopped, inactivated or component vaccines should be given when the therapy is at the lowest possible level. Live vaccines are generally contraindicated, although the risk-to-benefit ratio for several of these vaccines can favour immunization if only low doses of immunosuppressive drugs are required and there is significant risk of wild-type infection (e.g., varicella vaccine in seronegative individuals).

Children with acute lymphocytic leukemia may be vaccinated with the varicella vaccine if the disease has been in remission for $\geq$ 12 months, the patient's total lymphocyte count is $\geq 1.2 \times 10^9$/L, the patient is not receiving radiation therapy, and maintenance chemotherapy can be withheld for at least 1 week before to 1 week after immunization. Two doses of the vaccine are recommended, 1-3 months apart, since North American studies suggest that two doses are more immunogenic than a single dose in these patients. For more information refer to the *Varicella Vaccine* chapter, page 327.

♦ **High dose steroids:**

High-dose, systemic steroids (e.g., a prednisone dose of $\geq$ 2 mg/kg per day or $\geq$ 20 mg per day for $\geq$ 14 days) can interfere with vaccine-induced immune responses. Of course, reasonable clinical judgment must be exercised in the risk-to-benefit review of each case. Topical, inhaled and locally injected (intra-articular, bursal or tendon injection) steroids do not have an impact on vaccines unless there is clinical or laboratory evidence of immunosuppression from such therapy. A period of at least 1 month should elapse between high-dose steroid use and the administration of both inactivated and component vaccines (to establish immunogenicity, unless needed for post-exposure or outbreak management) and live vaccines (to reduce the risk of dissemination). Children with adrenogenital syndrome and those receiving physiologic replacement doses of glucocorticoids can follow the routine immunization schedule without restriction.

Hematopoietic stem cell transplantation

If time permits, careful consideration must be given to the pre-ablation immunization status of the patient and, in the case of allogenic bone marrow transplantation (BMT), the donor. It is well established that disease and immunization histories in both the host and the donor (i.e., in adoptive transfer) can influence immunity after ablation or transplantation. Antibody titres to vaccine-preventable diseases decline after allogenic or autologous hematopoietic stem cell transplantation if the recipient is not re-vaccinated. Hematopoietic stem cell transplant recipients are at increased risk of certain vaccine-preventable diseases (e.g., pneumococcal and Hib infections).

Recommendations for post-transplantation immunizations in this setting include the following:

◆ DTaP (< 7 years old) or one dose of Tdap followed by two doses of Td (persons ≥ 7 years old) should be given starting 12 months after transplantation. Three doses are required, at 12, 14 and 24 months after transplantation.

◆ Hib vaccine is recommended 12 months after transplantation. Three doses are required (12, 14 and 24 months after transplantation).

◆ Inactivated polio vaccine (IPV) should be given 12 months after transplantation. Three doses are required, 12, 14 and 24 months after transplantation.

◆ Pneumococcal vaccine is recommended for all persons 12 months after transplantation. Adults and children > 5 years of age should receive the Pneu-P-23. Children < 5 years should be immunized with the Pneu-C-7 according to the recommended schedule for their age, as if they had not been previously immunized. Children 2 to 5 years of age should receive both conjugate and polysaccharide vaccine (see *Pneumococcal Vaccine* chapter, page 267, for recommended schedules). Because antibody response to pneumococcal vaccination is known to be poor in these patients, some experts recommend that all transplant patients > 2 years of age receive a booster dose of polysaccharide vaccine 1 year after their initial Pneu-P-23 immunization.

◆ Meningococcal vaccine should be given 12 months after transplantation if indicated (see meningococcal chapter, page 237, for age-specific recommendation). At this time, there are a number of choices for immunization to prevent meningococcal disease, and new conjugate vaccines are being developed (see NACI Web site for future updates).

◆ Inactivated influenza vaccine should be given annually during early autumn, starting at least 6 months after transplantation.

◆ Hepatitis B vaccine should be given to all patients. Vaccination should be started 12 months after transplantation, and three doses are required, at 12, 14 and 24 months after transplantation.

◆ MMR should be given at least 2 years after the transplantation and only if the recipient is deemed to be immunocompetent by the transplant specialist. It should not be given to those with chronic graft-versus-host disease or those taking immunosuppressive therapy for chronic-graft-versus host disease. A second dose should be given 6-12 months later.

◆ Varicella vaccination of recipients at ≥ 2 years after transplantation may be considered, provided there is minimal immunosuppression and no graft-versus-host disease. Until further data are available, the same age-appropriate dosage schedule as for healthy children may be followed. Currently, the only varicella vaccine approved in Canada for use in select immunocompromised people is Varilrix®.

◆ Other live vaccines (BCG, yellow fever and oral typhoid vaccine) are usually contraindicated in hematopoietic stem cell recipients with active graft-versus-host diseases or immunosuppression. If such vaccines are required, consultation with a specialist is recommended.

◆ Non-immune household contacts should be immunized against measles, mumps, rubella, varicella and influenza. IPV and hepatitis A vaccine should be administered if indicated.

Solid organ transplantation

The ideal is to immunize all recipients before transplantation. However, many children undergo solid organ transplantation before completion of their immunization schedule. Solid organ recipients usually receive lifelong immunosuppression. No formal recommendations have been developed about when to resume immunization. In general, vaccination should not be re-initiated until at least 6-12 months after transplantation.

Recommendations in this setting include the following:

◆ IPV: recommended in children and adults before or after transplantation to complete the routine immunization schedule.

◆ DTaP in children < 7 years old and Td (first dose as Tdap) in persons ≥ 7 years old: recommended in children and adults before or after transplantation to complete the routine immunization schedule.

◆ Hib vaccine: recommended in children before or after transplantation to complete the routine immunization schedule. Hib vaccine should be administered to all lung transplant recipients.

◆ Pneumococcal vaccine: recommended before or after transplantation because of the increased risk of invasive pneumococcal disease in these patients. See the schedule described in the section on asplenic patients. A booster with Pneu-P-23 should be given once after 3-5 years (see *Pneumococcal Vaccine* chapter).

◆ Meningococcal vaccine: recommended before or after transplantation if routinely indicated (see *Meningococcal Vaccine* chapter for age-specific recommendation). At this time, there are a number of choices for immunization to prevent meningococcal disease, and new conjugate vaccines are being developed (see NACI Web site for future updates).

- MMR vaccine: recommended before transplantation for children, contraindicated after transplantation. Some experts consider using MMR in seronegative females before pregnancy ≥ 2 years after transplantation, when the patient is deemed to be taking minimal immunosuppressive therapy.

- Inactivated influenza vaccine is recommended yearly.

- Hepatitis B vaccine: recommended in children and adults before or after transplantation to complete the immunization schedule (see *Hepatitis B Vaccine* chapter).

- Hepatitis A vaccine: recommended for all transplant candidates with chronic liver diseases and for other transplant candidates if indicated. It can be considered for all solid organ transplant candidates before or after transplantation.

- Varicella vaccine: recommended before transplantation for non-immune (as determined by serology) children and adults but not recommended after transplantation. However, it may be considered ≥ 2 years after transplantation, when the patient is deemed to be taking minimal immunosuppressive therapy. Until further data are available, the same age-appropriate dosage schedule as for healthy children may be followed. Children awaiting renal and liver transplants may be immunized with one to two doses of varicella vaccine (depending on their age), the last dose being given at least 4-6 weeks prior to transplantation. They should not be receiving immunosuppressive treatment at the time of vaccination. As there is currently insufficient information regarding varicella immunization of cardiac and lung transplant candidates, no firm recommendation can be made at this time for these patients.

Other live vaccines are usually contraindicated after transplantation. However, if some live vaccines are needed, consultation with a specialist is recommended.

Household contacts who do not have immunity should be immunized against Hib, measles, mumps, rubella, varicella and influenza. IPV, hepatitis A and hepatitis B and any other vaccines should be administered if indicated.

Illnesses that progressively weaken the immune system (e.g., Human Immunodeficiency Virus (HIV), myelodysplasia)

With the exception of BCG, there are no contraindications to the use of any vaccine (including MMR) early in the course of these illnesses. With progression of these conditions, the risk of using live vaccines increases. Therefore, the risks and benefits of a particular vaccine (and the alternative therapies available) need to be carefully considered.

Early immunization is not only safer but is also more effective in these conditions. There is no contraindication to the use of inactivated or component vaccines at any time. Particular attention should be paid to the completion of childhood immunizations, pneumococcal immunization (see *Pneumococcal Vaccine* chapter), annual influenza immunization and possibly booster doses against Hib. In the case of HIV, consensus "cut-offs" have been determined for the use of some live vaccines. Infants infected with HIV who are asymptomatic should receive routine MMR vaccination. In addition, MMR is recommended for most symptomatic HIV-infected persons, including children who are symptomatic without evidence of severe immunosuppression. Please consult an infectious disease specialist/immunologist for more specific advice on MMR immunization for HIV-infected people.

Varicella vaccine should be considered in children > 12 months of age with asymptomatic or mildly symptomatic HIV infection (CDC class N1 or A1) and with age-specific CD4 percentages of > 25%. Two doses need to be given 3 months apart. Although theoretical concerns have been raised about increases (probably transient) in HIV viral load, which can occur after a number of routine immunizations, these changes are transient and should not influence the decision regarding immunization.

Immunocompromised travellers

Although the degree and range of infectious disease risks can increase dramatically when an immunocompromised individual travels to other countries or continents, the basic principles already outlined still apply. Evidence is accumulating to suggest that several live vaccines (including yellow fever vaccine) can be considered for people with HIV infection whose CD4+ T cell count is > 200/mm^3. However, the risks and benefits of each live vaccine must be carefully evaluated for every traveler. When a certificate of yellow fever vaccination is required but this vaccine is contraindicated, a letter of deferral should be supplied to the patient.

Selected references

American Society of Transplantation. *Guidelines for vaccination of solid organ transplant candidates and recipients.* American Journal of Transplantation 2004;4(Suppl 10): S160-63.

Ballout A, Goffin E, Yombi JC et al. *Vaccinations for adult solid organ transplant recipients: current recommendations.* Transplantation Proceedings 2005;37(6):2826-27.

Campbell AL, Herold BC. *Immunization of pediatric solid-organ transplantation candidates: immunizations in transplant candidates.* Pediatric Transplantation 2005;9(5):652-61.

Castagnola E, Fioredda F. *Prevention of life-threatening infections due to encapsulated bacteria in children with hyposplenia or asplenia: a brief review of current recommendations for practical purposes.* European Journal of Haematology 2003;71(5):319-26.

Centers for Disease Control and Prevention. *Guidelines for preventing opportunistic infections among hematopoietic stem cell transplant recipients.* Morbidity and Mortality Weekly Report 2000;49(RR-10):1-125.

Centers for Disease Control and Prevention. *Recommendations of the Advisory Committee on Immunization Practices (ACIP): use of vaccines and immune globulins*

Table 8. Vaccination of Individuals with Immunodeficiency

Vaccine	HIV/AIDS	Severe immunodeficiency	Solid organ transplantation	Post-BMT	Chronic renal disease/dialysis	Hyposplenism or asplenia
Inactivated/component vaccines						
DTaP, Tdap, Td°	Routine use*	Routine use	Routine use	Recommended†	Routine use	Routine use
IPV	Routine use	Routine use	Routine use	Recommended	Routine use	Routine use
Hib	Routine use	Routine use	Routine use	Recommended	Routine use	Recommended for children < 5 years. Consider for all
Influenza	Recommended	Recommended	Recommended	Recommended	Recommended	Recommended
Pneumococcal	Recommended	Recommended	Recommended	Recommended	Recommended	Recommended
Meningococcal	Routine use	Recommended	Routine use	Routine use	Routine use	Recommended
Hepatitis A	Recommended (MSM, IDU)	Use if indicated**	Use if indicated**	Use if indicated	Use if indicated	Use if indicated
Hepatitis B	Recommended (MSM, IDU)	Routine use	Routine use	Recommended	Recommended (higher dosage)	Routine use
Live vaccines						
MMR	Routine use‡ (if no significant compromise)	Contraindicated	Recommended before transplantation. Contraindicated after***	Consider at 24 mo (no suppressive Rx, no GVHD)	Routine use	Routine use

Table 8. Vaccination of Individuals with Immunodeficiency

Vaccine	HIV/AIDS	Severe immunodeficiency	Solid organ transplantation	Post-BMT	Chronic renal disease/dialysis	Hyposplenism or asplenia
Varicella	Consider in asymptomatic and mildly symptomatic disease	Contraindicated	Recommended before transplant. Consider at 24 mo (min suppressive Rx)	Consider at 24 mo (no suppressive Rx, no GVHD)	Recommended	Use if indicated
Oral typhoid	Contraindicated (use IM vaccine instead)	Contraindicated (use IM vaccine instead)	Contraindicated (use IM vaccine instead)	Contraindicated (use IM vaccine instead)	If indicated use IM	If indicated use IM
BCG	Contraindicated	Contraindicated	Contraindicated	Contraindicated	Use if indicated	Use if indicated
Yellow fever	Contraindicated	Contraindicated	Contraindicated	Contraindicated	Use if indicated	Use if indicated
Oral cholera	Contraindicated	Contraindicated	Contraindicated	Contraindicated	Use if indicated	Use if indicated

BMT: Bone marrow transplantation; MSM: Men who have sex with other men; IDU: intravenous drug users; GVHD: graft-versus-host disease; IM: intramuscular.

○ Product used would depend on age.

* Routine vaccination schedules should be followed with age-appropriate booster doses.

† Vaccination and/or re-vaccination recommended with or without verification of serologic response.

** Recommended for transplant candidates with chronic liver diseases.

‡ Most HIV-positive children can receive the first MMR vaccine without significant risk. Administration of the second MMR dose (particularly in adults) must be evaluated on a case-by-case basis.

*** Consider at 24 mo (no suppressive therapy, no GVHD) in seronegative females before pregnancy.

Part 3 — Recommended Immunization

129

for persons with altered immunocompetence. Morbidity and Mortality Weekly Report 1993;42(RR-4):1-18.

Committee to Advise on Tropical Medicine and Travel. *Statement on travellers and HIV/AIDS.* Canada Communicable Disease Report 1994;20(17):147-49.

Duchini A, Goss JA, Karpen A et al. *Vaccinations for adult solid-organ transplant recipients: current recommendations and protocols.* Clinical Microbiology Reviews 2003;16(3):357-64.

Fivush BA, Neu AM. *Immunization guidelines for pediatric renal disease.* Seminars in Nephrology 1998;18(3):256-63.

Gershon AA, Steinberg SP. *Persistence of immunity to varicella in children with leukemia immunized with live attenuated varicella vaccine.* New England Journal of Medicine 1989;320(14):892-97.

Keeffe EB. *Acute hepatitis A and B in patients with chronic liver disease: prevention through vaccination.* American Journal of Medicine 2005;118(Suppl 10A):S21-27.

LaRussa P, Steinberg S, Gershon AA. *Varicella vaccine for immunocompromised children: results of collaborative studies in the United States and Canada.* Journal of Infectious Diseases 1996;174(Suppl 3):S320-23.

McFarland E. *Immunizations for the immunocompromised child.* Pediatric Annals 1999;28(8):487-96.

Melles DC, de Marie S. *Prevention of infections in hyposplenic and asplenic patients: an update.* Netherlands Journal of Medicine 2004;62(2):45-52.

Mileno MD, Bia FJ. *The compromised traveler.* Infectious Disease Clinics of North America 1998;12(2):369-412.

Molrine DC. *Recommendations for immunizations in stem cell transplantation.* Pediatric Transplantation 2003;7(Suppl 3):S76-85

Molrine DC, Hibberd PL. *Vaccines for transplant recipients.* Infectious Disease Clinics of North America 2001;15(1):273-305.

National Advisory Committee on Immunization. *Statement on recommended use of meningococcal vaccines.* Canada Communicable Disease Report 2001;27(ACS-6):2-36.

National Advisory Committee on Immunization. *Statement on recommended use of pneumococcal conjugate vaccines.* Canada Communicable Disease Report 2002;28(ACS-2):1-32.

Neuhauss TJ. *Immunization in children with chronic renal failure: a practical approach.* Pediatric Nephrology 2004;19(12):1334-39.

Rangel MC, Coronado VG, Euler GL et al. *Vaccine recommendations for patients on chronic dialysis.* Seminars in Dialysis 2000;13(2):101-107.

Sartori AM. *A review of the varicella vaccine in immunocompromised individuals.* International Journal of Infectious Diseases 2004;8(5):259-70.

Somani J, Larson RA. *Reimmunization after allogeneic bone marrow transplantation.* American Journal of Medicine 1995;98(4):389-98.

Weber DJ, Rutala WA. *Immunization of immunocompromised persons.* Immunology and Allergy Clinics of North America 2003;23(4):605-34.

Yeung CY, Liang DC. *Varicella vaccine in children with acute lymphoblastic leukemia and non Hodgkins lymphoma.* Pediatric Hematology and Oncology 1992;9(1):29-34.

Immunization of Persons with Neurologic Disorders

The Institute of Medicine (IOM) has conducted evidence-based reviews and has rejected any causal associations between the following vaccines and neurological disorders:

◆ Measles, mumps and rubella (MMR) or thimerosal-containing vaccines and autism spectrum disorders in children;

◆ influenza vaccine and demyelinating neurological disorders in children aged 6-23 months (the age group studied);

◆ hepatitis B or influenza vaccines and incident or relapse of multiple sclerosis in adults.

The IOM concluded that the evidence supported a causal relation between the 1976 swine influenza vaccine and Guillain-Barré syndrome (GBS) in adults. The data they reviewed were insufficient to either refute or support any association between GBS and influenza vaccines used after 1976. However, a study by other investigators has estimated the vaccine-associated GBS incidence in adults as one extra case of GBS per million influenza vaccine doses administered. Data on GBS incidence after influenza vaccination in children are not available.

For the purposes of immunization, people with neurologic disorders may be considered according to the following two categories: those with pre-existing neurologic conditions and those in whom the onset of symptoms of a new condition followed immunization.

Pre-existing neurologic conditions

Disorders that usually begin during infancy, such as cerebral palsy, spina bifida, seizure disorder, neuromuscular diseases and inborn errors of metabolism, may have symptom onset before the administration of the vaccines routinely recommended in the first year of life. Other conditions, such as autism spectrum disorders, acute demyelinating encephalomyelitis, transverse myelitis, multiple sclerosis and GBS, often appear later in childhood or adulthood and may occur before or after the administration of the vaccines given to adolescents and adults (e.g., hepatitis B, tetanus, diphtheria and acellular pertussis (Tdap)).

Neurological disorders whose onset clearly precedes immunization are not contraindications to subsequent immunization. People with these disorders are at risk of added morbidity and mortality from vaccine-preventable infections due to *Haemophilus influenzae* type b, *Neisseria meningitidis* serogroup C, *Streptococcus pneumoniae* (vaccine serotypes), pertussis, measles

131

and rubella. Recent studies have demonstrated that children with neurologic conditions are at risk of varicella and influenza infections severe enough to require hospitalization. Consequently, people with pre-existing neurologic disorders should receive all routinely recommended immunizations without delay. In addition, adults and children ≥ 6 months of age with neurologic conditions that compromise clearance of respiratory secretions should receive yearly influenza vaccination. Please refer to the *National Advisory Committee on Immunization Statement on Influenza Vaccination* available at www.naci.gc.ca for more information.

Neurologic events following immunization

Rarely, neurologic events occur in the 8 weeks following immunization. Because these occur so close in time to the vaccine administration they are said to be "temporally associated". This temporal association alone is not evidence that the vaccine caused the neurologic events. Please refer to the *Vaccine Safety* chapter, page 59, for more information. Children who experience hypotonic-hyporesponsive events (HHE), febrile and non-febrile seizures or prolonged, inconsolable crying after receiving acellular pertussis vaccines or any other vaccine may receive the next dose(s) of vaccines without delay, as these events are not associated with any long-term problems and therefore are not considered contraindications to further immunization. Such events have occurred with equal frequency after either DTaP or DT vaccines, and children have received acellular pertussis vaccines safely after previous HHE episodes.

People with encephalopathy or encephalitis that develops within 7 days after immunization should be investigated. Those who have an alternative etiology for the encephalopathy (e.g., viral infection) or who recover fully by the next scheduled vaccination may be immunized without deferral. People with encephalopathy that persists or who have no alternative etiology should be referred to a specialist for further consultation and may be immunized if their condition is stable and found not to relate to immunization.

Children admitted for investigation of encephalopathy at the 12 participating pediatric tertiary care centres in Canada are captured by the Immunization Monitoring Program ACTive (IMPACT) surveillance system. IMPACT identified four children between 1997 and 2002 with encephalopathy that began within 7 days after immunization with acellular pertussis vaccines. All had concomitant infections or conditions that could have accounted for the encephalopathy. Two of the cases had concomitant influenza A infections, one had a diarrheal illness without any identified pathogen, and the last case was due to hypoglycemia secondary to adrenal insufficiency. Thus, encephalopathy temporally associated with whole cell or acellular pertussis vaccines appears to be very rare in Canada, and these data indicate that an alternative etiology is usually established.

A causal association has not been established between tetanus or currently available influenza vaccines and GBS. However, at the present time it is prudent to withhold tetanus vaccinations from children and adults in whom GBS developed within 8 weeks of a previous tetanus vaccine and to withhold influenza vaccination from children and adults whose GBS developed within 8 weeks of a previous influenza vaccine dose. People who have GBS that developed outside this interval or who have an alternative cause identified (e.g., *Campylobacter jejuni* infection) may receive subsequent tetanus and influenza vaccinations.

Since the IOM has rejected any causal association between the vaccines identified above and autism spectrum disorders or demyelinating disorders (including multiple sclerosis), children and adults with these disorders may receive further immunization with MMR, hepatitis B and influenza vaccines, as well as other routinely recommended vaccines, without deferral.

Immunization of Persons with Bleeding Disorders

While certain factors must be considered before immunizing individuals with bleeding disorders, these persons should receive all the recommended immunizations according to routine schedules. For all children, before giving the first immunization at 2 months of age, clinicians should ensure that there are no symptoms or signs compatible with an undiagnosed bleeding disorder. If these are present, a diagnosis should be established before commencing immunization.

Individuals receiving low doses of acetylsalicylic acid therapy and long-term anticoagulation with either coumadin or heparin are not considered to be at higher risk of complications and may be safely immunized through either the intramuscular or subcutaneous route without discontinuation of their anticoagulation therapy.

Route of administration of immunization

The risks and benefits of administering intramuscular injections to individuals with a bleeding disorder must be weighed before choosing the route of administration. In general, subcutaneous injections are preferred over intramuscular injections in this population and should be considered when the efficacy is known to be the same for both routes, especially if an individual has a bleeding disorder that is not correctible. For more information on immunizations that are available for subcutaneous administration please refer to Table 1, in the *General Considerations* chapter, page 7. In individuals with non-correctible bleeding disorders intramuscular gluteal injections should be avoided if possible.

Correction of bleeding disorder

When immunizations are to be given by the intramuscular route or when there is a concern that injection may stimulate bleeding, the immunization should be given following anti-haemophilia therapy or correction of the bleeding disorder when possible.

Method of immunization

Immunization should be carried out using a fine-gauge needle of appropriate length. After the injection, firm pressure should be applied, without rubbing, to the injection site for at least 5 minutes.

Immunizations to be considered in individuals with bleeding disorders

Although currently available plasma-derived products are all tested for viral contamination prior to administration, any patient with a bleeding disorder should still be considered at higher risk of contracting hepatitis A or B and should be offered these vaccines. Even when recombinant therapeutic products are being used, immunization is still recommended in case the recombinant supply is unavailable and patients are required to switch to plasma-derived products at short notice. Please refer to the *Hepatitis A* chapter, page 179, and *Hepatitis B* chapter, page 189, for information on dosage.

Selected references

Makris M, Conlon CP, Watson HG. *Immunization of persons with bleeding disorders.* Haemophilia 2003;9(5):541-46.

Part 3 — Recommended Immunization

Immunization of Travellers

A detailed discussion of immunization and other preventive measures recommended for travellers to other countries is beyond the scope of this *Guide*. Current information on immunization requirements and recommendations should be obtained from travel health clinics or public health agencies.

Readers are referred to the Travel Medicine Program section on the Public Health Agency of Canada (PHAC) Web site, http://www.travelhealth. gc.ca. This Program provides extensive information, including statements on travel medicine and tropical medicine, from CATMAT (Committee to Advise on Tropical Medicine and Travel).

Readers are also referred to *Health Information for International Travel* (U.S. Centers for Disease Control and Prevention, www.cdc.gov/travel) and *International Travel and Health: Vaccination Requirements and Health Advice* (World Health Organization, www.who.int/ith).

There is no single schedule for the administration of immunizations to travellers. Each schedule must be personalized. The immunization recommendations for travellers will vary according to the traveller's age, immunization history, existing medical conditions, countries to be visited, the duration and nature of travel (whether the traveller is staying in urban hotels or visiting remote rural areas), the legal requirements for entry into countries being visited and the amount of time available before departure.

With some notable exceptions, most immunizing agents can be given simultaneously at different sites. Concerns about individual vaccines and their potential compatibility with other vaccines or antimicrobials (including antimalarials) are dealt with in the specific vaccine chapters of the *Guide*.

A health care provider or travel medicine clinic ideally should be consulted 2 to 3 months in advance of travel in order to allow sufficient time for optimal immunization schedules to be completed. Even if a traveller is leaving at short notice, a pre-travel consultation will be beneficial. A listing of travel clinics across Canada can be found in the Travel Medicine Program section of the PHAC Web site, http://www.travelhealth.gc.ca.

It must be emphasized that the most frequent health problems faced by international travellers are not preventable by immunizing agents. As well, immunization is not a substitute for careful selection and handling of food and water.

Travel is a good opportunity for the health care provider to review the immunization status of infants, children, adolescents and adults. Unimmunized or incompletely immunized travellers should be offered vaccination as recommended in the specific vaccine chapters in this *Guide*. A pre-travel assessment is also a good opportunity to review safer sex practices.

Immunizations related to travel can be divided into three general categories: those that are considered **routine** (part of the primary series of immunizations or routine booster dose), those **required** by international law and those **recommended** for maintenance of health while travelling.

Routine immunizations

The following section specifically discusses the indication for "extra" or booster doses of routine immunizations or a change in the routine immunization schedule as it applies to travellers.

Accelerated primary vaccination schedule — infants

For infants embarking on travel, the primary vaccination series with diphtheria, tetanus, acellular pertussis, polio, *Haemophilus influenzae* type b (DTaP-IPV-Hib) and pneumococcal conjugate can be started as young as 6 weeks of age.

Hepatitis B — adults

Travel is a good opportunity to offer hepatitis B immunization to adults who have not been previously vaccinated. It should be recommended particularly to travellers who will be residing in areas with high levels of endemic hepatitis B or working in health care facilities, and those likely to have contact with blood or to have sexual contact with residents of such areas.

Hepatitis B — infants and children

The age at which infants, children and adolescents are offered hepatitis B vaccine varies from jurisdiction to jurisdiction in Canada. Since hepatitis B carrier rates are much higher in developing countries, every effort should be made to arrange full hepatitis B immunization for children of any age who will live in an area where hepatitis B is endemic.

Measles, mumps, rubella — adults

Measles, mumps and rubella are endemic in many countries. Protection against measles is especially important for people planning foreign travel, including adolescents and adults who have not had measles disease and have not been adequately immunized. Two doses of measles-containing vaccine (MMR) are recommended for all unimmunized adult travellers who were born in or after 1970 and who are en route to a measles-endemic area, unless there is serologic proof of immunity or physician documentation of prior measles. Similarly, protection against rubella is especially important for women of childbearing age who are not immune to the disease.

Part 3 — Recommended Immunization

Measles — infants and children

Measles vaccine should be given at an earlier age than usual for children travelling to countries where measles is endemic. Measles-containing vaccine (MMR) may be given as early as 6 months of age, but then the routine series of two doses must still be re-started after the child is 12 months old.

Pertussis

For adults who have not previously received a dose of acellular pertussis vaccine, it is recommended that the tetanus and diphtheria booster dose (Td) be replaced by the combined Tdap vaccine.

Poliomyelitis

The risk of polio for travellers has substantially decreased as we move towards global polio eradication. A single booster dose of poliomyelitis vaccine (IPV) in adulthood is recommended for international travellers who plan to visit regions of the world where poliovirus continues to circulate in either epidemic or endemic fashion. The need for subsequent boosters of poliovirus vaccine has not been established.

Tetanus and diphtheria — adults

Adult travellers should be vaccinated against tetanus and diphtheria with a Td vaccine booster dose every 10 years for optimal protection.

Required immunizations

The following may be a requirement of international law, or proof of immunization may be considered a visa requirement.

Cholera

Cholera vaccine has not been required for border crossing under International Health Regulations since 1973. Some travellers to parts of Africa have reported being asked to provide a certificate of immunization against cholera. This "requirement" is not usually the policy of the national government but, rather, of local authorities. Given the related risks of immunization in some countries, certain travel clinics provide a cholera "exemption certificate", which is used to help travellers avoid being given cholera vaccine while abroad.

Meningococcal disease

As a condition of entry, Saudi Arabia requires proof of meningococcal immunization for pilgrims to Mecca during the Hajj. Quadrivalent polysaccharide vaccine is recommended. For other indications for this vaccine see the Recommended Usage section in the *Meningococcal Vaccine* chapter, page 237.

Yellow fever

Yellow fever is the only vaccine required as a condition of entry under the World Health Organization's International Health Regulations. A valid International Certificate of Vaccination, issued within the previous 10 years, is mandatory for entry into certain countries in Africa and South America. Other countries have requirements for proof of immunization from travellers who have passed through yellow fever endemic zones. Please refer to the maps in the *Yellow Fever Vaccine* chapter, page 343, for more information.

The period of validity of the International Vaccination Certificate for yellow fever is 10 years, beginning 10 days after primary vaccination and immediately after re-vaccination. Only Yellow Fever Vaccination Centre clinics designated by PHAC can provide the International Certificate of Vaccination in Canada. A list of these centres can be obtained from PHAC's Travel Medicine Program Web site (http://www.travelhealth.gc.ca).

The decision to immunize against yellow fever will depend on the itinerary of the individual traveller and the specific requirements of the country to be visited (including stopovers). As well as being necessary for entry into certain countries, immunization against yellow fever is recommended for all travellers who are visiting or living in countries in Africa and South America where yellow fever infection is officially reported. It is also recommended for travel outside of urban areas in countries that do not officially report yellow fever but lie in the yellow fever endemic zones (see maps, page 344-345).

Recommended Immunizations

On the basis of a risk assessment of the itinerary, the style of travel and the traveller's underlying health, the following vaccines should be considered in consultation with a health care provider.

Bacille Calmette-Guérin (BCG)

Immunization with BCG may be considered for travellers planning extended stays in areas of high tuberculosis prevalence, particularly where a program of serial skin testing and appropriate chemoprophylaxis may not be feasible or where primary isoniazid resistance of *Mycobacterium tuberculosis* is high. Travellers are advised to consult a specialist in travel medicine or infectious diseases when considering a decision for or against BCG immunization. Please refer to the *Bacille Calmette-Guérin Vaccine* chapter, page 149, for more information.

Cholera

In specific, limited circumstances (e.g., high-risk ex-patriots such as relief and aid workers or health professionals working in endemic countries), the oral cholera vaccine (Chol-Ecol-O, Dukoral™) may be considered. A detailed, individual risk assessment should be made in order to determine which travellers may benefit from immunization.

The Chol-Ecol-O vaccine has been shown to provide limited, short-term protection against diarrhea caused by enterotoxigenic *Escherichia coli*. A detailed, individual risk assessment should be made in order to determine which travellers may benefit the most from this vaccine as a preventive strategy for travellers' diarrhea. Please refer to the *Cholera Vaccine* chapter, page 158, for more information.

Hepatitis A

Hepatitis A is the most common vaccine-preventable disease in travellers. Protection against hepatitis A is highly recommended for all travellers to developing countries, especially to rural areas or places with inadequate sanitary facilities in countries where the disease is endemic. Protective antibodies are detectable within 2 weeks of administration. Given the long incubation period of hepatitis A (2 to 7 weeks), the vaccine can be administered up to the day of departure and still protect the majority of travellers.

The advent of active immunizing agents has made the use of immune globulin virtually obsolete for the purposes of travel prophylaxis. The only exceptions would be people for whom hepatitis A immunization is contraindicated or may not be effective (e.g., immunocompromised travellers and infants < 1 year of age). Immune globulin provides protection for only 3 to 5 months and should be given immediately before departure.

Influenza

People at high risk of influenza complications embarking on foreign travel to destinations where influenza is likely to be circulating should be immunized with the most current available vaccine. Influenza transmission is enhanced in the crowded conditions associated with air travel, cruise ships and tour groups. In the tropics, influenza can occur throughout the year. In the southern hemisphere, peak activity occurs from April through September and in the northern hemisphere from November through March. Vaccines prepared specifically against strains that are predicted to circulate in the southern hemisphere are not currently available in Canada.

Japanese encephalitis

Japanese encephalitis is the leading cause of viral encephalitis in Asia, but the disease is rare in travellers. Its incidence has been decreasing in China, Korea and Japan but increasing in Bangladesh, India, Nepal, Pakistan, northern Thailand and Vietnam. It occurs in epidemics in late summer and early fall in temperate areas and sporadically throughout the year in tropical areas of Asia. Immunization should generally be considered for those who will spend 1 month or more in endemic or epidemic areas during the transmission season, especially if travel will include rural areas. In special circumstances, immunization should be considered for some people spending < 1 month in endemic areas, e.g., travellers to areas where there is an epidemic, travellers making repeated short trips or people with extensive outdoor rural exposure.

Meningococcal disease — adults

Quadrivalent meningococcal polysaccharide vaccine is recommended for travellers planning a prolonged stay in areas with a high incidence of meningococcal disease. Short-term travellers (< 3 weeks) on business or holiday (including safaris) who will have little contact with local populations are at minimal risk, and therefore immunization is not routinely recommended. When doubt about the nature of exposure exists, it may be prudent to offer immunization. However, in special circumstances, immunization should be considered for short-term travellers if (a) there will be close contact with the local population in endemic areas, (b) there will be travel to epidemic areas or (c) the traveller will be providing health care to others.

As noted previously, proof of meningococcal immunization may be required by certain countries e.g., Saudi Arabia for pilgrims to Mecca during the Hajj. Outbreaks of meningococcal disease have affected these pilgrims in the past, involving serogroup A in 1987, and both serogroups A and W135 in 2000 and 2001.

Meningococcal conjugate C vaccine was approved in Canada in 2001. This vaccine only protects against serogroup C and therefore is not appropriate for protection of travellers, as it does not protect against serogroups A, Y or W135. Travelers should therefore receive a quadrivalent vaccine that provides protection against serogroups A, C, Y and W135.

Meningococcal disease — infants and children

Because of the relative inability of very young children to respond to polysaccharide vaccine, infants aged 2 to 12 months should be immunized with the appropriate doses of meningococcal C conjugate based on age and vaccine manufacturer, if not previously received. However, bivalent meningococcal polysaccharide AC vaccine or quadrivalent ACYW135 may be considered for children as young as 3 months who are travelling to regions where broader protection is needed. Please refer to the *Meningococcal Vaccine* chapter, page 237, for more information.

Rabies

Pre-exposure immunization should be considered for travellers intending to live or work in areas where rabies is enzootic and rabies control programs for domestic animals are inadequate, or where adequate and safe post-exposure management is not available. Children, particularly those who are too young to understand the need to avoid animals or to report bites, should also be considered for pre-exposure immunization. After exposure to a rabid animal, administration of two additional doses of rabies vaccine is imperative as soon as possible. For someone who has received a full course of pre-exposure immunization, rabies immune globulin is not indicated. Please refer to the *Rabies Vaccine* chapter, page 285, for more information.

Typhoid

Typhoid vaccine is recommended for travellers who will have prolonged exposure (> 4 weeks) to potentially contaminated food and water, especially those travelling to smaller cities and villages or rural areas off the usual tourist itineraries in countries with a high incidence of disease. Individuals billeted with or visiting families in such areas may be at particularly high risk. Immunization should also be considered for travellers with reduced or absent gastric acid secretion. Immunization is not routinely recommended for business travel or short-term (< 4 weeks) holidays in resort hotels in such countries. Parenteral inactivated and live oral vaccines are available.

Travellers who are immunodeficient

In general, live vaccines should be avoided in individuals who are immunodeficient. These vaccines include yellow fever, oral typhoid, varicella, MMR and BCG. For more detailed information, see the *Immunization of Immunocompromised Persons* chapter, page 117, for recommendations on the use of vaccines in individuals who are immunodeficient.

Travellers who are pregnant

In general, live vaccines should be avoided in pregnancy, whereas inactivated (killed) vaccines are considered safe. For more detailed information, see the chapter on *Immunization in Pregnancy and Breast-Feeding*, page 107, as well as the individual vaccine chapters for recommendations for and contraindications to vaccines in pregnancy.

Malaria prophylaxis

There is no approved vaccine against malaria currently available.

Four components of malaria protection should be discussed with travellers: (a) the risk of acquiring malaria, (b) personal protective measures to prevent mosquito bites, (c) chemoprophylactic drugs (where appropriate) and (d) the need to seek early diagnosis and treatment of a febrile illness. Information concerning malaria, drug-resistant strains of *Plasmodium* and recommended drugs for prophylaxis and other preventive measures is regularly updated by CATMAT and published in the Canada Communicable Disease Report. Information is also available from local health departments, travel clinics and the Travel Medicine Program section on the PHAC Web site, http://www.travelhealth.gc.ca.

All travellers should be informed that malaria should be suspected if fever occurs during or after travel. Medical attention should be sought as soon as possible, and the traveller should request that a blood film be examined for malarial parasites.

Selected references

Centers for Disease Control and Prevention. *Travelers' health: yellow book. Health information for international travel 2005-2006.* Atlanta, GA: US Department of Health and Human Services, Public Health Service, 2005.

World Health Organization (WHO). *International travel and health: vaccination requirements and health advice.* Geneva: WHO, 2005.

Immunization of Persons New to Canada

Immunization of persons who have newly arrived in Canada is challenging, since immunization records may not exist, records that exist may be difficult to interpret because of language barriers, and immunization schedules and products may differ from those used in Canada. New immigrants, refugees and internationally adopted children may be lacking immunizations and/or immunization records because of their living conditions before arriving in Canada or because the vaccines are not available in their country of origin. Only written documentation of vaccination given at ages and intervals comparable with the Canadian schedule should be considered valid. See the section on *Immunization of Children and Adults with Inadequate Immunization Records*, page 105, for additional information.

Although the potency of vaccines administered in other countries can be generally assumed to be adequate, immunization schedules vary. The age at immunization (e.g., 9 months of age for immunization against measles in some countries), the number of doses and the intervals between doses should be carefully reviewed and compared with Canadian and provincial/territorial recommendations in determining the need for additional doses of vaccines. In many countries outside of Canada, mumps and rubella vaccines are in limited use, and measles vaccine alone is generally given. *Haemophilus influenzae* type b conjugate, hepatitis B, varicella, pneumococcal conjugate and meningococcal C conjugate vaccines are also in limited use. Information on vaccination schedules in other countries can be found on the following website: http://www.who.int/vaccines/GlobalSummary/Immunization/ScheduleSelect.cfm.

Some studies of internationally adopted children have shown that, despite written documentation of adequate immunizations, serologic evidence of protection against diphtheria and tetanus is lacking in some children. Recommendations regarding an approach to vaccinating these children vary and range from the following:

- ignoring the written record and repeating the vaccinations, especially when there is doubt about the authenticity of the records or vaccines used;
- accepting the written record provided it appears valid in terms of age of administration and timing of doses; or
- judiciously using serologic tests to ensure that good protection is present when there is concern regarding the adequacy of immunization records.

The epidemiology of some infectious diseases varies in different countries. For example, compared with temperate climates, in the tropics a higher proportion of varicella infections occurs in adults. Therefore, adolescents and adults from these countries are more likely to be susceptible to varicella and require vaccination than those who are Canadian-born. Individuals born in developing countries are more likely to be carriers of hepatitis B, necessitating vaccination of their sexual and household contacts. Hepatitis A immunity is also more likely in some foreign-born individuals, therefore testing for immunity before administering the hepatitis A vaccine to persons from hepatitis A-endemic countries should be considered.

Immigration medical examinations (IMEs) are required for children and adults seeking permanent residence in Canada. These are done within the 12 months preceding arrival in Canada for new immigrants and those seeking refugee status from abroad. In-Canada refugee claimants must undergo an IME within 60 days of claiming refugee status.

It is important to note what the IME does not routinely include:

◆ a review of immunization status;
◆ tuberculin skin testing;
◆ hepatitis B serologic testing.

Therefore health care providers in Canada who see persons newly arrived in the country should make the assessment and updating of immunizations a priority. As well, they should perform a complete health assessment (including comprehensive testing for a variety of chronic and non-vaccine-preventable diseases) as outlined in the references below. As part of this assessment, the following tests are particularly relevant in determining the need for some vaccines or contraindications to vaccination:

◆ Hepatitis B surface antigen (HBsAg), hepatitis B surface antibody, hepatitis B core antibody. Should any member of the family be found to be positive for HBsAg, the entire family should be tested for hepatitis B markers and vaccinated as appropriate.

◆ Hepatitis C antibody. Persons chronically infected with hepatitis C should be vaccinated against hepatitis A and hepatitis B (if not previously infected with these agents).

◆ Human immunodeficiency virus (HIV) serologic testing for persons from countries with high rates of HIV (if HIV status not known). HIV testing is performed as part of the IME for those 15 years of age and older and some children (those who have received blood and blood products, those whose mother is known to be HIV positive and all potential adoptees). Persons with advanced HIV infection should not receive live vaccines. Please refer to the *Immunization of Immunocompromised Persons* chapter, page 117, for more information.

◆ Complete blood counts, sickle cell preparation test and hemoglobin electrophoresis for persons from areas of the world where sickle cell disease and genetic hemoglobinopathies (such as beta-thalassemia) are present. Persons with sickle cell disease are at risk of serious infections with encapsulated bacteria, such as *Streptococcus pneumoniae*, *Haemophilus influenzae* and *Neisseria meningitidis*. They should be immunized with pneumococcal conjugate and polysaccharide vaccines, *Haemophilus*

Part 3 — Recommended Immunization

influenzae type b conjugate vaccine, and meningococcal C conjugate and quadrivalent polysaccharide vaccines (see relevant chapters). Persons with sickle cell disease or thalassemia should receive yearly influenza vaccination.

Because families new to Canada may return to their country of origin to visit friends and relatives or may receive visitors from their country of origin, vaccination against hepatitis A and/or B should be considered for all members of the family if they are from a country that is endemic for these diseases. A travel medicine consultation is recommended at least 6 to 8 weeks before travel. However, persons new to Canada may not perceive a return to their country of origin as a health risk and so may be less likely to seek pre-travel consultation.

Family members traveling outside of Canada to adopt a baby should also seek pre-travel advice and receive all appropriate travel immunizations. The adoption of a new baby into a family provides an opportunity to review the immunization status of all family members.

Selected references

Aronson J. *Medical evaluation and infectious considerations on arrival.* Pediatric Annals 2000;29(4):218-23.

Barnett ED. *Infectious disease screening for refugees resettled in the United States.* Clinical Infectious Diseases 2004;39(6):833-41.

Canadian Paediatric Society. *Children and youth new to Canada: a health care guide.* Ottawa: CPS, 1999. URL (for purchase): <http://www.cps.ca/english/publications/Bookstore/ChildrenNewToCanada.htm>.

Centers for Disease Control and Prevention. *Travelers' health: yellow book. Health information for international travel, 2005-2006.* Atlanta, GA: US Department of Health and Human Services, Public Health Service, 2005; chapter 8. URL: <http://www2.ncid.cdc.gov/travel/yb/utils/ybGet.asp?section=children&obj=adoption.htm&cssNav=browseoyb>.

Chen LH, Barnett ED, Wilson ME. *Preventing infectious diseases during and after international adoption.* Annals of Internal Medicine 2003;139:371-78.

Stauffer WM, Kamat D, Walker PF. *Screening of international immigrants, refugees and adoptees.* Primary Care 2002;29(4):879-905.

Part 4

Active Immunizing Agents

Bacille Calmette-Guérin (BCG) Vaccine

Tuberculosis (TB), a communicable bacterial disease caused by *Mycobacterium tuberculosis*, results in diverse clinical manifestations, including pneumonia, meningitis, osteomyelitis and disseminated infection. Latent infection that reactivates later in life can also occur. BCG vaccine, derived from an attenuated strain of living bovine tubercle bacillus, is one of the mostly widely used vaccines in the world and is currently given at or soon after birth to children in over 100 countries to minimize the potential for serious forms of TB disease.

Since the publication of the 2002 *Canadian Immunization Guide*, in which BCG vaccine was recommended for infants and children in groups with rates of new infection in excess of 1% per year, case review of adverse events associated with BCG vaccine has raised concerns that routine neonatal vaccination in First Nations and Inuit communities could be associated with unacceptable health risks. The National Advisory Committee on Immunization (NACI) subsequently revised its recommendation for usage of BCG vaccine in 2004 (see Recommended Usage).

Epidemiology

The reported incidence of TB in Canada has been in significant decline since a peak in the early 1940s (Figure 1). In 2003, 1,630 cases of TB were reported, representing an incidence rate of 5.1 per 100,000. In that year 4.8% of cases (78/1630) were < 15 years of age, and the corresponding age-specific incidence of these cases was 1.3 per 100,000 (Centre for Infectious Disease Prevention and Control, Public Health Agency of Canada [PHAC], Ottawa).

TB is a leading cause of morbidity and mortality worldwide. There is growing global concern about the emergence of drug-resistant strains, which are threatening to make TB incurable again; moreover, the resurgence of the disease is being accelerated by the spread of human immunodeficiency virus (HIV). In 1993, the World Health Organization (WHO) declared tuberculosis to be a "global emergency".

The distribution of risk for TB disease in the Canadian population has changed over recent decades. The Canadian-born non-Aboriginal population is generally at low risk, as TB now occurs in certain geographic areas and demographic groups that can be considered "high risk groups". These include homeless persons and illicit drug users, immigrants from areas with a high incidence of infectious TB, and Canadian-born Aboriginal peoples.

TB control measures include 1) early identification of people with active (infectious) disease and treatment of each case until cured using directly observed therapy (DOT); 2) treatment of latent TB infection in those who

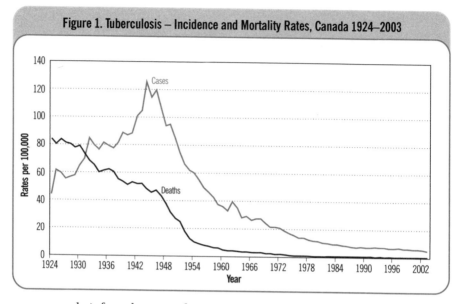

Figure 1. Tuberculosis – Incidence and Mortality Rates, Canada 1924–2003

are recently infected or are otherwise at high risk to progress from infection to disease; (3) infection prevention and control measures in health care facilities and other institutions to prevent nosocomial/institutional spread; and (4) BCG vaccination of selected population groups to prevent serious complications of infection.

Preparations approved for use in Canada

This chapter will deal only with vaccines that are currently marketed in Canada:

◆ BCG Vaccine (bacillus Calmette-Guérin vaccine, freeze-dried), Sanofi Pasteur Ltd.

BCG vaccine is made from a culture of an attenuated strain of living bovine tubercle bacillus (bacille Calmette-Guérin). It is supplied in a multidose vial as a freeze-dried product, which is reconstituted with a supplied diluent of sterile phosphate-buffered saline.

Efficacy and immunogenicity

Although there are many BCG vaccines available in the world, all are derived from the original strain. These vaccines may vary in immunogenicity, efficacy and reactogenicity. No laboratory markers exist that correlate with protection against TB infection or disease. As well, neither the presence nor the size of the tuberculin skin test reaction predicts protection. The efficacy of BCG vaccine is estimated from prospective clinical trials and retrospective case-control studies. Although clinical trials have demonstrated conflicting results with regard to estimating BCG vaccine efficacy, meta-analytic reviews have estimated the vaccine efficacy to be 51% (95% confidence interval [CI] 30%-66%) in preventing any TB disease. In newborns the protective effect of BCG vaccine against TB compared with that in unvaccinated children is estimated at 74% (95% CI 62%-83%) and 64% (95% CI 30%-82%) for meningitis, and up to 78% (95% CI 58%-88%) for disseminated disease.

The protective effect of immunization increases with increased distance from the equator. The significance of this finding is unclear at present. Many factors have been considered to explain variations among studies, including BCG strain, infection with non-tuberculous mycobacteria, climate, storage of vaccine, vitamin D intake, sunlight exposure, and population genetics. BCG strain differences were not an independent risk factor in the meta-analyses.

BCG vaccine does not provide permanent or absolute protection against TB. The disease should be considered as a possible diagnosis in any vaccinee who presents with a suggestive history, or signs or symptoms of TB, regardless of immunization history.

Lyophilized preparations of BCG for intravesical use in the treatment of primary and relapsed carcinoma *in situ* of the urinary bladder are formulated at a much higher strength and must **not** be used for TB vaccination purposes.

Recommended usage

Because BCG immunization usually results in a significant (positive) tuberculin skin test, the benefits gained by immunization must be carefully weighed against the potential loss of the tuberculin test as a primary tool to identify infection with *M. tuberculosis*. In Canada, TB rates are relatively low, and the tuberculin skin test (Mantoux 5 tuberculin units of purified protein derivative) has become increasingly useful as an epidemiologic, case-finding and latent TB infection diagnostic tool. BCG should be given only to people with a non-significant (negative) tuberculin skin test. Infants < 6 weeks of age do not need to be tuberculin tested before receiving BCG vaccine, since reactivity does not develop before this age. BCG immunization will not prevent the development of active TB in individuals who are already infected with *M. tuberculosis*.

NACI does not recommend routine use of BCG vaccine in any Canadian population. However, in the following settings, consideration of local TB epidemiology and access to diagnostic services may lead to the decision to offer BCG vaccine:

1. BCG vaccine may be considered for infants in First Nations and Inuit communities or infants residing among groups of persons with an average annual rate of smear-positive pulmonary TB greater than 15 per 100,000 population (all ages) during the previous 3 years, or infants

residing in populations with an annual risk of TB infection greater than 0.1%, if early identification and treatment of TB infection are not available. Human immunodeficiency virus (HIV) antibody testing in the mother of the child should be negative, and there should be no evidence or known risk factors for immunodeficiency in the child being vaccinated, including no family history of immunodeficiency. This rate of smear-positive pulmonary TB, 15 per 100,000, is the same rate as that recommended by the Canadian Tuberculosis Committee and the PHAC for designating geographic areas outside Canada as having a high incidence of infectious TB. It is approximately five times higher than the general Canadian smear-positive pulmonary TB rate as estimated by the WHO. For information on international smear-positive pulmonary TB incidence rates, refer to <http://www.phac-aspc.gc.ca/tbpc-latb/>.

The annual risk of TB infection quoted above, of > 0.1%, is the incidence below which the International Union Against Tuberculosis and Lung Disease recommends that selective discontinuation of BCG vaccination programs be considered. If BCG vaccination is currently offered to all infants in a community that does not meet one of the above criteria, the vaccination program should be discontinued as soon as a program of early detection and treatment of latent TB infection can be implemented.

2. Individuals, including health care workers and laboratory workers, repeatedly exposed to persons with untreated, inadequately treated or drug-resistant active TB or tubercle bacilli in conditions where protective measures against infection are not feasible (although primary treatment of the source, removal from the source or prophylaxis of the exposed person is generally preferred) may benefit from BCG vaccine. Consultation with a TB and/or infectious disease expert is recommended.

3. BCG vaccine may be considered for travelers planning extended stays in areas of high TB incidence, particularly when a program of serial tuberculin skin testing and appropriate chemotherapy is not possible or where the prevalence of drug resistance, particularly multidrug-resistant (MDR) TB, is high. This decision should be made in consultation with an infectious disease or travel medicine specialist. Those planning to live for more than 12 months in a high prevalence area may opt for skin testing on an annual basis or 8-12 weeks after returning home. Preventive therapy according to current guidelines should be considered if tuberculin skin test conversion occurs. Factors that favour the BCG option might include poor access to repeat skin testing, personal preference against taking isoniazid (INH), contraindications to taking INH such as liver disease or previous intolerance to INH, and the limited number of treatment options if infected with an MDR strain. The efficacy of BCG vaccine in adults is uncertain. Travelers with medical conditions, particularly HIV infection, that may be associated with an increased risk of progression of latent TB infection to

active disease should carefully weigh, with their physician, the risk of travel to a high-incidence area in determining the most appropriate means of prevention.

Schedule and dosage

The recommended dose is 0.05 mL (0.05 mg) in infants < 12 months of age. In persons > 12 months of age the dose is 0.1 mL (0.1 mg). Instructions in the manufacturer's product insert for suspending and administering vaccine should always be followed.

Route of administration

BCG vaccine is given as a single intradermal injection over the deltoid muscle of the arm. It is administered in a 1.0 mL syringe with a 26-gauge needle, the bevel facing upwards.

Booster doses and re-immunization

Re-immunization with BCG is not recommended. Tuberculin skin testing should not be used as a method to determine whether previously administered BCG immunization was effective.

Serologic testing

There is no indication for pre- or post-immunization serology.

Storage requirements

Before reconstitution, BCG vaccine should be kept in a refrigerator at +2° to +8° C. The vaccine is reconstituted by introducing the supplied diluent into the vaccine vial using aseptic technique. Detailed instructions for maintaining aseptic technique while handling the multidose vial are provided in the product insert. Reconstituted product must be maintained at +2° to +8° C and used within 8 hours or discarded. Neither freeze-dried nor reconstituted vaccine should be exposed to direct or indirect sunlight, and exposure to artificial light should be minimized.

Simultaneous administration with other vaccines

BCG should not be given within 4 weeks after administration of any live vaccine, since these vaccines are known to suppress the immune response, resulting in lowered immunogenicity. Live vaccines (e.g., MMR) may be given simultaneously with BCG, administered at a different site. Simultaneous administration of the inactivated vaccines against diphtheria, pertussis, tetanus and polio does not interfere with the immune response to BCG vaccine, therefore these vaccines may be given at the same time at a different site.

Adverse reactions

Serious adverse events are rare following immunization and, in most cases, data are insufficient to determine a causal association.

The usual response to (intradermal) administration of BCG vaccine is the development of erythema and either a papule or ulceration, followed by a scar at the immunization site.

Most reactions are generally mild and do not require treatment. Adverse reactions are more common in young vaccinees (infants versus older children) and are frequently related to improper technique in administration (mainly improper dilution). Reactions may include persistent or spreading skin ulceration at the immunization site, regional lymphadenopathy and keloid formation.

Moderately severe reactions, such as marked lymphadenitis or suppurative adenitis, occur in 0.2 to 4.0 per 1,000 vaccinees. Rates of adverse reactions appear to vary with the strain of vaccine, dose and method of immunization, and the age of the recipient. A review of published and unpublished data, including a survey sponsored by the International Union Against Tuberculosis and Lung Disease, recorded 10,371 complications following almost 1.5 billion BCG vaccinations in adults and children. The most serious complication of BCG vaccination was disseminated BCG infection, which occurred in 3.0 per 1 million recipients. In that review dissemination was fatal in 0.02 per 1 million vaccine recipients and occurred in children who had had primary immunodeficiencies.

A review of adverse events associated with BCG vaccine in Canada was conducted by the PHAC's Advisory Committee on Causality Assessment (ACCA) after case reports of disseminated BCG infection had been identified by the IMPACT (Immunization Monitoring Program ACTive) system of hospital-based surveillance. IMPACT identified 21 BCG vaccine-related adverse events between 1993 and 2002, which were reviewed by ACCA. Fifteen of these were designated as serious (patient died or was in hospital for 3 or more days), consisting of six cases of disseminated BCG disease (five in First Nations and Inuit children, all of whom subsequently died), two cases of osteomyelitis, five abscesses and two cases of adenitis. In assessing causality, 14 of the 21 cases were deemed "very likely-certainly" associated with the vaccine (including the six disseminated cases), five were probably associated with the vaccine, one was possibly associated with the vaccine and one could not be classified. An additional fatal case of disseminated BCG was identified in 2003 and assessed by ACCA as "very likely-certainly" associated with the vaccine.

Contraindications and precautions

BCG immunization is contraindicated in persons with immune deficiency diseases, including congenital immunodeficiency, HIV infection, altered immune status due to malignant disease, and impaired immune function secondary to treatment with corticosteroids, chemotherapeutic agents or radiation. Extensive skin disease or burns are also contraindications. BCG is contraindicated for individuals with a positive tuberculin skin test, although immunization of tuberculin reactors has frequently occurred without incident. Before a newborn is vaccinated with BCG vaccine the mother must be known to be HIV negative, and there should be no family history of immunodeficiency. Clues that an inherited immunodeficiency may be present in a family include a history of neonatal or infant deaths in the immediate or extended family. Immunization of pregnant women should preferably be deferred until after delivery, although harmful effects on the fetus have not been observed. The vaccine should not be administered to individuals receiving drugs with antituberculous activity, since these agents may be active against the vaccine strain.

Other considerations

When interpreting tuberculin skin test results, there are at least three considerations: 1) size of the reaction; 2) predictive value of a positive test based on the relative likelihood of true-positive and false-positive reactions; and 3) risk of development of active TB. The following is based on the *Canadian Tuberculosis Standards*, produced by the Canadian Lung Association/Canadian Thoracic Society and PHAC (2006 edition; in press).

Previous BCG vaccination may be the cause of a false-positive result. Vaccine may have been received by several population groups, including immigrants from many European countries and most developing countries. In Canada, many Aboriginal Canadians and persons born in Quebec and Newfoundland and Labrador from the 1940s until the late 1970s were vaccinated. For information on current and historical BCG vaccine usage in Canada by province/territory, refer to <http://www.phac-aspc. gc.ca/tbpc-latb>.

Studies conducted in Canada and in several other countries reveal that if BCG vaccine is received in infancy (the first year of life), it is very unlikely to cause tuberculin skin test reactions of 10 mm or more in persons aged ≥ 5 years. Therefore, a history of BCG immunization received in infancy can be ignored in all persons in this age range when interpreting a tuberculin skin test result of 10 mm or greater. If the BCG immunization was received between the ages of 1 and 5 years, persistently positive tuberculin skin test reactions will be seen in 10% to 15% of subjects even 20 to 25 years later. Among subjects vaccinated at the age of ≥ 6 years, up to 40% will have persistent positive reactions. BCG-related reactions may be as large as 25 mm or even greater. Therefore, if BCG immunization was received after the first year of life, it can be an important cause of false-positive tuberculin skin test reactions, particularly in populations in which the expected prevalence of TB infection (i.e., true positive reactions) is less than 10%.

In summary, BCG immunization can be ignored as a cause of a positive tuberculin skin test under the following conditions:

♦ BCG vaccine was given during infancy, and the person tested is now aged ≥ 5 years;

♦ the person is from a group with a high prevalence of TB infection (true positives), e.g., close contacts of an infectious TB case, Aboriginal Canadians from a high-risk community, immigrants from countries with a high incidence of TB;

♦ the person has a high risk of progression to disease if infected (refer to *Canadian Tuberculosis Standards* for further details).

BCG should be considered the likely cause of a positive tuberculin skin test if BCG vaccine was given after 12 months of age AND there has been no known exposure to an active TB case or other risk factors AND the person is either Canadian-born non-Aboriginal OR an immigrant from a country with low TB incidence (e.g., Western Europe, USA, etc.).

Selected references

Brewer TF, Colditz GA. *Relationship between bacille Calmette-Guérin (BCG) strains and the efficacy of BCG vaccine in the prevention of tuberculosis.* Clinical Infectious Diseases 1995;20(1):126-35.

Canadian Lung Association/Canadian Thoracic Society, Public Health Agency of Canada. *Canadian tuberculosis standards,* 6th edition. Ottawa (Canada): Canadian Lung Association and Government of Canada; in press.

Ciesielski SD. *BCG vaccination and the PPD test: what the clinician needs to know.* Journal of Family Practice 1995;40(1):76-80.

Colditz GA, Berkey CS, Mosteller F et al. *The efficacy of bacillus Calmette-Guérin vaccination of newborns and infants in the prevention of tuberculosis: meta-analyses of the published literature.* Pediatrics 1995;96:29-35.

Colditz GA, Brewer TF, Berkey CS et al. *Efficacy of BCG vaccine in the prevention of tuberculosis. Meta-analysis of the published literature.* Journal of the American Medical Association 1994;271(9):698-702.

Deeks SL, Clark M, Scheifele D et al. *Serious adverse events associated with bacille Calmette-Guérin vaccine in Canada.* Pediatric Infectious Disease 2005;24(6):538-41.

Fine PE. *Bacille Calmette-Guérin vaccines: a rough guide.* Clinical Infectious Diseases 1995;20(1):11-14.

Houston S, Fanning A, Soskolne CL et al. *The effectiveness of bacillus Calmette-Guérin (BCG) vaccination against tuberculosis: a case-control study in Treaty Indians, Alberta, Canada.* American Journal of Epidemiology 1990;131(2):340-48.

Lotte A, Wasz-Hockert O, Poisson N et al. *BCG complications. Estimates of the risks among vaccinated subjects and statistical analysis of their main characteristics.* Advances in Tuberculosis Research 1984;21;107-93.

National Advisory Committee on Immunization. *Statement on Bacille Calmette-Guérin (BCG) vaccine.* Canada Communicable Disease Report 2004;30(ACS-5):1-12.

O'Brien KL, Ruff AJ, Louis MA et al. *Bacille Calmette-Guérin complications in children born to HIV-1 infected women with a review of the literature.* Pediatrics 1995;95(3):414-18.

Pabst HF, Godel J, Grace M et al. *Effect of breast-feeding on immune response to BCG vaccination.* Lancet 1989;1(8633):295-97.

World Health Organization. *Global tuberculosis programme and global programme on vaccines. Statement on BCG revaccination for the prevention of tuberculosis.* Weekly Epidemiological Record 1995;70(32):229-31.

Cholera Vaccine

Cholera is an acute bacterial infection that presents as profuse, watery diarrhea. It is associated with rapid dehydration and occasionally hypovolemic shock, which may be life-threatening. The spectrum of disease is wide, with mild and asymptomatic illness occurring more frequently than severe disease. Cholera is caused by an enterotoxin produced by *Vibrio cholerae*. Two serogroups, 01 and 0139 (Bengal), have been implicated in human epidemics. Currently, serogroup 01 predominates worldwide. Within serogroup 01 are the classical and El Tor biotypes.

Case fatality ranges from 50% or more without treatment to less than 1% among adequately treated patients. Treatment consists mainly of oral or parenteral rehydration. Cholera infection is associated with poor sanitation and is generally acquired from contaminated water or food, particularly undercooked or raw shellfish and fish.

The ratio of symptomatic to asymptomatic cases varies from strain to strain. In El Tor infections, the ratio of symptomatic to asymptomatic cases (1:50) is much lower than in cholera infection due to the classical biotype (1:5). Humans are the only known natural host.

Changes since the publication of the 2002 *Canadian Immunization Guide* include 1) changes in preparations approved for use in Canada; 2) additional recommended usage for travellers' diarrhea; 3) new schedule and dosage table for the protection against cholera and enterotoxigenic *Escherichia coli* (ETEC); 4) changes to booster doses and re-immunization indications; and 5) information on the simultaneous administration with antibiotics or antimalarials.

Epidemiology

The seventh cholera pandemic began in 1961, when *V. cholerae* of the El Tor biotype spread through Southern Asia, the Middle East, Eastern Europe and, in 1970, Africa. In 1991, the El Tor biotype caused an outbreak in Peru, which led to an extensive epidemic in other Amazonian and Central American countries. In recent years there have been multiple cholera outbreaks related to mass population movement, especially at times of strife, such as within refugee camps in resource-poor countries.

During the 1990s in Asia, beginning in India and Bangladesh around the Bay of Bengal, there was an epidemic caused by a new strain of cholera, serogroup 0139. This epidemic spread to other countries in Asia but not outside the region.

In Canada, cholera cases are very uncommon. There were five cases of cholera 01/0139 reported in 2003 and three cases reported in 2004. All were related to travel or immigration. No secondary transmission was noted. The risk of transmission is low in countries such as Canada that have modern sanitation, good hygiene and clean water supplies.

For travellers, prevention relies primarily on care in the choice of food and water supply and in the use of good hygienic measures rather than on immunization.

Preparations approved for use in Canada

This chapter will deal only with vaccines that are currently marketed in Canada.

◆ Dukoral™ (oral, inactivated travellers' diarrhea and cholera, [Chol-Ecol-O]), Sanofi Pasteur Ltd (distributor).

Dukoral™ was approved for use in Canada in 2003 for children 2 years of age and older, and adults. This vaccine consists of killed *V. cholerae* and the non-toxic recombinant cholera toxin B-subunit. Through its beta-subunit (BS), Chol-Ecol-O vaccine has been shown to provide moderate, short-term protection against diarrhea caused by ETEC.

For a list of all approved products in Canada, please refer to Table 1 in the *General Considerations* chapter, page 7.

Efficacy and immunogenicity

Protection against cholera

A clinical trial in adult US volunteers (using an early formulation of the vaccine) demonstrated an overall efficacy against challenge with *V. cholerae* 01 El Tor of 64% but complete (100%) protection against moderate to severe diarrhea. A large, double-blind, placebo-controlled field trial (using an early formulation of the vaccine) was undertaken in Bangladesh, which demonstrated an efficacy of 85% against El Tor disease for the initial 6 months and 50% for the 3 year follow-up period. A double-blind, placebo-controlled field trial in Peru (using the currently licensed recombinant BS component of the vaccine) demonstrated an efficacy of 86% against epidemic cholera.

Of note is the observation that there is no efficacy against the 0139 Bengal strain of cholera.

Protection against ETEC diarrhea

Many ETEC strains produce a heat-labile enterotoxin that is similar to cholera toxin. As a result, through the B-subunit, the Chol-Ecol-O vaccine has been shown to provide moderate, short-term protection against diarrhea caused by ETEC.

In the Bangladesh oral cholera vaccine field trial, the Chol-Ecol-O vaccine demonstrated 67% protection against ETEC for 3 months.

A prospective, double-blind study involving US students in Mexico demonstrated that the vaccine had a protective efficacy of approximately 50% against ETEC diarrhea. Given the proportion of travellers' diarrhea caused by ETEC, the overall protection against this condition would be expected to be approximately 25%. This was demonstrated in another prospective, double-blind study of the Chol-Ecol-O vaccine conducted among tourists who went to Morocco from Finland. The study showed efficacy against ETEC diarrhea of 52% and an overall protection against travellers' diarrhea of 23%.

Recommended usage

Cholera

Travellers should take all the necessary precautions to avoid contact with or ingestion of potentially contaminated food or water since not all recipients of the vaccine will be fully protected against cholera. This is particularly true for travellers to areas where the 0139 Bengal strain is endemic.

The World Health Organization indicates that, since 1992, no country or territory has required a certificate of vaccination against cholera from international travellers. Most travellers following the usual tourist itineraries in countries affected by cholera are at extremely low risk of acquiring cholera infection.

Travellers who may be at significantly increased risk (e.g., high-risk expatriots such as relief and aid workers or health professionals working in endemic countries) may benefit from immunization. A detailed, travel-related risk assessment should be made to determine which travellers are most likely to benefit.

Travellers' diarrhea

Indications for the Chol-Ecol-O vaccine to prevent diarrhea are limited because 1) most episodes of travellers' diarrhea are usually mild and self-limited; 2) therapeutic options (oral rehydration, dietary management, antimotility and antibiotic treatment) are available if prevention fails; 3) less than 50% (range 25% to 50%) of travellers' diarrhea cases are caused by ETEC; 4) the protection against ETEC diarrhea is approximately 50%; and 5) vaccinated travellers may gain a false sense of security and may not be as strict in observing food and water precautions.

In summary, vaccination with the Chol-Ecol-O vaccine as a prevention strategy against travellers' diarrhea is of limited value and is not routinely recommended for the majority of travellers.

Chol-Ecol-O vaccine may be considered for selected high-risk, short-term travellers. These individuals would include people 2 years of age and over:

◆ with chronic illnesses (e.g., chronic renal failure, congestive heart failure, insulin-dependent diabetes mellitus, inflammatory bowel disease) for whom there is an increased risk of serious consequences from travellers' diarrhea;

◆ with an increased risk of acquiring travellers' diarrhea (e.g., young children 2 years of age and over, and people with gastric hypochlorhydria);

◆ who are immunosuppressed because of human immunodeficiency virus (HIV) infection or other immunodeficiency states;

◆ with a history of repeated severe travellers' diarrhea.

In addition, individuals for whom a brief illness cannot be tolerated (i.e., elite athletes, business or political travellers) may want to consider immunization.

A detailed, individual, travel-related risk assessment should be made to determine which travellers may benefit the most from Dukoral™ vaccination as a prevention strategy for travellers' diarrhea.

As noted previously, the Chol-Ecol-O vaccine provides only short-term protection (approximately 3 months) against ETEC diarrhea, so for the traveller who has been vaccinated but is at ongoing risk, the need for booster doses should also be considered

Schedule and dosage

The schedule varies by whether protection is sought against cholera or ETEC and by age, as shown in Table 1.

Protection against cholera and ETEC diarrhea can be expected approximately 1 week after completion of the primary immunization.

Route of administration

Chol-Ecol-O vaccine consists of a whitish suspension in a single-dose glass vial along with a sodium hydrogen carbonate effervescent granule buffer that has a raspberry flavour. The buffer granules should be dissolved in a glass of water that is at a temperature between +2° and +27° C. Do not use milk, juice or other beverages. The vaccine vial should be shaken, and the entire contents should be added to the buffer solution. Food and drink must be avoided for 1 hour before and 1 hour after vaccine administration. If the vaccine and buffer mixture is not used immediately, it can be stored at room temperature (but below + 27° C) for up to 2 hours.

Table 1. Summary of Schedule and Dosage of Chol-Ecol-O vaccine

| | Cholera | | ETEC | |
	Adults and children > 6 yrs	Children 2-6 yrs	Adults & children ≥ 2 yrs	General instructions
Primary immunization	2 doses at least 1 week but less than 6 weeks apart	3 doses at least 1 week but less than 6 weeks apart	2 doses at least 1 week but less than 6 weeks apart	If more than 6 weeks elapses between doses, the primary immunization should be restarted. Children 2 to 6 years of age: half the amount of buffer solution is discarded, and the remaining part is mixed with the entire contents of the vaccine vial.
Booster	1 dose after 2 years	1 dose after 6 months	1 dose every 3 months if ongoing risk	If more than 5 years have passed since primary immunization or last booster dose, restart primary series.

Booster doses and re-immunization

Cholera

An optimal booster dose or interval has not been established. However, if indicated, the manufacturer recommends a single booster after 2 years for adults and children older than 6 years. For children 2 to 6 years of age, a single booster dose after 6 months is recommended.

ETEC travellers' diarrhea

An optimal booster dose or interval has not been established. However, if indicated, the manufacturer recommends a single booster dose every 3 months for those at ongoing risk.

Serologic testing

There is no indication for pre- or post-immunization serology.

Storage requirements

The Chol-Ecol-O vaccine should be kept refrigerated (at a temperature of +2° to +8° C) until used. The vaccine can be stored at room temperature, but below + 27° C, for up to 2 weeks on one occasion only. The buffer sachet may be stored at room temperature.

Simultaneous administration with other vaccines

The administration of the Chol-Ecol-O vaccine and oral typhoid capsules should be separated by at least 8 hours. The administration of oral typhoid vaccine available in sachet form does not need to be separated from Chol-Ecol-O vaccine, but the two vaccines should not be mixed in the same glass of water because they use a different buffer solution.

There are limited data, but the Chol-Ecol-O vaccine is an inactivated vaccine, and there is no known interaction between it and other commonly used travel vaccines, such as hepatitis A, hepatitis B, meningococcal and yellow fever vaccines.

Adverse reactions

In field trials of Chol-Ecol-O vaccine in Bangladesh and Peru, the side effect profile for the vaccine group was similar to that of the placebo group. The most commonly reported adverse events included abdominal pain (16%), diarrhea (12%), nausea (4%) and vomiting (3%). Serious adverse events, such as dizziness and dyspnea, have been reported very rarely (< 1/100,000 doses distributed), and a causal relation has not been established.

Contraindications and precautions

A history of an anaphylactic reaction to a previous dose of the vaccine or hypersensitivity to any component of the vaccine is an absolute contraindication to vaccination. The buffer solution uses an artificial raspberry flavouring, and therefore a history of allergy to raspberry is not a contraindication.

Vaccination should be deferred in the presence of any acute febrile illness or acute gastrointestinal illness.

Pediatric use

Chol-Ecol-O vaccine has been given to children between 1 and 2 years of age in studies of safety and immunogenicity, but because the protective efficacy has not been studied in children less than 2 years of age, it is not recommended in this age group.

Use in pregnant and nursing women

Although the inactivated, Chol-Ecol-O vaccine would not be expected to have any adverse effects, its safety in pregnancy has not been directly studied. Therefore, the benefits of vaccine must be carefully weighed against any potential adverse effects before it is given to pregnant women.

Although there are no data, it is reasonable to assume that this vaccine can be used safely in nursing mothers.

Use in immunocompromised persons

The Chol-Ecol-O vaccine can be given to immunocompromised persons, including those with HIV. However, immunocompromised persons may not obtain the expected immune response.

Other considerations

Simultaneous administration with antibiotics or antimalarials

Since the Chol-Ecol-O vaccine is not a live vaccine there is no anticipated interaction or interference when co-administered with antibiotics or antimalarials.

Selected references

Clemens JD, Sack DA, Harris JR et al. *Cross-protection by B subunit-whole cell cholera vaccine against diarrhea associated with heat-labile toxin-producing enterotoxigenic Escherichia coli: results of a large-scale field trial.* Journal of Infectious Diseases 1988;158(2):372-77.

Clemens JD, Sack DA, Harris JR et al. *Field trial of oral cholera vaccines in Bangladesh: results from three-year follow-up.* Lancet 1990;335(8684):270-73.

Committee to Advise on Tropical Medicine and Travel (CATMAT). *Statement on new oral cholera and travellers' diarrhea vaccination.* Canada Communicable Disease Report 2005;31(ACS7):1-12.

Committee to Advise on Tropical Medicine and Travel (CATMAT). *Statement on travellers' diarrhea.* Canada Communicable Disease Report 2001;27(ACS3):1-12.

Ericsson CD, DuPont HL. *Travelers' diarrhea: approaches to prevention and treatment.* Clinical Infectious Diseases 1993;16(5):616-24.

Peltola H, Siitonen A, Kyronseppa H et al. *Prevention of travellers' diarrhoea by oral B-subunit/whole-cell cholera vaccine.* Lancet 1991;338(8778):1285-89.

Pitzinger B, Steffen R, Tschopp A. *Incidence and clinical features of traveler's diarrhea in infants and children.* Pediatric Infectious Disease Journal 1991;10(10):719-23.

Sanchez JL, Vasquez B, Begue RE et al. *Protective efficacy of oral whole-cell/recombinant-B-subunit cholera vaccine in Peruvian military recruits.* Lancet 1994;344(8932):1273-76.

Scerpella EG, Sanchez JL, Mathewson III JJ et al. *Safety, immunogenicity, and protective efficacy of the whole-cell/recombinant B subunit (WC/rBS) oral cholera vaccine against travelers' diarrhea.* Journal of Travel Medicine 1995;2(1):22-7.

Steffen R. *Epidemiologic studies of travelers' diarrhea, severe gastrointestinal infections, and cholera.* Reviews of Infectious Diseases 1986;8 (Suppl 2):S122-30.

World Health Organization. *Cholera vaccines.* Weekly Epidemiological Record 2001;76(16):117-24.

Diphtheria Toxoid

Diphtheria is an acute, communicable disease caused by exotoxin-producing strains of the bacterium *Corynebacterium diphtheriae*. Symptoms result from local infection of the respiratory tract, which may lead to breathing difficulties, or infection of the skin or mucosal surfaces, or from dissemination of diphtheria toxin, which damages the heart and central nervous system. The case-fatality rate remains at about 5% to 10%, the highest death rates occurring among the very young and the elderly. About 3%-5% of healthy persons may be asymptomatically colonized on the skin or in the nasopharynx with *C. diphtheriae*, making eradication of the disease difficult.

Since the publication of the 2002 *Canadian Immunization Guide* changes include 1) a recommendation for adolescents aged 14-16 years of age to be vaccinated with tetanus toxoid, diphtheria toxoid and acellular pertussis (Tdap); and 2) a new recommendation about subsequent vaccinations of persons known to have developed Guillain-Barré Syndrome (GBS) within 8 weeks of a previous tetanus vaccine dose.

Epidemiology

Routine immunization against diphtheria in infancy and childhood has been widely practised in Canada since 1930. In 1924, there were 9,000 cases reported, the highest annual number ever recorded in Canada (see Figure 2). At the same time diphtheria was one of the most common causes of death in children from 1 to 5 years of age. By the mid-1950s, routine immunization had resulted in a remarkable decline in the morbidity and mortality of the disease. Toxigenic strains of diphtheria bacilli are detected each year, although classic diphtheria is rare. In Canada, there are 0 to 5 isolates reported each year. In developed countries occasional cases of imported diphtheria are identified.

Serosurveys of healthy adult populations in Canada indicate that approximately 20% of those surveyed (higher in some age groups) do not have protective levels of antibody to diphtheria. The potential for disease re-emergence if immunization levels are allowed to fall was demonstrated during the 1990s in the Commonwealth of Independent States (former Soviet Union), where over 140,000 cases and 4,000 deaths were reported.

Preparations approved for use in Canada

This chapter will deal only with vaccines that are currently marketed in Canada.

♦ Adacel® (tetanus and diphtheria toxoids adsorbed combined with component pertussis vaccine, [Tdap]), Sanofi Pasteur Ltd.

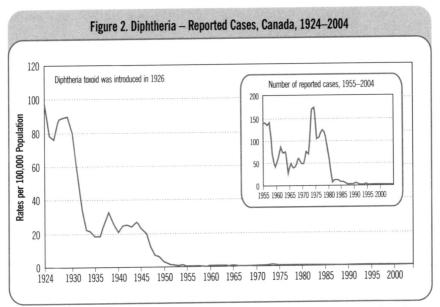

Figure 2. Diphtheria – Reported Cases, Canada, 1924–2004

Diphtheria toxoid was introduced in 1926

Number of reported cases, 1955–2004

- ◆ DT Polio Adsorbed (diphtheria and tetanus toxoids adsorbed and inactivated poliomyelitis vaccine), Sanofi Pasteur Ltd.

- ◆ Pentacel® (Act-HIB® [*Haemophilus* b conjugate vaccine (tetanus protein conjugate)] reconstituted with Quadracel®, [DTaP-IPV-Hib]), Sanofi Pasteur Ltd.

- ◆ Quadracel® (component pertussis vaccine and diphtheria and tetanus toxoids adsorbed combined with inactivated poliomyelitis vaccine, [DTaP-IPV]), Sanofi Pasteur Ltd.

- ◆ Td Adsorbed (tetanus and diphtheria toxoids [adult]), Sanofi Pasteur Ltd.

- ◆ Td Polio Adsorbed (tetanus and diphtheria toxoids and inactivated poliomyelitis vaccine adsorbed [adult]), Sanofi Pasteur Ltd.

- ◆ Tripacel® (component pertussis vaccine combined with diphtheria and tetanus toxoids adsorbed, [DTaP]), Sanofi Pasteur Ltd.

Diphtheria toxoid is a cell-free preparation of diphtheria toxin detoxified with formaldehyde. It is available as a preparation adsorbed with aluminum phosphate and combined with other toxoids or vaccines (e.g., tetanus [T], poliomyelitis [IPV], acellular pertussis [aP], *Haemophilus influenzae* type b [Hib]). The amount of toxoid present is measured in flocculating units (Lf). The amount of diphtheria toxoid varies with the specific product and manufacturer. Preparations containing from 15 to 25 Lf per 0.5 mL dose (commonly designated as "D") are intended for use in children < 7 years of age (pediatric formulation). Preparations containing 2 Lf per 0.5 mL dose (commonly designated as "d") are intended for use in persons ≥ 7 years of age (adolescent/adult formulation). This reduced amount is less likely to cause reactions in persons who have previously received the vaccine. Polysaccharide vaccines that are conjugated with the CRM (cross-reacting material) diphtheria protein do not provide immunity to diphtheria.

For a list of all approved products in Canada, please refer to Table 1, in the *General Considerations* chapter, page 7.

Efficacy and immunogenicity

The immunity conferred by diphtheria vaccine is antitoxic, not antibacterial. Vaccination thus protects against the potentially lethal systemic effects of diphtheria toxin but not directly against local infection. After the primary series over 99% of persons develop antibody levels that are considered protective against disease (antitoxin titres of > 0.1 IU/mL). The antitoxin is believed to persist at protective levels for 10 years or more. Titres decline slowly with time but are boosted by additional doses. Carriage of *C. diphtheriae* can occur in immunized individuals, but the rate has been observed to be lower in immunized populations.

Recommended usage

Routine immunization against diphtheria is recommended for everyone, regardless of the age at which immunization is begun.

Primary immunization of children < 7 years of age

The primary immunizing course of diphtheria toxoid consists of three doses of a combination vaccine beginning at 2 months of age, followed by a booster dose administered approximately 1 year after the third dose. Diphtheria toxoid is most conveniently given as part of the recommended routine immunization schedule. Please refer to the *Recommended Immunization Schedules* chapter, page 93. It is preferable to use products in which diphtheria toxoid is combined with acellular pertussis vaccine and tetanus toxoid (DTaP), with or without inactivated poliomyelitis vaccine (DTaP-IPV) and Hib conjugate vaccine (DTaP-IPV-Hib).

Primary immunization of persons ≥ 7 years of age

The recommended agent is a combined adsorbed tetanus, diphtheria and pertussis preparation (Tdap) containing less diphtheria toxoid than preparations given to younger children.

Schedule and dosage

Children < 7 years of age should be immunized with 0.5 mL of the pediatric formulation of diphtheria toxoid-containing vaccine, DTaP-IPV-Hib, at 2, 4, 6 and 18 months of age. If for any reason this schedule is delayed, three doses of 0.5 mL should be administered with an interval of 4 to 8 weeks between doses, followed by a fourth dose of 0.5 mL administered approximately 1 year after the third dose.

A booster dose of 0.5 mL of DTaP-IPV should be administered between 4 and 6 years of age (school entry). This booster dose is unnecessary if the fourth primary immunizing dose has been administered after the fourth birthday.

A booster dose with the adolescent/adult formulation of tetanus, diphtheria toxoid and acellular pertussis (Tdap) should be administered at 14-16 years of age.

The schedule for routine immunization of persons $\geq$ 7 years of age is a three-dose series of adolescent/adult formulation of diphtheria toxoid-containing vaccine, as noted in the *Recommended Immunization Schedules* chapter, page 93. The second dose is given 2 months after the first, with a third dose 6 to 12 months later to complete the course.

Please refer to the *Immunization of Immunocompromised Persons* chapter, page 117, for recommendations on hematopoietic stem cell and solid organ transplant recipients.

Route of administration

Diphtheria vaccines are prepared as adsorbed products. It is important to ensure that adsorbed vaccines are given intramuscularly because subcutaneous injection of adsorbed products produces a much higher rate of local reactions.

Booster doses and re-immunization

To maintain immunity to diphtheria it is recommended that all Canadians receive a primary immunizing course of diphtheria vacccine (combined with other vaccines), as already described, followed by booster doses at 18 months, 4 to 6 years of age, at 14-16 years of age and then every 10 years.

Additional indications include the following:

◆ Persons travelling to areas where they are likely to be exposed to diphtheria should be offered a booster dose of Td or Tdap if > 10 years has elapsed since their most recent booster.

◆ If a case of diphtheria occurs, close contacts (household, classroom or similar) should be given a dose of a toxoid preparation appropriate for their age unless they are known to have been fully immunized and the last dose was given in the previous 10 years. The remaining doses required to provide full immunization should be given to any contacts who were previously unimmunized or incompletely immunized. Patients convalescent from diphtheria should be given a complete primary course of diphtheria toxoid using an appropriate product for their age and immunization history, unless serologic testing indicates protective levels of antitoxin, since diphtheria infection does not always confer immunity.

Persons requiring a booster dose of tetanus toxoid for wound management should receive Td or Tdap as a convenient means of reinforcing their diphtheria protection. The current National Advisory Committee on Immunization recommendation for Tdap in adults is one dose (please refer to the *Pertussis Vaccine* chapter, page 257).

Serologic testing

There is no indication for routine pre- or post-immunization serology.

Storage requirements

The package insert should be consulted for the storage requirements for the appropriate combination product being used.

Simultaneous administration with other vaccines

Diphtheria vaccine should always be administered in a combined formulation appropriate to age and prior immunization history (e.g., pertussis, polio, tetanus, Hib). Other vaccines may be given at the same time at a different site (e.g., pneumococcal conjugate vaccine).

For details of usage and precautions to be taken with individual vaccines, see relevant sections of the *Guide*.

Adverse reactions

Serious adverse events are rare following immunization and, in most cases, data are insufficient to determine a causal association. The most common adverse reaction following administration of combination vaccines containing diphtheria toxoid that are given in childhood are redness, swelling and pain at the injection site. Systemic reactions such as fever and irritability are less common. Redness and swelling of > 3.5 cm diameter, with minimal pain, are more common in children receiving the fifth consecutive dose of vaccine at 4 to 6 years of age and have been reported in up to 16% of children. In older persons receiving the Td booster, injection site reactions are reported by about 10% of recipients.

Contraindications and precautions

Individuals ≥ 7 years of age should be given only those preparations formulated for older children and adults (Td or Tdap). Before any combined vaccine is given, it is very important to ensure that there are no contraindications to the administration of any of the other components.

As diphtheria vaccine is given in combination with tetanus vaccine, withholding tetanus (e.g. in persons who develop GBS within 8 weeks of a previous tetanus vaccine dose – see *Tetanus Vaccine* chapter, page 309) would necessitate withholding the diphtheria component as well.

Selected references

David ST, Hemsley C, Pasquali PE et al. *Enhanced surveillance for vaccine-associated adverse events: dTap catch-up of high school students in Yukon.* Canada Communicable Disease Report 2005;31(11):117-26.

Dittmann S, Wharton M, Vitek C et al. *Successful control of epidemic diphtheria in the states of the former Union of Soviet Socialist Republics: lessons learned.* Journal of Infectious Diseases 2000;181(Suppl 1):S10-22.

Galazka AM, Robertson SE. *Immunization against diphtheria with special emphasis on immunization of adults.* Vaccine 1996;14(9):845-57.

Halperin SA, Sweet L, Baxendale D et al. *How soon after a prior tetanus-diphtheria vaccination can one give adult formulation tetanus-diphtheria-acellular pertussis vaccine?* Pediatric Infectious Disease Journal 2006;25(3):195-200.

National Advisory Committee on Immunization. *Interval between administration of vaccines against diphtheria, tetanus, and pertussis.* Canada Communicable Disease Report 2005;31(ACS- 9).

Plotkin SA, Orenstein WA. *Vaccines,* 4th edition. Philadelphia: W.B Saunders Company, 2003: 211-228.

Varughese P. *Diphtheria in Canada – surveillance summary.* Canada Diseases Weekly Report 1978;4:65-8.

Haemophilus Vaccine

Haemophilus influenzae type b (Hib) was the most common cause of bacterial meningitis and a leading cause of other serious invasive infections in young children before the introduction of Hib vaccines. About 55% to 65% of affected children had meningitis, the remainder suffering from epiglottitis, bacteremia, cellulitis, pneumonia or septic arthritis. The case-fatality rate of meningitis is about 5%. Severe neurologic sequelae occur in 10% to 15% of survivors and deafness in 15% to 20% (severe in 3% to 7%). *H. influenzae* is also commonly associated with otitis media, sinusitis, bronchitis and other respiratory tract disorders. However, since type b organisms seldom cause these disorders, Hib vaccines have not affected their incidence.

Universal immunization against Hib has led to a significant reduction in the incidence of invasive Hib disease in Canada. The protection resulting from infant immunization appears to be long lasting, and no cases have been reported to date in fully immunized, healthy adolescents.

Since the publication of the 2002 *Canadian Immunization Guide*, the changes that have occurred have been in the preparations approved for use in Canada and recent studies suggesting that vaccine failures may be associated with underlying immune deficiency.

Epidemiology

Since the introduction of Hib vaccines in Canada in 1988, the overall incidence of reported disease has decreased from 2.6 per 100,000 (686 cases) in 1988 to 0.3 per 100,000 (81 cases) in 2004. During this period, the number of reported cases among children < 5 years of age has fallen by almost 97%, from 526 to 17 cases. In 2004, the incidence was 2.4 per 100,000 children < 1 year of age and 0.7 per 100,000 children between the ages of 1 and 5 years. The majority of pediatric cases occur in unimmunized children or in children too young to have received their primary series.

Between 2001 and 2003 only 29 Hib cases were reported in children < 16 years of age by the 12 centres involved in the Immunization Monitoring Program, ACTive (IMPACT) enhanced surveillance program across the country. Only two cases occurred in fully vaccinated, previously healthy children. Twenty of the 29 cases had received no or incomplete primary vaccination, of whom 11 were children < 6 months of age. In addition, eight cases were in children with either an immunodeficiency or other chronic illness.

Non-typeable *H. influenzae* as well as other non-b typeable *H. influenzae* can rarely cause invasive disease. In Canada, only invasive Hib disease is under national surveillance. Between 2000 and 2004, 51 cases of invasive *H. influenzae* were detected in northern Canadian regions participating in the

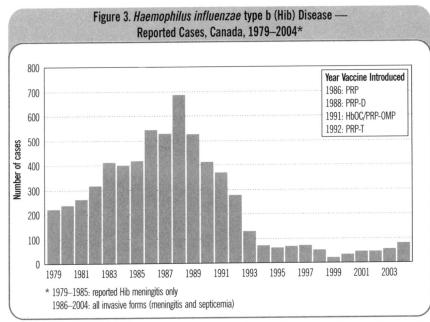

Figure 3. *Haemophilus influenzae* type b (Hib) Disease —
Reported Cases, Canada, 1979–2004*

Year Vaccine Introduced
1986: PRP
1988: PRP-D
1991: HbOC/PRP-OMP
1992: PRP-T

Number of cases

* 1979–1985: reported Hib meningitis only
1986–2004: all invasive forms (meningitis and septicemia)

International Circumpolar Surveillance (i.e., Yukon, Northwest Territories, Nunavut and northern regions of Quebec and Labrador). Of these, only five cases (11% of 47 with serotype information) were due to serotype b. Fifty-five percent of cases were caused by serotype a, and 28% of invasive disease involved non-typeable isolates. Serotypes c, d and e were isolated in one case each of invasive disease.

The risk of Hib meningitis is at least twice as high for children attending full-time day care as for children cared for at home. The risk is also increased among children with splenic dysfunction (e.g., sickle cell disease, asplenia) or antibody deficiency, and among Inuit children. In 2002, a possible association between receipt of a cochlear implant and development of bacterial meningitis was identified. Persons who have received a cochlear implant should also be considered at high risk of invasive Hib disease.

Preparations approved for use in Canada

This chapter will deal only with vaccines that are currently marketed in Canada.

The vast majority of the Hib conjugate vaccines currently used in Canada contain purified polyribosylribitol phosphate (PRP) capsular polysaccharide of Hib covalently bound to tetanus protein (PRP-T) and are available as part of combination vaccine products. PRP-T vaccines include the following:

◆ Act-HIB® (*Haemophilus* b conjugate vaccine [tetanus protein conjugate]), Sanofi Pasteur Ltd.

- Pentacel® (Act-HIB® [*Haemophilus* b conjugate vaccine (tetanus protein conjugate)] reconstituted with Quadracel® [component pertussis vaccine and diphtheria and tetanus toxoids adsorbed combined with inactivated poliomyelitis vaccine]), Sanofi Pasteur Ltd.

There is one PRP-outer membrane protein (OMP) conjugate vaccine available in Canada, purified PRP capsular polysaccharide of Hib covalently bound to an outer membrane protein complex of a strain of serogroup B *Neisseria meningitidis*. No reconstitution is necessary.

- Liquid PedvaxHIB® (*Haemophilus* b conjugate vaccine [meningococcal protein conjugate]), Merck Frosst Canada Ltd.

For a list of all approved products in Canada, please refer to Table 1 in the *General Considerations* chapter, page 7.

All Canadian provinces and territories include Hib conjugate vaccine in their immunization program for children. Hib polysaccharide-protein conjugate vaccines are the second generation of vaccines against Hib disease, having replaced an earlier polysaccharide product. Polysaccharide-protein conjugate antigens have the advantage of producing greater immune response in infants and young children than purified polysaccharide vaccine. The latter stimulates only B-cells, whereas the former activates macrophages, T-helper cells and B-cells, resulting in greatly enhanced antibody responses and establishment of immunologic memory.

The Hib conjugate vaccines differ in a number of ways, including the protein carrier, polysaccharide size, and types of diluent and preservative. PRP-OMP is unique among the Hib conjugate vaccines in its ability to induce a strong antibody response in young infants with the first dose. A third dose of PRP-OMP at 6 months of age does not boost levels or the proportion of responders, and therefore only a two-dose primary series has been recommended for infants. However, as of 1997, all Canadian provinces and territories use the PRP-T vaccine, as it is the only currently approved Hib conjugate vaccine that is combined with acellular pertussis vaccine, diphtheria and tetanus toxoids, and inactivated polio vaccine.

The protein carriers used in Hib conjugate vaccines should not be considered as immunizing agents against diphtheria, tetanus or meningococcal disease.

Efficacy and immunogenicity

PRP-T and PRP-OMP stimulate good antibody responses after primary immunization in infants starting at 2 to 3 months of age and prime them for an excellent booster response at 15 to 18 months. The booster response can be elicited by any of the conjugate Hib vaccines.

Several studies have demonstrated a reduction in the antibody responses to the Hib component when it is given as a combination vaccine with pertussis. However, with each of the products currently available in Canada, the

Hib antibody levels are all in the range of what is considered protective, the functional antibodies are not reduced, and the immunologic memory is unchanged.

When given as a single dose to previously unimmunized children ≥ 15 months of age, PRP-T and PRP-OMP stimulate excellent antibody responses (> 1 μg/mL) in 80% to 100% of children. The duration of immunity following completion of age-appropriate immunization is unknown and warrants ongoing study. Current data suggest that protection will be long lasting.

Capsular polysaccharide antigen can be detected in the urine of vaccinees for up to 2 weeks after vaccination with conjugate vaccine. This phenomenon could be confused with antigenuria associated with invasive Hib infections, and therefore this method alone should not be used to diagnose invasive disease in a recently immunized child.

Hib conjugate vaccine failure, defined as onset of confirmed invasive Hib infection more than 28 days after completion of the primary immunization series, can occur but is rare with the products in current use. Recent studies suggest that vaccine failures may be associated with underlying immune deficiency. It is therefore recommended that children who have invasive Hib disease after completing the 2, 4 and 6 month immunization series be evaluated for evidence of an underlying immune deficiency, although it is expected that this would only be a rare finding.

Recommended usage

Routine immunization with Hib conjugate vaccine is recommended for all infants beginning at 2 months of age. It is preferable to use the same product for all doses in the primary series. However, available data suggest that a primary immunization series consisting of three doses of different Hib conjugate vaccine products results in adequate antibody responses.

Children in whom invasive Hib disease develops before 24 months of age should still receive vaccine as recommended, since natural disease may not induce protection.

Infections due to encapsulated bacteria, including *H. influenzae*, occur more commonly in those with primary and secondary disorders of the humoral immune system, including disorders of antibody production or function, lymphoreticular or hematopoietic malignancies, antibody dyscrasias, protein wasting syndromes, anatomic or functional asplenia, bone marrow transplantation and HIV infection. For previously unimmunized adults and children > 5 years of age who have these underlying conditions the efficacy of Hib immunization is unknown. Despite limited efficacy data, Hib vaccination is commonly given to those with anatomic or functional asplenia and may be considered in other immunocompromised persons at increased risk of invasive Hib infection. Please refer to the *Immunization of Immunocompromised Persons* chapter, page 117, for more information on the recommendations related to provision of this vaccine for stem cell and solid organ transplant recipients. Individuals with cochlear implants are also considered at high risk of invasive Hib disease and should be immunized. Consultation with an infectious disease expert may be helpful in these cases.

The role of chemoprophylaxis in the management of contacts is not discussed in detail here. Rifampin or other appropriate chemoprophylaxis is not required for household contacts of cases of invasive Hib infection when the contacts are completely immunized against Hib. Complete immunization is defined as receipt of the primary Hib vaccination series and booster dose as presented in Table 2. When contacts < 48 months of age are not completely immunized, consultation with the local public health unit is advised.

Schedule and dosage

The recommended Hib vaccination schedule is shown in Table 2. The dose of Hib conjugate vaccine is 0.5 mL. Infants and children starting a primary series of Hib vaccine after 2 months of age should be immunized as soon as possible according to the schedules shown in the Table.

Hib conjugate vaccines that are supplied as a lyophilized powder (e.g., Pentacel®) should be reconstituted only with products supplied by the same manufacturer, as recommended in the package insert. Liquid PedvaxHIB® does not require reconstitution.

Table 2. Detailed Vaccination Schedule for *Haemophilus b* Conjugate Vaccines*

Hib vaccine	Age at 1st dose (months)	Primary series	Age at booster dose** (months)
PRP-T (Sanofi Pasteur Ltd)	2-6	3 doses, 2 months apart	15-18
	7-11	2 doses, 2 months apart	15-18
	12-14	1 dose	15-18
	15-59	1 dose	
PRP-OMP (Merck Frosst Ltd)	2-6	2 doses, 2 months apart	12
	7-11	2 doses, 2 months apart	15-18
	12-17	1 dose	18
	18-59	1 dose	

* Schedule for Hib vaccination. As Hib vaccine is given as part of a combination product, the schedule for children vaccinated after 6 months of age for other antigens included in the combination product may differ, and additional doses may be required to complete the series.

** The booster dose should be given at least 2 months after the previous dose.

Route of administration

Conjugate vaccines should be administered intramuscularly.

Booster doses and re-immunization

Protective serum antibody (anti-PRP) concentrations are achieved in 99% of children after completion of the primary PRP-T immunization series of three doses. Antibody levels subsequently decline, and a booster dose is recommended at 15 to 18 months of age with any of the Hib conjugate vaccines approved for use in infants.

For children who have conditions that predispose them to infection with encapsulated bacteria and who have already received the primary Hib immunization series plus booster, it is not known whether additional doses of Hib vaccine are beneficial. For further information, please see chapter on *Immunization of Immunocompromised Persons*, page 117.

Serologic testing

There is no indication for pre- or post-immunization serology

Storage requirements

Hib conjugate vaccines should be stored between +2° and +8° C and should not be frozen. Following reconstitution, vaccine should be used immediately.

Simultaneous administration with other vaccines

In Canada, Hib vaccines are usually administered as components of combination products. Combined vaccine products allow the administration of multiple antigens with the use of a single needle and have safety profiles similar to those of separately administered vaccines.

Any of the Hib conjugate vaccines may be given simultaneously with polio, measles, mumps, rubella, hepatitis B, polysaccharide and conjugate pneumococcal and meningococcal vaccines, and varicella. There are no data on administration of Hib conjugate vaccines with influenza vaccine, but expert opinion recommends that the two may be given concomitantly. Concomitant vaccines must be administered at separate sites and with separate syringes.

Part 4 — Active Immunizing Agents – Haemophilus Vaccine

Adverse reactions

Serious adverse events are rare following immunization and, in most cases, data are insufficient to determine a causal association.

A temperature of > 38.3° C has been reported in a minority of infants given Hib conjugate vaccine either alone or in combination with other vaccines. A local reaction at the site of injection, including pain, redness and swelling, occurs in 5% to 30% of immunized children. These symptoms are mild and usually resolve within 24 hours. A meta-analysis, which included 257,000 infants, reported no serious adverse events following administration of Hib conjugate vaccine.

Contraindications and precautions

Vaccination is contraindicated in people who are allergic to any component of the vaccine.

Selected references

Anderson EL, Decker MD, Englund JA et al. *Interchangeability of conjugated Haemophilus influenzae type b vaccines in infants.* Journal of the American Medical Association 1995;273(11):849-53.

Eskola J. *Analysis of Haemophilus influenzae type b conjugate and diphtheria-tetanus-pertussis combination vaccines.* Journal of Infectious Diseases 1996;174(Suppl 3):S302-305.

Friede A, O'Carroll PW, Nicola RM et al. Centers for Disease Control and Prevention. *CDC prevention guidelines. A guide to action.* Baltimore: Williams and Wilkins, 1997:394-492.

National Advisory Committee on Immunization. *Interchangeability of diphtheria, tetanus, acellular pertussis, polio, Haemophilus influenzae type b combination vaccines presently approved for use in Canada for children < 7 years of age.* Canada Communicable Disease Report 2005;(ACS-1):1-10.

Scheifele DW. *Recent trends in pediatric Haemophilus influenzae type b infections in Canada. Immunization Monitoring Program, ACTive (IMPACT) of the Canadian Paediatric Society and the Laboratory Centre for Disease Control.* Canadian Medical Association Journal 1996;154(7):1041-47.

Scheifele D, Halperin S, Law B et al. *Invasive Haemophilus influenzae type b infections in vaccinated and unvaccinated children in Canada, 2001-2003.* Canadian Medical Association Journal 2005;172(1):53-56.

Swingler G, Fransman D, Hussey G. *Conjugate vaccines for preventing Haemophilus influenzae type b infections.* Cochrane Database Systematic Reviews 2003(4):CD001729.

Hepatitis A Vaccine

Hepatitis A virus (HAV) is an RNA virus of a single serotype. Infection usually causes clinical hepatitis in adults and school-aged children but is often asymptomatic in younger children. Jaundice develops in < 10% of children 6 years and under. Typical symptoms of illness include anorexia, nausea, fatigue, fever and jaundice. The severity of the illness increases with age. Recovery often takes 4 to 6 weeks but may take months. Recurrent hepatitis for up to a year occurs in about 15% of cases, but longer chronic infection is not known to occur. About 25% of reported adult cases require hospitalization. Fulminant disease with liver necrosis is rare but can be fatal. Individuals with pre-existing chronic liver disease are at increased risk of serious complications from HAV infection. The overall estimated case fatality rate associated with hepatitis A is 0.1% to 0.3%, but this rises to 1.8% in persons over the age of 50. It reaches 12.5% in patients over the age of 60 who are hospitalized because of the disease.

Since the publication of the 2002 *Canadian Immunization Guide*, new data have been obtained on the epidemiology of hepatitis A in Canada and on the immunization coverage of travellers to endemic countries.

Epidemiology

HAV is most frequently transmitted by the fecal-oral route, through direct contact with infected people or indirectly through ingestion of contaminated water or foods. On rare occasions, transmission has been reported after exposure to HAV-contaminated blood or blood products. It also occurs through sexual activities that include direct or indirect oro-anal contact but not through exposure to saliva, semen or urine. The virus may persist for days or weeks in the environment. Shedding of the virus in feces and thus maximum infectiousness occurs during the latter part of the incubation period with peak levels in the 2 weeks before clinical illness. Infectiousness diminishes rapidly thereafter and ends shortly after the onset of jaundice. Humans are the principal reservoir for HAV. Persistent infection does not occur. The incubation period ranges from 15 to 50 days with an average of 20 to 30 days. Lifelong immunity usually follows infection.

In Canada, between 1990 and 2004 the number of cases of HAV infection reported annually varied from 3,562 (1991) to 396 (2003), representing rates of 10.8 and 1.2 per 100,000 population respectively. During this period, there have been outbreaks involving men who have sex with men (MSM) in major Canadian cities. Since the introduction of the vaccine in 1996, no new major outbreak has occurred, and the incidence rate has slowly decreased. It is not known whether this is due to the impact of the targeted immunization programs. There is no information on the proportion of targeted groups being immunized, but it is likely low. The estimated

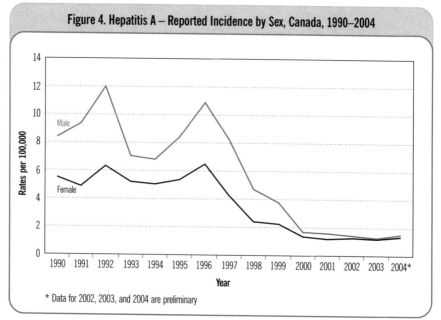

Figure 4. Hepatitis A – Reported Incidence by Sex, Canada, 1990–2004

* Data for 2002, 2003, and 2004 are preliminary

coverage in MSM at the end of the massive immunization campaign during the Montreal outbreak was only 35%. Within Canada, there have been considerable geographic variations in the reported incidence, and this is observed even during periods of decline nationally. In the 5 year period of 1999 to 2004, no substantial sex difference in reported rates was observed. In 2004, the reported rate was 1.4 among females and 1.6 among males per 100,000 population. Age-specific incidence was highest among those 15-24 years old with a rate of 2.3 per 100,000 population, followed closely by those aged 5-14 (2.2 per 100,000 population).

Given asymptomatic infection, underdiagnosis and underreporting, the actual number of cases has been estimated to be 10 times higher than the number of notifications. A nationwide Canadian seroprevalence study has shown a seroprevalence of 2.0% in unvaccinated 8- to 13-year-olds. In this same study, HAV antibody prevalence was 1.1% in non-vaccinated, non-Aboriginal children born in Canada who did not travel to endemic countries. There are no other nationwide seroprevalence data. A systematic review of all seroprevalence studies conducted in Canada has been published recently and demonstrates an increase with age, which is probably due both to the cumulative incidence with increasing age and a cohort effect attributable to higher incidence rates in the past.

Risk factors for HAV infection in Canada include the following:

♦ Sexual behaviours involving anal contact, particularly between men (MSM). This resulted in the major outbreaks of the 90s.

♦ Travel to or residence in countries with endemic hepatitis A. In recent years 40% of all notified hepatitis A cases have been in travelers. Among those, 40% are taking low-risk trips (staying for short periods of time in luxury hotels where meals are provided). More than 5 million Canadians go to an HAV-endemic country in a year. Over 5 years, 30% of Canadians will travel to an endemic country, yet less than 15% of these travelers go to a travel clinic and receive hepatitis A vaccine.

◆ Immigrants or children of new Canadians who return to their country of origin to visit friends and relatives.

◆ Household contacts of an acute case.

◆ Residence in certain communities in rural or remote areas lacking adequate sanitation or a secure supply of potable water.

◆ Residence in certain institutions, such as correctional facilities and those for developmentally challenged individuals.

◆ Illicit drug use. In this group, transmission is seldom related to contaminated injection material. It is rather associated with a number of risk factors: low hygiene standards, contaminated drugs, and sharing of materials for oral or nasal use of drugs.

More than 25% of cases have no identifiable risk factor. Food handlers are not at higher risk of hepatitis A because of their occupation. However, food handlers may belong to a demographic group with a higher incidence of hepatitis A and thus cause major outbreaks. They may also trigger very extensive public health interventions that become necessary when a food handler is found to be contagious, even if the number of secondary cases is ultimately small.

Preparations approved for use in Canada

This chapter will deal only with vaccines that are currently marketed in Canada.

◆ Avaxim® (hepatitis A vaccine inactivated), Sanofi Pasteur Ltd.
◆ Avaxim® Pediatric, Sanofi Pasteur Ltd.
◆ Havrix® (hepatitis A vaccine, inactivated), GlaxoSmithKline Inc.
◆ Vaqta® (hepatitis A vaccine, inactivated), Merck Frosst Canada Ltd.

There is some evidence that these vaccines may be used interchangeably, despite different schedules and systems of measuring antigen content.

In these vaccines, various strains of cell-culture-adapted virus are propagated in human fibroblasts, purified from cell lysates, inactivated with formalin and adsorbed to an aluminum hydroxide adjuvant.

Immune globulin (Ig) may be used for short-term protection against HAV in infants and in people who are immunocompromised (who may not respond fully to HAV vaccine), and in people for whom HAV vaccine is contraindicated. Please refer to the *Passive Immunizing Agents* chapter, page 353, for more information.

Formulations combining antigens against both HAV and HBV are also marketed in Canada. Please refer to the *Hepatitis Vaccines Combined* chapter, page 205, for more information.

For a list of all approved products in Canada, please refer to Table 1 in the *General Considerations* chapter, page 7.

Efficacy and immunogenicity

All the HAV vaccines have shown high levels of immunogenicity and at least 85% to 90% efficacy in preventing clinical illness. Epidemiologic studies of hepatitis A outbreaks have shown repeatedly that the use of vaccine in the susceptible population interrupts the outbreak, suggesting that receipt of vaccine before exposure is almost invariably protective. This conclusion is also supported by an Italian study, in which the use of vaccine in household contacts, after exposure, prevented secondary cases. Protection appears to occur rapidly within 2 weeks after immunization. Given the long incubation period of hepatitis A (2 to 7 weeks), vaccine given a few days after exposure can still elicit an adequate immune response to protect the vaccinee. In serologic studies of all HAV vaccines, 95% to 100% of individuals consistently developed protective levels of serum antibody against HAV 4 weeks after a single dose of any inactivated hepatitis A vaccine.

In the countries where universal immunization is in place, a decrease in incidence far in excess of the vaccine coverage has been demonstrated. This is indicative of herd immunity.

Recommended usage

Pre-exposure prophylaxis

Hepatitis A vaccine is recommended for pre-exposure prophylaxis of individuals at increased risk of infection or increased risk of severe hepatitis A:

- travelers to countries where hepatitis A is endemic;
- residents of communities that have high endemic rates of HAV or are at risk of HAV outbreaks;
- members of the Canadian armed forces, emergency relief workers and others likely to be posted abroad at short notice to areas with high rates of HAV infection;
- people with life-style risks for infection, including people engaging in illicit drug use and MSM;
- people who have chronic liver disease or who are receiving hepatotoxic medications, including persons infected with hepatitis C who may not

be at increased risk of infection but are at increased risk of fulminant hepatitis A, should infection occur;

- people with other conditions for which hepatotoxic medications are likely to be prescribed in the future;

- people with hemophilia A or B receiving plasma-derived replacement clotting factors; the solvent-detergent method used to prepare all the present plasma-derived factor VIII and some factor IX concentrates does not reliably inactivate HAV, since the virus does not have an envelope;

- zoo-keepers, veterinarians and researchers who handle non-human primates;

- workers involved in research on HAV or production of hepatitis A vaccine who may be exposed to HAV.

The National Advisory Committee on Immunization (NACI) also encourages all those who wish to decrease their risk of acquiring HAV to be vaccinated.

Post-exposure prophylaxis

HAV vaccine has been shown in one randomized study to be as effective as immune globulin (Ig) for the prevention of HAV. Although more studies of its use in post-exposure prophylaxis are needed to document its effect fully, HAV vaccine used in the first week after exposure appears to be highly effective as a post-exposure measure to prevent infection in identified contacts. It is recommended for this use in preference to Ig. Therefore, one dose of HAV vaccine should be given to contacts of HAV within 1 week of exposure. It should also be considered if > 1 week has elapsed since exposure, as there are no data on the outer limit of efficacy.

Post-exposure immunoprophylaxis should be undertaken for household and other intimate contacts of proven or suspected cases of HAV. It should be given when hepatitis A occurs in day care centres and kindergartens. Post-exposure prophylaxis is not necessary for other contacts, such as school, workplace or health care workers caring for HAV cases unless an outbreak is suspected or likely (see *Outbreak Control*, below).

If HAV vaccine is unavailable for post-exposure prophylaxis, Ig may be used as a substitute. Ig is still the recommended immunoprophylactic agent for infants < 1 year of age, immunocompromised people, who may not respond fully to the vaccine, and those for whom vaccine is contraindicated. Please refer to the *Passive Immunizing Agents* chapter, page 353, for information on dosage.

Outbreak control

There have been several outbreaks in which HAV vaccine has been used to arrest the transmission of the virus in communities. This observation supports its use in outbreak control. The outbreaks in which the vaccine has been used successfully include those in Toronto and Vancouver in 2002, in Kitchener-Waterloo in 1997, in Montreal in 1997-98 and on Vancouver Island in 1995-96. In accordance with the data and experience documented in these reports, HAV vaccine should be considered as an important control measure in a coordinated public health response to hepatitis A outbreaks in the community and also in institutions (correctional facilities, institutions for the developmentally challenged, etc). When a food handler is infected, co-workers and clients should receive post-exposure prophylaxis.

Universal immunization

Universal immunization programs against HAV are possible because of the availability of safe and effective vaccines. In the United States, universal immunization of 2-year-old children started in states in which the incidence of HAV exceeded the national average. Since these states now have incidence rates lower than the formerly low-incidence states, universal immunization has been extended to the whole country. Israel and provinces of Spain and Italy have also introduced universal programs.

Universal immunization programs against HAV should be considered in Canada, but the decision to implement such programs will depend on circumstances in each jurisdiction.

The establishment of a universal program would benefit people who may be at risk but who do not seek pre-exposure immunization. For example, more than 85% of travelers to endemic areas do not go to a travel clinic to obtain the vaccine. Because of their large numbers and high turnover, a universal program is also the only feasible way to achieve high immunization rates among food handlers.

In Canada, it is also possible to give the vaccine efficiently by using combined hepatitis A and B vaccines. Please refer to the *Hepatitis Vaccines Combined* chapter, page 205, for more information.

Schedule and dosage

The dosage schedules of the three HAV vaccines for adults and children are listed in Table 3, along with antigen content and volumes of doses.

If the second dose in the hepatitis A vaccine series is missed, it can be given at a later time without repeating the first dose.

Table 3. Doses and Schedules for Monovalent Hepatitis A Vaccines

Vaccine	Antigen*	Volume	Schedule (booster)	Age†
Avaxim®	160 antigen units HAV	0.5 mL	0, (6-12) months	12 years and older
Avaxim® Pediatric	80 antigen units HAV	0.5 mL	0, (6-12) months	1 to 15 years
Havrix® 1440	1440 ELISA units HAV	1.0 mL	0, (6-12) months‡	19 years and older
Havrix® 720 Junior	720 ELISA units HAV	0.5 mL	0, (6-12) months	1 to 18 years
Vaqta®	50 units HAV	1.0 mL	0, (6-18) months	18 years and older
Vaqta® Pediatric/Adolescent	25 units HAV	0.5 mL	0, (6-18) months	2 to 17 years

* There is no international standard for HAV antigen measurement. Each manufacturer uses its own units of measurement.

† Ages for which the vaccine is approved for use.

‡ Studies have shown that 720 ELISA units provides an effective booster dose in those over 19 years of age.

Because each of the HAV vaccines approved for use in Canada has similar HAV antigen and because each vaccine alone has been shown to induce high levels of protective antibody, it is likely that any HAV vaccine will provide an effective second dose after a first dose of one of the others. Lack of availability of the identical product, therefore, should not be considered an impediment to administering the second dose of HAV vaccine, nor is there a need to repeat the first dose of vaccine in these circumstances. The timing of the second dose in this situation should be based on the vaccine used for the second dose.

Route of administration

Hepatitis A vaccines should be administered intramuscularly.

Booster doses and re-immunization

Although the duration of protection and thus the need for additional booster doses after two doses of HAV vaccine are unknown, kinetic models of antibody decline suggest that protective levels of antibody will likely persist for at least 20 years. Immune memory has been demonstrated in a number of studies, with the implication that protection may persist even when antibodies are no longer measurable, as is the case for hepatitis B vaccine. Should future study results indicate the need for booster doses, recommendations will be made at that time.

Serologic testing

Pre-immunization

Pre-immunization serologic testing is only cost-effective in populations that have a high level of immunity. Variations in the cost of testing and of vaccine will affect these analyses and the specific level of population immunity at which testing will become cost-effective. Nevertheless, pre-immunization testing for immunity against HAV should be considered in populations with the potential for higher levels of pre-existing immunity. Older Canadians and people from HAV-endemic areas of the world are examples of these populations. In addition, people with a history of hepatitis or jaundice that may have been caused by HAV should be considered for assessment of immunity before immunization is undertaken.

Post-immunization

The high response rate to immunization makes routine serologic testing unnecessary. Moreover, commercial assay kits are not universally reliable for detecting vaccine-induced antibody.

Storage requirements

Hepatitis A vaccine should be stored at a temperature between +2° C and +8° C and should not be frozen.

Simultaneous administration with other vaccines

Concomitant administration of other vaccines at other injection sites is unlikely to interfere with the immune response to HAV vaccine. There have been studies on concomitant administration of some of the HAV vaccines with various other vaccines, such as yellow fever, typhoid and cholera, which demonstrated no immune interference; however, complete data on all HAV vaccines are not available.

Adverse reactions

Side effects reported in vaccine recipients are generally mild and transient, and limited to soreness and redness at the injection site. Other less frequent side effects include headache, malaise, fever, fatigue and gastrointestinal symptoms. Local side effects in children appear to be less frequent than in adults. No significant difference in reactions is evident between initial and subsequent doses or in the presence of pre-existing immunity. Rare cases of anaphylaxis have been reported.

Contraindications and precautions

HAV vaccine should not be given to any person who has had an anaphylactic reaction to any component of the vaccine preparation. Since each HAV vaccine has different components, it is important to ascertain the specific cause of previous anaphylaxis, if possible, and refer to the package insert.

The safety of HAV vaccine given during pregnancy has not been studied in clinical trials. Since the vaccine is prepared from inactivated virus, however, there is no apparent risk to the developing fetus. Therefore, HAV vaccine may be given to pregnant women when indicated. HAV vaccine can be used safely in breast-feeding women.

HAV vaccine can also be used safely in those with chronic illnesses or immunosuppression. Although the efficacy of the vaccine may be reduced in those who are immunosuppressed, the vaccine still provides some protection against HAV in these populations and should be considered for pre-exposure use when there is an indication for the vaccine. Ig is still recommended for immunosuppressed persons for post-exposure immunoprophylaxis.

Selected references

Bryan JP, Henry CH, Hoffman AG et al. *Randomized, cross-over, controlled comparison of two inactivated hepatitis A vaccines.* Vaccine 2000;19(7-8):743-50.

Dagan R, Leventhal A, Anis E et al. *Incidence of hepatitis A in Israel following universal immunization of toddlers.* Journal of the American Medical Association 2005;294(2):202-10.

De Serres G, Duval B, Shadmani R et al. *Ineffectiveness of the current strategy to prevent hepatitis A in travelers.* Journal of Travel Medicine 2002;9(1):10-6.

De Serres G, Laliberte D. *Hepatitis A among workers from a waste water treatment plant during a small community outbreak.* Occupational and Environmental Medicine 1997;54(1):60-2.

Deshaies D, Dion R, Valiquette L et al. *Immunization against hepatitis A during an outbreak in a Jewish orthodox community Quebec 1997-1998.* Canada Communicable Disease Report 1998;24(18):145-51.

Duval B, De Serres G, Ochnio J et al. *Nationwide Canadian study of hepatitis A antibody prevalence among children eight to thirteen years old.* Pediatric Infectious Disease Journal 2005;24(6):514-19.

Fiore AE. *Hepatitis A transmitted by food.* Clinical Infectious Diseases 2004;38(5):705-15.

Hockin J, Isaacs S, Kittle D et al. *Hepatitis A outbreak in a socially contained religious community in rural southern Ontario.* Canada Communicable Disease Report 1997;23(21):161-66.

McMahon BJ, Beller M, Williams J et al. *A programme to control an outbreak of HAV in Alaska by using an inactivated hepatitis A vaccine.* Archives of Pediatrics and Adolescent Medicine 1996;150(7):733-39.

Pham B, Duval B, De Serres G et al. *Seroprevalence of hepatitis A infection in a low endemicity country: a systematic review.* BioMed Central Infectious Diseases 2005;5:56. URL: <http://www.biomedcentral.com/1471-2334/5/56>.

Sagliocca L, Amoroso P, Stroffolini T et al. *Efficacy of hepatitis A vaccine in prevention of secondary hepatitis A infection: a randomised trial.* Lancet 1999;353(9159):1136-39.

Scheifele DW. *Hepatitis A vaccines: the growing case for universal immunisation of children.* Expert Opinion on Pharmacotherapy 2005;6(2):157-64.

Vento S, Garofano T, Renzini C et al. *Fulminant hepatitis associated with hepatitis A virus superinfection in patients with chronic hepatitis C.* New England Journal of Medicine 1998;338(5):286-90.

Werzberger A, Kuter B, Shouval D et al. *Anatomy of a trial: a historical view of the Monroe inactivated hepatitis A protective efficacy trial.* Journal of Hepatology 1993;18(Suppl. 2): S46-S50.

Wu J, Zou S, Giulivi A. *Hepatitis A and its control.* In: Health Canada. *Viral hepatitis and emerging bloodborne pathogens in Canada.* Canada Communicable Disease Report 2001;27(S3):7-9.

Hepatitis B Vaccine

Hepatitis B virus (HBV) is one of several viruses that cause hepatitis. HBV is a double-stranded DNA virus with three major antigens, known as hepatitis B surface antigen (HBsAg), hepatitis B e antigen (HBeAg) and hepatitis B core antigen (HBcAg). HBsAg can be detected in serum 30 to 60 days after exposure and persists until the infection resolves. Any person positive for HBsAg is considered infectious. In most cases, anti-HBs appears after HBsAg has disappeared and the infection has resolved. In severe acute HBV infections, anti-HBs may be present simultaneously with HBsAg. In a proportion that varies inversely with age, infection persists. Anti-HBs confers long-term immunity.

HBcAg never appears in serum. Anti-HBc develops in all HBV infections, is not protective and persists indefinitely as a serologic marker, both in chronic active infection and in resolved infection after clearance of HBsAg. Anti-HBc IgM is a marker of recent HBV infection. It appears during the first week of acute hepatitis illness and is usually present for 6-12 months. It can be used to diagnose recent acute hepatitis B. In 10%-15% of cases of chronic hepatitis B infection, IgM anti-HBc may also be detected, particularly when a replication HBV is present. HBeAg is associated with viral replication and high infectiousness. Anti-HBe usually indicates a reduction in replicating virus and lower infectiousness. Methods of quantification of HBV DNA in serum are available to assist in determining both infectiousness and prognosis.

Initial infection with HBV may be asymptomatic in up to 50% of adults and 90% of children. The incubation period is 45 to 160 days, with an average of 120 days. When symptoms occur, they include an insidious onset of anorexia, vague abdominal pain, nausea, vomiting and jaundice. Acute illness may last up to 3 months and has a case fatality rate of 1% to 2%, which increases with age. Fulminant hepatitis and death may also occur in pregnant women and in infants born to infected mothers.

An individual with either acute symptomatic or asymptomatic HBV infection may become a chronic carrier. A chronic carrier is an individual from whom serum samples taken 6 months apart are HBsAg positive or a single serum sample is HBsAg positive and anti-HBc IgM negative. The risk of becoming a chronic carrier varies inversely with the age at which infection occurs (infants: 90% to 95%; children < 5 years: 25% to 50%; adults: 3% to 10%). The risk of becoming a chronic carrier is also greater in immunocompromised patients. Chronic carriers often do not have overt disease but over time are at increased risk of developing hepatic cirrhosis and primary hepatocellular carcinoma. All carriers should be considered infectious.

Since the publication of the 2002 *Canadian Immunization Guide* the major change is the continuous decline in the incidence of hepatitis B with the increased use of the vaccine. New combination vaccines and new schedules have been approved. Research results have confirmed the safety of the vaccine.

Epidemiology

The epidemiology of the disease has been considerably modified by the introduction of the universal program of immunization and the increased use of vaccine in targeted groups. The incidence of hepatitis B has been decreasing in all age groups in recent years, coinciding with the increasing use of the vaccine (see Figure 5). HBV infection has virtually disappeared in the cohorts that have benefited from the universal immunization programs.

HBV is found mainly in the blood, vaginal secretions, semen and serous fluids of an infected person. It is present in the saliva at concentrations 1,000-10,000 times less than in blood. HBV is transmitted through percutaneous or mucosal contact with infectious biological fluids. It is transmitted from infected mothers to newborns and in settings of close personal contact through unrecognized contact with infectious bodily fluids. It is transmitted through sexual contact, both heterosexual and homosexual, and through contact with blood (needle stick, intravenous drug use with needle sharing). The risk of transfusion-related hepatitis B is extremely low because of routine HBsAg and anti-HBc screening of donated blood and exclusion of donors at risk of infection. The precise role of saliva in the transmission of HBV is not clearly known. Saliva is considered infectious in bite wounds with broken skin involving the percutaneous inoculation of saliva, or when it is visibly tainted with blood. In Canada, like elsewhere,

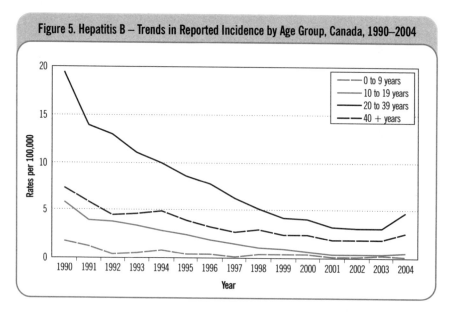

Figure 5. Hepatitis B – Trends in Reported Incidence by Age Group, Canada, 1990–2004

almost one-third of infections have no identified risk factors, despite thorough enquiries.

The regions of the world with the highest prevalence of infection are South-East Asia and Africa, but the use of vaccine in some of these countries for the last 20 years has reduced drastically the incidence of hepatitis B. Although there are no national data on the prevalence of chronic HBV infection for the whole Canadian population, Canada is considered an area of low endemicity. It is estimated that < 5% of residents have markers of past infection, and < 1% are HBsAg carriers. This will vary in different subgroups of the population according to the presence of the factors listed earlier and the vaccine coverage achieved.

Preparations approved for use in Canada

This chapter will deal only with vaccines that are currently marketed in Canada.

- Engerix®-B (hepatitis B vaccine, recombinant), GlaxoSmithKline Inc.

- Recombivax HB® (hepatitis B vaccine, recombinant), Merck Frosst Canada Ltd.

Both vaccines contain purified HBsAg produced from a genetically engineered yeast strain. Recombivax HB® vaccine contains 10 µg/mL and Engerix®-B vaccine 20 µg/mL of purified HBsAg. A preparation of Recombivax HB® containing 40 µg/mL is available for use in hemodialysis patients and others in whom hyporesponsiveness is likely. Trace amounts of yeast antigens are present in the vaccines, but no increase in yeast antibody titres has been observed following administration of either vaccine.

The antigen is adsorbed onto aluminum hydroxide. In some preparations thimerosal is used as preservative. Thimerosal has been shown not to be associated with chronic neurological disease despite theoretical concerns raised a few years ago that resulted in the marketing of thimerosal-free HBV vaccines. It is to be emphasized strongly that post-exposure immunoprophylaxis for infants born to infected mothers must be undertaken without delay, regardless of the type of vaccine available, because of the high risk of long-term complications if infection occurs.

Hepatitis B vaccines are approved for use in Canada for pre-exposure and post-exposure prophylaxis.

Hepatitis B immune globulin (HBIg) is prepared from pooled human plasma from selected donors who have a high level of anti-HBs and are seronegative for blood-borne infections. It provides immediate short-term passive immunity. HBIg administered concurrently with vaccine, but at a different site, does not interfere with the antibody response of the vaccine.

Formulations combining antigens against both HAV and HBV are also marketed in Canada. Please refer to the *Hepatitis Vaccines Combined* chapter, page 205, for more information.

For a list of all approved products in Canada, please refer to Table 1 in the *General Considerations* chapter, page 7.

Efficacy and immunogenicity

Antigenic subtypes of HBV exist, but immunization provides immunity to all subtypes because of the presence of a common antigen. Seroconversion (anti-HBs ≥ 1 mIU/mL), seroprotection (anti-HBs ≥ 10 mIU/mL) and geometric mean titre (GMT) are used to assess the immune response. There is a general consensus that a titre of 10 mIU/mL of anti-HBs is an indication of protection. People who reach that titre after immunization are considered protected for life. The GMT reaches a peak 1 month after the last dose of the schedule, drops rapidly up to 6 months and decreases slowly thereafter. The anti-HBs will eventually disappear in most vaccinees, more quickly if the initial titre was low. Fortunately, many studies have demonstrated the persistence of an immune memory, despite the disappearance of anti-HBs. An anamnestic response can be detected 3-5 days after exposure to HBsAg.

The duration of the protection induced has not yet been fully determined since the vaccines began to be used 20 years ago. In endemic regions, the protection has been shown to persist for at least 15 years in most of the vaccinees. A large 15-year cohort study was started in Quebec in 1995 to assess the protection conferred by immunization in the schoolchildren universal programs. At the 5-year follow-up, the protection as measured by an anamnestic response to a booster dose had persisted in more than 99% of children who initially had anti-HBs titres ≥ 10 mIU/mL.

The major determinant of seroprotection rates achieved is the age at vaccination, but outcome also varies with the schedule used, the dosage and the underlying health status of the vaccinee. Children < 2 years of age have a 95% response rate with relatively low GMTs. The best response is observed in children between the ages of 5 and 15 years with 99% seroprotection rates and very high GMTs. On average, the response rate for older individuals is as follows:

◆ 20 to 29 years: 95%;
◆ 30 to 39 years: 90%;
◆ 40 to 49 years: 86%;
◆ 50 to 59 years: 71%;
◆ ≥ 60 years: 50% to 70%.

The immune mechanisms for suboptimal response to hepatitis B vaccine are only partially understood. The antibody response is lower in patients with diabetes mellitus (70% to 80%), renal failure (60% to 70%) and chronic liver disease (60% to 70%). Immunization of obese people, smokers and those with alcoholism may also produce lower antibody titres. Immunocompromised patients, such as those infected with HIV, will have a diminished response in proportion to the level of immune deficiency. Patients undergoing dialysis are particularly vulnerable because they do not respond well to the vaccine and do not develop an immune memory. For these reasons and because of their frequent contact with blood, they need a vaccine formulation with a much higher concentration of HBsAg and regular monitoring of their anti-HBs titre.

Recommended usage

Hepatitis B prevention should include programs for universal immunization of children, universal screening of all pregnant women for HBsAg, pre-exposure immunization of high-risk groups and post-exposure intervention for those exposed to HBV, particularly infants born to HBV-infected mothers.

Universal immunization

Universal immunization against HBV is now part of the publicly funded vaccine programs offered in all provinces and territories. The age at which children and adolescents are offered HBV vaccine varies from jurisdiction to jurisdiction. The National Advisory Committee on Immunization (NACI) supports the use of available combination vaccines, including hepatitis B and other childhood vaccines, for the immunization of infants.

Pre-exposure prophylaxis

♦ **Health care and emergency service workers and other occupational exposure:**

Immunization with hepatitis B vaccine is recommended for people who are at increased risk of occupational infection, namely, those exposed frequently to blood, blood products and bodily fluids that may contain the virus. This group includes all health care workers and others who will be or may be exposed to blood or are at risk of injury by instruments contaminated by blood. For these workers, a series of hepatitis B immunizations should be initiated at the first opportunity. Students in these occupations should complete their vaccine series before possible occupational exposure to blood or sharps injuries. Emergency service workers, such as police and firefighters, may also be at higher risk of exposure, although there are currently no data to quantify their risk. Workers who have no contact with blood or blood products are at no greater risk than the general population.

♦ **Others at increased risk:**

• residents and staff of institutions for the developmentally challenged;

- men having sexual contact with men;

- those who have unprotected sex with new partners or have had more than one sexual partner in the previous 6 months, those with a history of sexually transmitted infections (STI), and persons attending an STI clinic or who otherwise engage in risky sexual practices;

- injection drug users;

- hemophiliacs and others receiving repeated infusions of blood or blood products;

- hemodialysis patients (40 µg of vaccine antigen per dose should be used);

- staff and inmates of correctional facilities;

- household and sexual contacts of acute HBV cases and HBV carriers;

- populations or communities in which HBV is highly endemic;

- children < 7 years of age whose families have immigrated to Canada from areas where there is a high prevalence of hepatitis B and who may be exposed to HBV carriers through their extended families or when visiting friends and relatives in their country of origin;

- travelers to hepatitis B endemic areas;

- children in child care settings in which there is an HBV-infected child.

◆ **Others for whom the vaccine is recommended:**

- people who have chronic liver disease or are taking hepatotoxic drugs, including persons infected with hepatitis C, who may not be at an increased risk of infection but may be at risk of more severe acute hepatitis B infection, should infection occur;

- people with other conditions for which hepatotoxic medications are likely to be prescribed in the future;

- people who have undergone hematopoietic stem cell transplantation (please refer to the *Immunization of Immunocompromised Persons* chapter, page 117, for more information).

NACI also recommends that any person who wishes to decrease his or her risk of acquiring HBV be immunized.

Post-exposure prophylaxis

◆ **Infants:**

Because of the importance of preventing hepatitis B infection in infants, all pregnant women should be routinely tested for HBsAg. All infants born to infected mothers should be given the initial dose of HBV vaccine within 12 hours of birth. The second and third dose of the vaccine series should be given 1 and 6 months after the first. An intramuscular dose of 0.5 mL HBIg should also be given immediately after birth, since its efficacy decreases sharply after 48 hours. Vaccine and HBIg may be given at the same time but at different sites. If exceptional circumstances prevent immediate administration of vaccine and HBIg, they should be given at the first possible opportunity.

The response to hepatitis B vaccine may be diminished in infants with birth weights below 2000 g. Routine immunization of infants of mothers known to be negative for HBsAg should be delayed until the infant reaches 2000 g or 1 month of age. Premature infants born to women who are HBsAg positive should receive HBIg and the appropriate dose of vaccine within 12 hours of birth. These latter infants require a fourth dose of hepatitis B vaccine and assessment of anti-HBs response after the series has been completed.

If maternal testing has not been conducted during pregnancy, it should be done at the time of delivery. If maternal HBV status is not available within 12 hours of delivery, serious consideration should be given to administering vaccine and HBIg while the results are pending, *taking into account the mother's risk factors* and erring on the side of providing vaccine and HBIg if there is any suspicion that the mother could be infected. If the mother is ultimately shown to have HBV infection, vaccination should be completed, as described earlier. Should the mother's infection be recognized during the infant's first year of life, the infant's HBV status should be assessed urgently and the infant started immediately on full immunoprophylaxis, which should be completed if the infant is found not to be already infected or immune.

When a mother is infected with HBV, testing of the infant for HBsAg and anti-HBs is recommended 1 month after completion of the vaccine series to monitor the success of immunoprophylaxis. If HBsAg is found, the child is likely to become a chronic carrier. If the infant is negative for both HBsAg and anti-HBs (i.e., a non-responder), additional doses up to a second full course of vaccine should be given, with repeated serologic testing for antibody response.

Accountability mechanisms should be in place to ensure that every infant born to an infected mother receives a full course of vaccine and HBIg expeditiously as well as testing for serologic response to the vaccine (see *Serologic Testing*).

- **Percutaneous (needlestick, bite) or mucosal exposure:**

Figures 6 and 7 outline the management of vaccinated or unvaccinated individuals after potential exposure to hepatitis B, including injury by needles found on the street or deep bites associated with bleeding. The management of potential percutaneous or mucosal exposure to HBV should be based on the immunization and antibody status of the injured person and the infectious status, if known, of the source. It is critically important to ascertain whether the exposed individual has received a full and properly administered course of hepatitis B vaccine and to assess the post-vaccination anti-HBs antibody level. Therefore, all health care workers and health care students should have their antibody status assessed and documented after immunization. For those who were immunized in the school-based program, their antibody status should be assessed when they begin training in a health care profession. Those found to be negative should receive one dose of the vaccine and be tested 1 month later to document anamnestic response. If found negative again, they should complete the vaccination schedule.

Testing of the source should be conducted according to the Health Canada/Public Health Agency of Canada guidelines *An integrated protocol to manage health care workers exposed to bloodborne pathogens* available at: http://www.phac-aspc.gc.ca/publicat/ccdr-rmtc/97vol23/23s2/index.html, with informed consent and respect for confidentiality. If the assessment results of the injured person and the source are not available within 48 hours, management of the injured person should assume possible exposure.

◆ **Sexual and household contacts of hepatitis B:**

All non-immune and non-infected sexual and household contacts of acute cases and chronic carriers should be immunized with hepatitis B vaccine. HBIg is not indicated for household contacts of an acute HBV case. An exception is made for infants < 12 months of age when the mother is acutely or chronically infected. For sexual contacts, a single dose of HBIg (0.06 mL/kg) should also be given within 14 days of the last sexual contact with the HBV-infected person. Unimmunized sexual assault victims should be managed in the same manner, i.e., with both vaccine and HBIg, if the assailant is infected with HBV or cannot be assessed. All sexual partners of people with HBV infection should be counselled that protection from infection cannot be ensured until the course of vaccine has been completed and protective levels of anti-HBs demonstrated. Counselling on the use of condoms and their ability to reduce but not eliminate the risk of transmission should be provided. People with identifiable exposure to the infected person's blood (sharing toothbrushes or razors) should be managed as described in the preceding section on mucosal exposure.

Schedule and dosage

Hepatitis B vaccines have a large number of different schedules and dosages, some of which have been officially approved, others have not. These schedules have been developed for a number of reasons: to accommodate immunization program constraints, to diminish either vaccine or administration costs, to provide protection to individuals with special needs in terms of accessibility of vaccine services, to accommodate the difference in immune response in specific groups, etc. It should be emphasized that the key element to evaluate a given schedule is the seroprotection rate

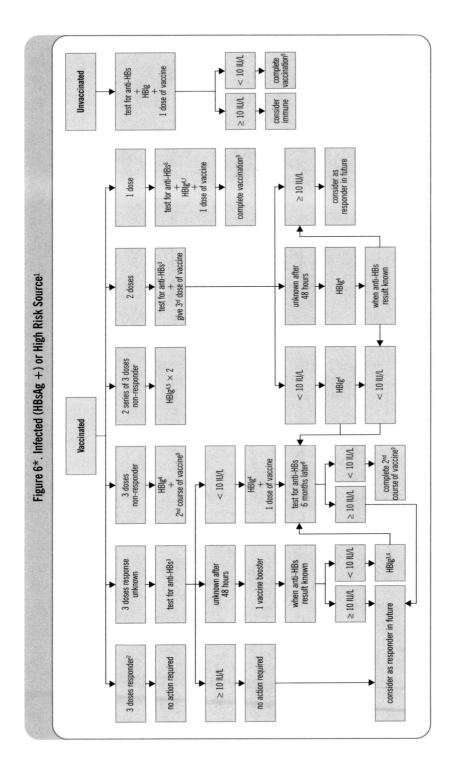

Figure 6*. Infected (HBsAg +) or High Risk Source¹

Part 4 — Active Immunizing Agents – Hepatitis B Vaccine

Figure 6*. Infected (HBsAg +) or High Risk Source[1]

1. A known source is high risk if the person comes from a highly endemic region for HBV, has sexual relations with multiple partners, has a partner infected with HBV or at high risk of being so, is in close family contact with an infected person, uses injection drugs, or received blood or blood products prior to 1970. Wherever possible, the source should be tested. In the case of an unknown source, background circumstances may provide some indication of the degree of risk, e.g., syringe found in the street, attendance at an STI clinic, detoxification or well baby clinic.

2. Responder known to have 10 IU/L anti-HBs. No measures are required if the person has developed an immunity following an infection.

3. Anti-HBs titre should be determined as soon as possible to avoid needless administration of HBIg and because efficacy is unknown if given after 7 days.

4. The administration of HBIg can be omitted if the high risk source can be tested within 48 hours and the result is negative. In that case, the non-infected source algorithm is followed.

5. The second dose of HBIg should be given 1 month after the first.

6. This test does not change the continuation of vaccination, but may reassure the exposed individual about the immediate risk of becoming infected.

7. If it is possible to quickly obtain anti-HBs titre confirming 10 IU/L, administration of HBIg should be omitted.

8. Determination of anti-HBs titre should be delayed for 6 months to allow HBIg antibodies to wane.

9. Test for anti-HBs 1 to 6 months after the course of vaccine.

* This figure has been adapted from *Protocole d'immunisation du Québec*, 3ᵉ édition, 1999, and published with the kind permission of the Ministère de la santé et des services sociaux.

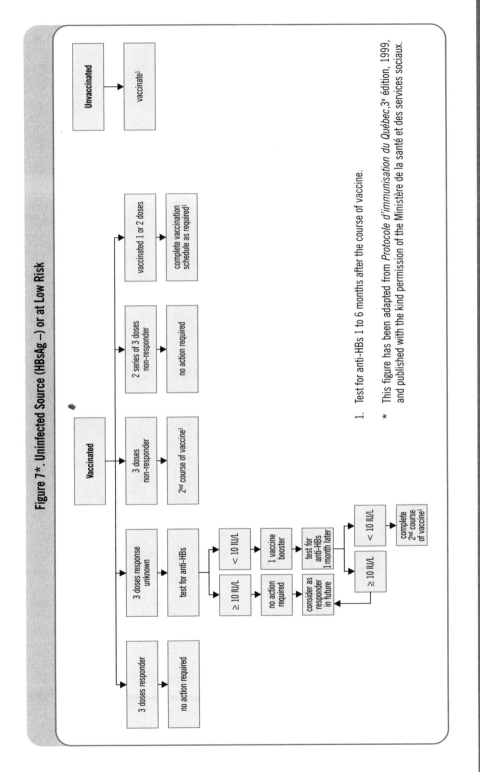

Figure 7*. Uninfected Source (HBsAg –) or at Low Risk

1. Test for anti-HBs 1 to 6 months after the course of vaccine.

* This figure has been adapted from *Protocole d'immunisation du Québec*, 3ᵉ édition, 1999, and published with the kind permission of the Ministère de la santé et des services sociaux.

achieved. High titres of anti-HBs bring longer persistence of antibodies. High titres of anti-HBs are also thought to be predictive of a longer duration of protection, although this has not been completely demonstrated yet (see section on *Efficacy and Immunogenicity*). A longer interval between doses will usually not change the seroprotection rates achieved but will increase the titres.

NACI's preferred schedule is 0, 1 and 6 months, with at least 1 month between the first and second dose, 2 months between the second and third dose and 4 months between the first and the third dose, particularly for children under 12 months of age. A schedule of 0 and 6 months with the pediatric dosage of Recombivax HB® has been tested with good results (94.5% seroprotection rate) in Canadian schoolchildren. Vaccines produced by different manufacturers can be used interchangeably even though

Table 4. Doses and Schedules for Monovalent Hepatitis B Vaccines

Recipients	Recombivax HB®			Engerix®-B		
	μg	mL	Schedule (months)	μg	mL	Schedule (months)
Infants of HBV-negative mothers or children < 11*	2.5	0.25	0, 1, 6**	10	0.5	0, 1, 6 or 0, 1, 2, 12
Infants of HBV-positive mothers*	5.0	0.5	0, 1, 6**	10	0.5	0, 1, 6 or 0, 1, 2, 12
11 to 15 years	10.0	1.0	0, 4-6	20	0.5	0, 6
11 to 19 years	5.0	0.5	0, 1, 6**	10†	0.5	0, 1, 6 or 0, 1, 2, 12
Over 19 years	10.0	1.0	0, 1, 6**	20	1.0	0, 1, 6, or 0, 1, 2, 12 or 0, 7, 21 and 365 days
Over 19 years in hemodialysis	40.0	1.0‡ or 4.0‡	0, 1, 6	40	2.0	0, 1, 2, 6

Individuals under 19 years of age who may be hyporesponsive: double the microgram dose for the age and use the three or four dose schedule only.

* The thimerosal preservative-free preparation is recommended. For the post-exposure schedule for children of HBV-infected mothers, please refer to Figure 6 and the text section on post-exposure prophylaxis.

** Although a schedule of 0, 1 and > 2 months is approved, the preferred schedule is 0, 1 and 6. Refer to text.

† The manufacturer recommends the standard adult dosage (20 μg, 1.0 mL) if it is unlikely that there will be compliance with this schedule.

‡ 1.0 mL of the dialysis formulation, 4.0 mL of the standard formulation.

their antigen content is not the same, provided that the dosage used is the one recommended by the manufacturer for the appropriate age group and schedule.

Route of administration

All hepatitis B vaccines should be injected into the deltoid muscle of children and adults, and into the anterolateral thigh muscle of infants. Gluteal administration should not be used because of poor immune response, possibly the result of inadvertent deposition into fatty tissue. Immune responses following intradermal injection have been variable, and this route of vaccine administration should not be used.

Booster doses and re-immunization

Routine boosters in immunocompetent persons are not needed. Persons who have had a previously demonstrated protective antibody level will not contract the disease when exposed to HBV, whether or not the antibody has waned. Absence of detectable anti-HBs in a person who has been previously demonstrated to have anti-HBs does not mean lack of protection, because immune memory persists. Studies of long-term protective efficacy, however, will determine whether booster doses of vaccine are ever needed.

Additional doses of vaccine (up to three doses) will produce a protective antibody response in 50% to 70% of otherwise healthy adults who fail to respond after the first series of vaccines. For most school-age children in this same situation, one additional dose will produce a protective titre. Administration of additional doses with testing for response after each dose should be undertaken when the response to vaccine needs to be ensured. Individuals who fail to respond to three additional doses of vaccine are unlikely to benefit from further immunization.

Immunocompromised people often respond suboptimally to the vaccine and may need additional antigen to respond. Should protection be achieved and then wane, however, subsequent HBV exposure in these individuals can result in acute disease or carrier state. Therefore, in this population boosters may be necessary for those who have responded initially. The optimal timing of booster doses for immunocompromised individuals (dialysis patients in particular) who are at continued risk of HBV exposure and have responded initially is not known. Periodic monitoring for the presence of anti-HBs should be considered, taking into account the severity of the compromised state and whether the risk of HBV is still present. Should antibody testing show subsequent suboptimal protection, a booster dose and re-testing should be undertaken as necessary.

Part 4 — Active Immunizing Agents – Hepatitis B Vaccine

Serologic testing

Pre-immunization

♦ **Pregnancy:**

All pregnant women should be routinely tested for HBsAg at the first prenatal visit. If testing has not been done during pregnancy, it should be done at the time of delivery. A pregnant woman who has no markers of acute or chronic HBV infection but who is at high risk of acquiring HBV should be offered the vaccine at the first opportunity during the pregnancy and tested for antibody response. Repeat testing before delivery may be considered in uninfected and unimmunized women with continuing high-risk behaviour. Infants born to HBsAg-positive mothers should receive post-exposure prophylaxis immediately after delivery.

♦ **Adopted children at high risk:**

Children adopted from countries, geographic regions or family situations in which there is a high prevalence of HBV infection should be screened for HBsAg, and if they are positive the household contacts of the adopting family should be immunized before adoption if possible, or as soon as possible thereafter.

♦ **Others at high risk of HBV infection:**

Routine pre-immunization serologic testing for hepatitis B, including HBsAg, anti-HBs or anti-HBc, is recommended for people at high risk of infection. This testing will identify those already infected or immune, for whom vaccine will provide no benefit. Testing will also assist in the medical management and contact follow-up of those individuals found to be infected and will prevent the mistaken belief that they pose no risk to others.

Post-immunization

Post-immunization testing for universal programs is not necessary. It is recommended, however, if it is important to ensure that there is protection against a continual known or repeated potential exposure to hepatitis B. People included in these circumstances are infants born to infected mothers, sexual partners and household contacts of chronic carriers, and those who have been immunized because of occupational exposure. If anti-HBs is < 10 mIU/mL, re-immunization should be conducted as described earlier (see *Boosters and Re-immunization*).

In particular, post-immunization testing for anti-HBs should be conducted among all health care workers and students in health care disciplines to establish antibody response and the need for re-immunization should the first course of vaccine fail to provide protection. Ideally, testing should be undertaken at least 1 month (but no later than 6 months) after the last dose of vaccine. If a health care worker has completed immunization against

HBV more than 6 months previously, testing for anti-HBs should still be done as part of the routine occupational health assessment or when a potential exposure occurs (see Figure 6). This type of routine assessment will be even more important as new professionals, immunized as adolescents, begin their training.

The results of post-immunization testing should be recorded in the individual's medical file and provided to the tested person. If protective antibody is documented, testing need not be repeated nor should further immunization be undertaken, even when a definite exposure occurs. If testing is done beyond the recommended 6-month window, a negative test may indicate primary vaccine failure or waning antibody as indicated previously. Re-immunization should be conducted as described in the section above.

Determination of antibody response *after re-immunization is complete* will identify those who do not respond to two courses of vaccine and who will need passive immunization after potential exposure to hepatitis B. In addition, those who are immunocompromised should be tested after the vaccine course is complete. If protective antibody is not present, the vaccine course should be repeated, and if protective antibody is still not present, the individual should receive counselling on alternative risk reduction measures. If an antibody response ultimately occurs in an immunocompromised person, periodic reassessment of antibody and booster doses may be indicated, as noted in the section on *Boosters and Re-immunization*.

Storage requirements

Hepatitis B vaccine should be stored at a temperature between +2° C and +8° C and should not be frozen.

Simultaneous administration with other vaccines

Hepatitis B vaccine may be administered simultaneously with other vaccines at different sites. A separate needle and syringe should be used for each vaccine.

Adverse reactions

Hepatitis B vaccines are well tolerated and safe to administer to adults and children. Reported side effects are usually mild, transient and generally limited to soreness at the injection site and temperature no greater than 37.7° C. Pain occurs no more frequently than with placebo.

As with all vaccines, anaphylaxis is very rare but can occur. A number of studies have demonstrated no link between hepatitis B vaccine and chronic fatigue syndrome, multiple sclerosis, Guillain-Barré syndrome (GBS), rheumatoid arthritis or sudden infant death syndrome.

Adverse reactions have not been observed when hepatitis B vaccines have been given to people who are immune to hepatitis B or who are hepatitis B carriers.

Contraindications and precautions

Hepatitis B vaccine is contraindicated if the person is allergic to any component of the vaccine or has had a previous anaphylactic reaction.

Hepatitis B vaccine can be used safely in pregnancy and during breast-feeding and should be administered when indicated, since acute hepatitis B in a pregnant woman may result in severe disease for the mother and chronic infection of the infant.

Selected references

Ascherio A, Zhang SM, Hernan MA et al. *Hepatitis B vaccination and the risk of multiple sclerosis.* New England Journal of Medicine 2001;344(5):327-32.

Banatvala J, Van Damme P, Oehen S et al. *Lifelong protection against hepatitis B: the role of vaccine immunogenicity in immune memory.* Vaccine 2000;19(7-8):877-85.

Confavreux C, Suissa S, Saddier P et al. *Vaccinations and the risk of relapse of multiple sclerosis.* New England Journal of Medicine 2001;344(5):319-26.

Duval B, Boulianne N, De Serres G et al. *Should children with isolated anti-HBs or anti-HBc be immunized against hepatitis B virus?* Journal of the American Medical Association 1997;287(13):1064.

Duval B, Gîlca V, Boulianne N et al. *Comparative long-term immunogenicity of two recombinant hepatitis B vaccines and the effect of a booster dose given after 5 years in a low endemicity country.* Pediatric Infectious Disease Journal 2005;24(3):213-18.

FitzSimons D, François G, Hall A et al. *Long-term efficacy of hepatitis B vaccine, booster policy, and impact of hepatitis B virus mutant.* Vaccine 2005;23(32):4158-66.

Health Canada. *An integrated protocol to manage health care workers exposed to blood-borne pathogens.* Canada Communicable Disease Report 1997;23S2. URL: <http://www.phac-aspc.gc.ca/publicat/ccdr-rmtc/97vol23/23s2/index.html>,

Jarrosson L, Kolopp-Sarda MN, Aguilar P et al. *Most humoral non-responders to hepatitis B vaccines develop HBV-specific cellular immune responses.* Vaccine 2004;22(27-28):3789-96.

McMahon BJ, Bruden DL, Petersen KM et al. *Antibody levels and protection after hepatitis B vaccination: results of a 15-year follow-up.* Annals of Internal Medicine 2005;142(5):333-41.

Watson B, West DJ, Chilkatowsky A et al. *Persistence of immunologic memory for 13 years in recipients of a recombinant hepatitis B vaccine.* Vaccine 2001;19(23-24):3164-68.

Zhang J, Zou S, Giulivi A. *Hepatitis B in Canada.* Canada Communicable Disease Report 2001;27(S3):10-12.

Zou S, Zhang J, Tepper M et al. *Enhanced surveillance of acute hepatitis B and acute hepatitis C in four health regions in Canada 1998-1999.* Canadian Journal of Infectious Diseases 2001;12(6):357-63.

Hepatitis Vaccines Combined

There are vaccine formulations for adults and children that protect against both hepatitis A and hepatitis B. The reader should consult the chapters on the monovalent hepatitis A and B vaccines for more information on epidemiology, efficacy and immunogenicity, recommended usage, pre- and post-immunization serologic testing and adverse reactions.

Since the publication of the 2002 *Canadian Immunization Guide*, the key change is the addition of a new table on schedule and dosage.

Epidemiology

Please refer to the *Hepatitis A Vaccine* chapter, page 179, and the *Hepatitis B Vaccine* chapter, page 189, for more information.

Preparations approved for use in Canada

This chapter will deal only with vaccines that are currently marketed in Canada.

◆ Twinrix® (hepatitis A and hepatitis B vaccine), GlaxoSmithKline Inc. Bivalent vaccine for individuals 19 years and over

◆ Twinrix® Junior (hepatitis A and hepatitis B vaccine), GlaxoSmithKline Inc. Reduced dose format for individuals aged 1 to 18 years

Each Twinrix® dose contains 20 µg of purified hepatitis B surface antigen (HBsAg) protein and 720 ELISA units of inactivated hepatitis A viral antigen (HM 175 strain) in 1 mL. Twinrix® Junior contains 10 µg of purified HBsAg and 360 ELISA units of inactivated hepatitis A antigen in 0.5 mL. These vaccines are made from the same bulk vaccines as are used in the monovalent formulations.

For a list of all approved products in Canada, please refer to Table 1 in the *General Considerations* chapter, page 7.

Efficacy and immunogenicity

There is no reduction and possibly even an increase in seroprotection rates and geometric mean titres (GMT) achieved by the combined vaccine compared with the monovalent vaccines for both hepatitis A and B components.

Part 4 — Active Immunizing Agents – Hepatitis Vaccines Combined

205

Recommended usage

Combined or bivalent hepatitis vaccine is the preferred vaccine for people with indications for immunization against both hepatitis A and hepatitis B:

- travellers to certain areas of Africa, Asia and the Americas where both hepatitis A and hepatitis B are endemic;

- persons engaging in illicit drug use;

- men who have sex with men (MSM);

- hemophiliacs receiving plasma-derived replacement clotting factors;

- populations and communities in which both hepatitis A and hepatitis B are endemic;

- people who have previously received hepatitis A vaccine and hepatitis B vaccine, and who require additional doses of both;

- people with clinically significant chronic liver disease, including persons infected with hepatitis C virus.

There are also situations in which different indications may apply for the two vaccine components. Under these circumstances, bivalent vaccine is an efficient way to protect against both diseases. Examples include:

- children who are scheduled to receive hepatitis B vaccine routinely in a universal program and who also have an indication for hepatitis A vaccine;

- inmates of correctional facilities who have not already received hepatitis B vaccine and who are in a facility with uncontrolled transmission of hepatitis A.

The combined vaccine is also used in some countries for efficient universal immunization against hepatitis A and B of pre-adolescents in school-based programs. This vaccine should be used for any person who wishes to decrease his or her risk of acquiring hepatitis A and B.

Schedule and dosage

As is the case for the monovalent hepatitis A and B vaccines, a large number of different schedules and dosages, both approved and unapproved, have been tested and are being used. The reader should consult the monovalent hepatitis B vaccine chapter for a discussion of the interpretation of this vaccine's immunogenicity and effectiveness.

There are a number of approved schedules for Twinrix® formulations in Canada. For individuals 19 years and over, the regular schedule is 0, 1 and 6 months. There is also a rapid schedule of 0, 7 and 21 days, followed by a fourth dose at 1 year. The dose of Twinrix® is 1.0 mL. For individuals from

Table 5. Schedule and Dosage for Combined Hepatitis A and B Vaccine

Vaccine	Antigen	Volume	Schedule	Age
Twinrix®	720 ELISA units HAV 20 µg HBsAg	1.0 mL	0, 1, 6 months	19 years and older
Twinrix® rapid schedule	720 ELISA units HAV 20 µg HBsAg	1.0 mL	0, 7 days, 21 days, 12 months later	19 years and older
Twinrix® Junior	360 ELISA units HAV 10 µg HBsAg	0.5 mL	0, 1, 6 months	1 to 18 years
Twinrix®	720 ELISA units HAV 20 µg HBsAg	1.0 mL	0, 6-12 months	1 to 15 years

1-18 years, the regular schedule of Twinrix® Junior is 0, 1 and 6 months. The dose of Twinrix® Junior is 0.5 mL. There is an alternative schedule for children 1-15 years of age consisting of two doses of Twinrix® given at 0, and 6-12 months. A dose of Twinrix® is 1.0 mL.

Clinical trials have shown that other schedules and dosages provide good seroprotection rates and GMT. A 0, 6 month schedule with Twinrix Junior® in Canadian schoolchildren (8-10 years) has been tested with good results (100% seroprotection rate for hepatitis A, 96.5% seroprotection rate for hepatitis B with very high GMTs).

Injection drug users have a reduced immune response but need a rapid protection. Some provinces use a rapid schedule combining a double dose of Twinrix® at 0 and 12 months with the hepatitis B dosage for immuno-compromised people at days 7 and 21.

Route of administration

Combined hepatitis vaccines should be given intramuscularly.

Booster doses and re-immunization

Booster doses are not needed for individuals who have completed a course of Twinrix® or Twinrix® Junior or their equivalent in the form of monovalent hepatitis vaccines.

Serologic testing

The same pre- and post-immunization indications as those for the monovalent vaccines apply.

Part 4 — Active Immunizing Agents – Hepatitis Vaccines Combined

Storage requirements

Twinrix® and Twinrix® Junior should be stored at a temperature between +2° C and +8° C and should not be frozen.

Simultaneous administration with other vaccines

Twinrix® Junior has been administered at the age of 2 years with DTaP-IPV-Hib or MMR without interference. Although it has not been tested in clinical trials, it is assumed that it can be given at the same time as other vaccines.

Adverse reactions

Serious adverse events are rare following immunization and, in most cases, data are insufficient to determine a causal association.

There is no increase in adverse events when combined vaccine is compared with the monovalent vaccines. When the adult dose is given to children in the two-dose schedule, there is also no increase in adverse events compared with those occurring after the children's dosage.

Contraindications and precautions

The only contraindication to bivalent hepatitis vaccines is previous anaphylaxis demonstrated to any component of the bivalent vaccine.

Selected references

Duval B, Gîlca V, Boulianne N et al. *Immunogenicity of two paediatric doses of monovalent hepatitis B or combined hepatitis A and B vaccine in 8-10-year-old children.* Vaccine 2005;23(31):4082-87.

Navas E, Salleras L, Gisbert R et al. *Efficiency of the incorporation of the hepatitis A vaccine as a combined A+B vaccine to the hepatitis B vaccination programme of preadolescents in schools.* Vaccine 2005;23(17-18): 2185-89.

Product Monograph. Twinrix®: combined hepatitis A and hepatitis B vaccine. GlaxoSmithKline Inc., 2004.

Roberton D, Marshall H, Nolan TM et al. *Reactogenicity and immunogenicity profile of a two-dose combined hepatitis A and B vaccine in 1-11-year-old children.* Vaccine 2005(43);23:5099-105.

Influenza Vaccine

The National Advisory Committee on Immunization (NACI) produces a *Statement on Influenza Vaccination* each year that contains specific information and recommendations regarding the vaccine to be used in the forthcoming season. It is published in the Canada Communicable Disease Report (CCDR) and is available at www.naci.gc.ca. The reader is referred to the latest annual CCDR statement for a more in-depth discussion of selected topics and for recommendations that have been updated after publication of this edition of the *Guide*.

Since the publication of the 2002 *Canadian Immunization Guide* changes include 1) a new recommendation for the immunization of healthy children aged 6-23 months; 2) changes in preparations approved for use in Canada; 3) a new recommendation for contacts capable of transmitting influenza to those at high-risk of influenza-related complications; 4) a new recommendation for the immunization of those directly involved in the culling of poultry infected with avian influenza; 5) a new recommendation on subsequent influenza vaccination of persons known to have developed Guillain-Barré syndrome (GBS) within 8 weeks of a previous influenza vaccination; and 6) a new recommendation for the immunization of those with conditions that compromise the management of respiratory secretions and are associated with an increased risk of aspiration.

Epidemiology

Influenza is caused by influenza A and B viruses and occurs in Canada every year, generally during late fall and the winter months. Influenza A viruses are the most common cause of annual influenza epidemics. Outbreaks of influenza B are generally more localized and in any one year may be restricted to one region of the country. An association between influenza outbreaks, especially those caused by type B virus, and cases of the rare, but serious, Reye syndrome has been noted.

The annual incidence of influenza varies widely, depending on the virulence of circulating strains and the susceptibility of the population, which is affected by antigenic changes in the virus, vaccine match and vaccine coverage. People at greatest risk of serious infections, complications, hospitalization and/or death are children aged 6-23 months, those with chronic medical conditions (especially cardiopulmonary diseases) and the elderly. Although many other respiratory viruses can cause influenza-like illness during the year, influenza virus is usually the predominant cause of serious respiratory infections in a community.

Influenza A viruses are classified into subtypes based on their hemagglutinin (H) and neuraminidase (N) antigens. Recently circulating strains have possessed one of three H and one of two N antigens, and the subtypes are designated accordingly (e.g., H3N2, H1N1). Antibodies to these antigens, particularly to H antigen, can protect an individual against a virus carrying the same antigen. During inter-pandemic periods, minor H antigen changes (referred to as drifts) are common, and the greater the change the less the cross-immunity will be to the previously circulating virus. It is this antigenic variation from one influenza virus subtype to another that is responsible for continued outbreaks of influenza, necessitating annual reformulation and administration of the influenza vaccine.

Since 1997, two influenza A subtypes, H3N2 and H1N1, have been circulating in the human population. Influenza B viruses have evolved into two antigenically distinct lineages since the mid-1980s, represented by B/Yamagata/16/88-like and B/Victoria/2/87-like viruses. The B/Victoria lineage first re-appeared in 2001 after an absence of more than 10 years in North America, and since that time viruses belonging to the two influenza B lineages have caused outbreaks in different influenza seasons. The antigens of influenza B viruses are much more stable than those of influenza A viruses and, although antigenic variation does occur, it is less frequent.

Between 1996 and 2005, six of the nine seasons (1997-98, 1998-99, 1999-2000, 2001-02, 2003-04, 2004-05) were predominantly influenza A seasons (84%-99% of laboratory detections being influenza A). Two seasons (1996-97 and 2002-03) were considered mixed seasons (61% and 58% of laboratory detections being influenza A and 39% and 42% being influenza B, respectively), and one season (2000-01) was a predominantly influenza B season (68% of laboratory detections being influenza B). Influenza A is typically associated with greater morbidity and mortality than influenza B and typically affects the elderly, whereas influenza B is more often seen in young children. As well, influenza A/H3N2-like viruses tend to be associated with more severe illness than influenza A/H1N1-like or influenza A/H1N2-like viruses.

In four of the six predominantly influenza A seasons, 41%-46% of laboratory-confirmed influenza cases were in persons 65 years of age and older. In those same seasons, children less than 5 years of age accounted for less than 20% of laboratory-confirmed cases. In the mixed seasons and influenza B season, children less than 5 years of age accounted for 24%-32% of laboratory-confirmed cases, whereas persons 65 years of age and older accounted for 7% to 19% of laboratory-confirmed cases.

Pandemic influenza is usually associated with a major antigenic change (referred to as a shift) and the rapid global spread of influenza A virus with a different H and possibly a different N antigen from strains circulating previously. Canada, like other countries, was affected by the major influenza pandemics that occurred in 1889-90, 1918-19, 1957-58 and 1968-69.

Preparations approved for use in Canada

This chapter will deal only with vaccines that are currently marketed in Canada.

- Fluviral® S/F (influenza trivalent split virion), ID Biomedical Corporation

- Influvac™ (influenza vaccine, inactivated, surface antigen), Solvay Pharma Inc.

- Vaxigrip® (inactivated influenza trivalent types A and B [split virion]), Sanofi Pasteur Ltd.

All three vaccines are sterile suspensions prepared from influenza viruses propagated in chicken embryos. The viruses are inactivated and purified.

Two products (Vaxigrip® and Fluviral®) are "split virus" vaccines, which are treated with an organic solvent to remove surface glycoproteins, producing a "split-virus" resulting in reduced vaccine reactogenicity. Influvac™ is a surface antigen, trivalent, inactivated subunit vaccine.

One dose (0.5 mL) of influenza vaccine contains 15 µg of hemagglutinin of each of three antigens. The antigens are selected from one strain of influenza A/H3N2, one strain of influenza A/H1N1 and one strain of influenza B. The virus strains chosen for inclusion in influenza vaccine are reviewed annually to ensure that they include antigens that are expected to provide the best protection during the following influenza season. The antigenic match between the vaccine strains recommended by the World Health Organization and subsequent circulating epidemic strains was appropriate during 12 of the 15 (80%) influenza seasons between 1982-1983 and 1996-1997.

As of 2005, Vaxigrip® and Fluviral® contain thimerosal, which is used as a preservative. Influvac™ does not contain thimerosal. Vaxigrip® may contain undetectable traces of neomycin, used during production. At this time, influenza vaccines derived from tissue culture and live attenuated viruses are not approved for use in Canada.

For a list of all approved products in Canada, please refer to Table 1 in the *General Considerations* chapter, page 7.

Efficacy and immunogenicity

Intramuscular administration of inactivated influenza vaccine results in the production of circulating IgG antibody to the viral hemagglutinin as well as a cytotoxic T lymphocyte response. Both humoral and cell-mediated responses are thought to play a role in immunity to influenza. Anti-hemagglutinin serum antibody is a predictor of total protection (acquisition of infection) and partial protection (disease after infection). The production and persistence of antibody after vaccination depends on several factors, including the age of the recipient, prior and subsequent exposure to antigens, and the presence of immunodeficiency states. Humoral antibody levels, which correlate with vaccine protection, are generally achieved 2 weeks after immunization, and immunity usually lasts less than 1 year. However, antibody levels in the elderly may fall below protective levels in 4 months or less. Data are not available at this time to support the administration of a second dose of influenza vaccine in elderly individuals within the same influenza season in order to boost immunity.

Repeated annual administration of influenza vaccine has not been demonstrated to impair the immune response of the recipient to influenza virus.

The effectiveness of influenza vaccine varies, depending upon the age and immunocompetence of the vaccine recipient, the endpoint studied, the incidence of infection and the degree of similarity ("match") between the vaccine strains and the circulating viral strain(s) during the influenza season. With a good match, influenza vaccination has been shown to prevent influenza illness in approximately 70% to 90% of healthy children and adults, whereas a vaccine efficacy of 30% to 60% has been demonstrated when there are significant antigenic differences between circulating and vaccine viral strains.

A double-blind, placebo controlled trial involving people > 60 years of age demonstrated vaccine efficacy of 58% in the prevention of laboratory-proven influenza illness. Pooled estimates from a meta-analysis of 20 cohort studies of influenza vaccine among the elderly demonstrated 56% effectiveness in preventing respiratory illness, 50% in preventing hospitalization for pneumonia and 68% in preventing death. Among residents of long-term care facilities, effectiveness in preventing influenza illness may be relatively low (30% to 40%), but vaccination may be 50% to 60% effective in preventing hospitalization and pneumonia, and up to 85% to 95% effective in preventing death.

Recommended usage

As is the case with other vaccines, recommendations for usage may change over time as new research becomes available. Recommended recipients for the influenza vaccine at the time of this publication are outlined below, but for up-to-date information, the reader is referred to the annual *Statement on Influenza Vaccination* published in the CCDR and at www.naci.gc.ca.

Recommended recipients (see Table 6)

Influenza vaccine may be administered to any healthy child, adolescent or adult for whom contraindications are not present. To reduce the morbidity and mortality associated with influenza and the impact of illness in our communities, immunization programs should focus on those at high risk of influenza-related complications, those capable of transmitting influenza to individuals at high risk of complications, and those who provide essential community services. However, significant morbidity and societal costs are also associated with seasonal interpandemic influenza illness and its complications occurring in healthy children and adults. For this reason, healthy children and adults should be encouraged to receive the vaccine.

People at high risk of influenza-related complications

- Adults and children with selected chronic health conditions. These include cardiac or pulmonary disorders (including bronchopulmonary dysplasia, cystic fibrosis and asthma), diabetes mellitus and other metabolic diseases, cancer, immunodeficiency, immunosuppression (due to underlying disease and/or therapy), renal disease, anemia and hemoglobinopathy, as well as conditions that compromise the management of respiratory secretions and are associated with an increased risk of aspiration. This category includes children and adolescents (age 6 months to 18 years) with conditions treated for long periods with acetylsalicylic acid (because of the potential increased risk of Reye syndrome associated with influenza). Pregnant women with any of these co-morbidities are also at increased risk of the complications of influenza and should be immunized.

- People of any age who are residents of nursing homes and other chronic care facilities.

- People ≥ 65 years of age.

- Healthy children aged 6-23 months.

People capable of transmitting influenza to those at high risk of influenza-related complications

People who are potentially capable of transmitting influenza to those at high risk should receive annual immunization, regardless of whether the high-risk person(s) has been immunized. These individuals include the following:

- Health care workers (HCWs) and other care providers in facilities and community settings who, through their activities, are potentially capable of transmitting influenza to those at high risk of influenza complications. This group includes regular visitors, emergency response workers, those who have contact with residents of continuing care facilities or residences, and those who provide home care for persons in high-risk groups. NACI considers the provision of influenza vaccination for these HCWs to be an essential component of the standard of care for influenza prevention for the protection of their patients. HCWs who have direct patient contact should consider it their responsibility to provide the highest standard of care, which includes undergoing annual influenza vaccination. In the absence of contraindications, refusal of HCWs who have direct patient contact to be immunized against influenza implies failure in their duty of care to patients.

- Household contacts (adults and children) of people at high risk of influenza complications. This group includes household contacts of children < 6 months of age (who are at high risk of complications from influenza but for whom there is no available effective vaccine) and of children aged 6-23 months whether or not they have been immunized. Pregnant women should be immunized in their third trimester if they are expected to deliver during influenza season, as they will become household contacts of their newborn.

- Those providing regular child care to children under 24 months of age, whether in or out of the home.

- Those who provide services within closed or relatively closed settings to persons at high risk (e.g., crew on cruise ships).

People who provide essential community services

Vaccination for these individuals should be encouraged in order to minimize the disruption of routine activities during annual epidemics. Employers and their employees should consider yearly influenza immunization for healthy working adults as this has been shown to decrease work absenteeism from respiratory and other illnesses.

People in direct contact with avian influenza-infected poultry during culling operations

These individuals may be at increased risk of avian influenza infection because of exposure during the culling operation. The theoretical rationale is that it may prevent the infection of these individuals with human influenza strains and thus reduce the potential for human-avian reassortment of genes should they become coinfected with avian influenza. Please refer to the current *Statement on Influenza Vaccination* in the Canada Communicable Disease Report and at www.naci.gc.ca for further information.

Further comments regarding influenza immunization

Immunization of healthy persons aged 2-64 years

Individuals in this age group should be encouraged to receive the vaccine, even if they are not in one of the aforementioned priority groups. In an analysis of randomized controlled trials of inactivated influenza vaccine among healthy adults, Demicheli et al. estimated vaccine efficacy to be 24% in preventing influenza-like illness (ILI) and 68% in preventing laboratory-confirmed influenza infections. Depending on whether infection was defined by serology or culture, in trials of inactivated trivalent influenza vaccine in children aged 2-5 years vaccine efficacy was estimated to be 31%-83%. Fifteen randomized controlled trials of healthy individuals aged 6 months to 19 years conducted over a period during which the recommended vaccine was both well matched and not well matched with circulating viral strains showed a relative risk reduction associated with influenza vaccination ranging from 0% to 93%.

Table 6. Recommended Recipients of Influenza Vaccine

People at high risk of influenza-related complications	• Adults and children with selected chronic medical conditions if significant enough to require regular medical follow-up or hospital care. These high risk conditions include: 　• cardiac or pulmonary disease (including bronchopulmonary dysplasia, cystic fibrosis, and asthma) 　• diabetes mellitus and other metabolic diseases 　• cancer, immunodeficiency, immunosuppression (due to underlying disease and/or therapy) 　• renal disease 　• anemia and hemoglobinopathy 　• conditions that compromise the management of respiratory secretions and are associated with an increased risk of aspiration 　• children and adolescents with conditions treated for long periods with acetylsalicylic acid • People of any age who are residents of nursing homes and other chronic care facilities • People ≥ 65 years of age • Healthy children aged 6 to 23 months
People capable of transmitting influenza to those at high risk of influenza-related complications	• Health care and other care providers in facilities and community settings who, through their activities, are potentially capable of transmitting influenza to those at high risk of influenza complications. • Household contacts (adults and children) of people at high risk of influenza complications, whether or not they have been immunized. These persons include household contacts of children < 6 months of age (who are at high risk of complications from influenza but for whom there is no currently licensed vaccine) and of children aged 6 to 23 months. Pregnant women should be immunized in their third trimester if they are expected to deliver during influenza season, as they will become household contacts of their newborn. • Those providing regular child care to children aged 0 to 23 months, whether in or out of the home. • Those who provide services within closed or relatively closed settings to persons at high risk (e.g. crew on cruise ships).
Others	• People who provide essential community services. • People in direct contact with avian influenza-infected poultry during culling operations. • Healthy persons aged 2-64 years should be encouraged to receive the vaccine, even if they are not in one of the aforementioned priority groups.

Travellers

People with selected chronic medical conditions should be immunized (see Table 6). Healthy persons should be encouraged to receive vaccine. Vaccines prepared specifically against strains that are predicted to circulate in the southern hemisphere are not currently available in Canada. For further information on advising travellers about influenza prevention the Committee to Advise on Tropical Medicine and Travel (CATMAT) statement should be consulted: http://www.phac-aspc.gc.ca/tmp-pmv/catmat-ccmtmv/index.html.

Immunization during pregnancy and during lactation

Influenza vaccination is recommended for pregnant and breast-feeding women who are characterized by any of the conditions listed under *Recommended Recipients* above, in particular those who have co-morbidities or who are close contacts of high-risk persons. Pregnant women with any of the selected chronic conditions putting them at high risk of the complications associated with influenza are a priority for immunization. Influenza vaccine is safe for pregnant women at all stages of pregnancy and for breast-feeding mothers.

Immunization of pregnant women has the advantage of potentially protecting the fetus through transplacental antibody passage or through breast milk. Among healthy pregnant women, the morbidity and mortality associated with influenza is increased during pandemics.

Healthy women who will be pregnant during influenza season and who wish to avoid morbidity associated with influenza should be encouraged to be vaccinated during any trimester of pregnancy. Pregnant women should be immunized in their third trimester if they are expected to deliver during influenza season, as they will become household contacts of their newborn.

Schedule and dosage

The recommended dosage schedule and type of influenza vaccine are presented in Table 7. Influenza vaccines in Canada are available as a split-virus (chemically disrupted) and an inactivated subunit preparation. Each 0.5 mL of vaccine contains 15 µg of hemagglutinin of each vaccine strain.

Previously unvaccinated children < 9 years of age require two doses of the split-virus influenza vaccine, with an interval of 4 weeks. The second dose of influenza vaccine is not needed if the child has received one or more doses of vaccine during a previous influenza season.

The subunit vaccine is currently approved for use only in those 18 years of age and older.

There are no data suggesting that administration of a second dose of influenza vaccine in the same influenza season in elderly individuals or

Table 7. Recommended Influenza Vaccine Dosage, by Age

Age	Vaccine type	Dose (mL)	No. of doses
6-35 months	Split-virus	0.25	1 or 2*
3-8 years	Split-virus	0.5	1 or 2*
≥ 9 years	Split-virus	0.5	1
≥ 18 years	Subunit**	0.5	1

* Previously unvaccinated children < 9 years require two doses of the split-virus influenza vaccine, with an interval of 4 weeks.

** Influvac™ is approved for use only in persons 18 years of age and older.

other individuals who may have an altered immune response will boost immunity.

Immunization with currently available influenza vaccines is not recommended for infants < 6 months of age.

Route of administration

The vaccine should be administered intramuscularly. The deltoid muscle is the recommended site in adults and children ≥ 12 months of age. The anterolateral thigh is the recommended site in infants under 12 months of age.

Serologic testing

There is no indication for pre- or post-immunization serology.

Storage requirements

Influenza vaccine should be stored at a temperature between +2° C and +8° C and should not be frozen.

Simultaneous administration of other vaccines

Influenza vaccine may be given at the same time as other vaccines. The same limb may be used if necessary, but different sites on the limb should be chosen. A separate needle and syringe must be used.

The target groups for influenza and pneumococcal immunization overlap considerably. Health care providers should take the opportunity to immunize eligible people against pneumococcal disease when influenza vaccine is given. Pneumococcal vaccine, in contrast to influenza vaccine, is not given annually.

Adverse reactions

Influenza immunization cannot cause influenza because the vaccine does not contain live virus. Soreness at the injection site lasting up to 2 days occurs in 10%-72% of patients but rarely interferes with normal activities. Fever, malaise and myalgia may occur within 6 to 12 hours after vaccination and last 1 to 2 days, especially in those receiving vaccine for the first time. Prophylactic acetaminophen may decrease the frequency of some side effects in adults. Healthy adults receiving the split-virus vaccine have shown no increase in the frequency of fever or other systemic symptoms compared with those receiving placebo.

Split-virus influenza vaccines are safe and well tolerated in healthy children. Mild local reactions, primarily soreness at the vaccination site, occur in ≤ 7% of healthy children who are < 3 years of age. Post-vaccination fever may be observed in ≤ 12% of immunized children aged 1 to 5 years.

Allergic responses are rare and are probably a consequence of hypersensitivity to some vaccine component, such as residual egg protein, which is present in minute quantities.

GBS occurred in adults in association with the 1976 swine influenza vaccine, and evidence favours a causal relation between the vaccine and GBS during that season. In an extensive review of studies since 1976, the Institute of Medicine in the United States concluded that the evidence is inadequate to accept or reject a causal relation between GBS in adults and influenza vaccines administered since 1976.

Influenza vaccine is not known to predispose vaccine recipients to Reye syndrome.

During the 2000-2001 influenza season, the Public Health Agency of Canada received an increased number of reports of vaccine-associated symptoms and signs that were subsequently described as oculorespiratory syndrome (ORS). The case definition is as follows: the onset of bilateral red eyes and/or respiratory symptoms (cough, wheeze, chest tightness, difficulty breathing, difficulty swallowing, hoarseness or sore throat) and/or facial swelling occurring within 24 hours of influenza immunization. The pathophysiologic mechanism underlying ORS remains unknown, but it is considered distinct from IgE-mediated allergy.

Since the 2000-2001 influenza season fewer ORS cases have been reported. In the province of Quebec the rate of ORS per 100,000 doses distributed declined from 46.6 in 2000, to 34.2 in 2001, 20.6 in 2002 and down to 9 per 100,000 in 2003. Surveillance for all adverse events following immunization, including ORS, is ongoing.

Contraindications and precautions

Influenza vaccine should not be given to people who had an anaphylactic reaction to a previous dose.

Persons with known IgE-mediated hypersensitivity to eggs, manifested as hives, swelling of the mouth and throat, difficulty breathing, hypotension or shock, should not be routinely vaccinated with influenza vaccine. If egg-allergic individuals are at risk of the complications of influenza they should be evaluated by an allergy specialist, as vaccination might be possible after careful evaluation, skin testing and graded challenge or desensitization. If such an evaluation is not possible, the risk of an allergic reaction to the vaccine must be weighed against the risk of influenza disease.

It is not known whether influenza vaccination is causally associated with increased risk of recurrent GBS in persons with a previous history of GBS. Avoiding subsequent influenza vaccination of persons known to have developed GBS within 8 weeks of a previous influenza vaccination appears prudent at this time.

Individuals with serious, acute febrile illness should not be immunized until their symptoms have abated. Those with mild, non-serious febrile illness (such as mild upper respiratory tract infections) may be given influenza vaccine. Opportunities for immunization should not be lost because of inappropriate deferral of immunization.

Other considerations

Strategies for reducing the impact of influenza

Immunization is recognized as the single most effective way of preventing or attenuating influenza for those at high risk of serious illness or death from influenza infection and related complications. Influenza vaccination programs should aim to vaccinate at least 90% of eligible recipients. Nevertheless, only 70% to 91% of residents of long-term care facilities and 20% to 40% of adults and children with medical conditions that put them at high risk of influenza complications receive the vaccine annually. Studies of HCWs in hospitals and long-term care facilities have shown immunization rates of 26% to 61%. This low rate of utilization is due both to failure of the health care system to offer the vaccine and to immunization refusal by people who fear adverse reactions or mistakenly believe that the vaccine is either ineffective or unnecessary.

The reader is referred to the most up-to-date annual NACI *Statement on Influenza Vaccination* for a discussion of strategies to increase vaccination coverage of target groups, as well as guidelines regarding prophylactic use of antivirals.

Selected references

Committee to Advise on Tropical Medicine and Travel (CATMAT). *Statement on travel, influenza, and prevention.* Canada Communicable Disease Report 2005;31(ACS-2):1-8.

Demicheli V, Rivetti D, Deeks JJ et al. *Vaccines for preventing influenza in healthy adults* (Cochrane Review). In: *The Cochrane Library.* Chichester: John Wiley and Sons Ltd., 2003:4.

Fukuda K, Levandowski RA, Bridges CB et al. *Inactivated influenza vaccines.* In: Plotkin SA, Orenstein WA, Offit PA (eds), *Vaccines,* 4th edition. Saunders: Philadelphia, 2003:339-70

Glezen WP, Alpers M. *Maternal immunization.* Clinical Infectious Diseases 1999;28(2):219-24.

Institute of Medicine. *Immunization safety review: influenza vaccines and neurological complications.* URL: <http://www.iom.edu/?id=15639>.

Jefferson T, Smith S, Demicheli V et al. *Assessment of the efficacy and effectiveness of influenza vaccines in healthy children: systematic review.* Lancet 2005;365(9461):773-80.

Langley JM, Faughnan ME. *Prevention of influenza in the general population.* Canadian Medical Association Journal 2004;171(10):1213-22.

National Advisory Committee on Immunization. *Supplementary statement for the 2002-2003 influenza season: update on oculorespiratory syndrome in association with influenza vaccination.* Canada Communicable Disease Report 2002;28(ACS-6):1-8.

Orr P. *Influenza vaccination for health care workers: a duty of care.* Canadian Journal of Infectious Diseases 2000;11(5):225-26.

Japanese Encephalitis Vaccine

Introduction

Japanese encephalitis (JE) virus is the leading cause of viral encephalitis in Asia, where more than 50,000 cases occur each year. Clinically apparent infection with JE virus is seen only rarely in travellers. Countries where the disease occurs are listed in Table 8. The incidence of JE varies widely from year to year and between regions within countries. JE virus is an arthropod-borne flavivirus, a group that also includes yellow fever virus, West Nile virus and St. Louis encephalitis virus. The principal vectors are *Culex* mosquitoes that breed mainly in rice fields. Swine and certain species of wild birds are intermediate hosts in the transmission cycle. Conditions that support transmission of JE virus are primarily rural agricultural ones, but occasionally cases are reported from urban areas. *Culex* mosquitoes tend to bite in the evening and night, but day-biting species predominate in some regions.

There are no key changes in the recommendations for JE immunization since the publication of the 2002 *Canadian Immunization Guide*.

Epidemiology

The disease occurs in epidemic form in temperate and northern tropical regions and is endemic in southern tropical regions of Asia. Cases occur chiefly during the summer and autumn in temperate zones and during the rainy season in tropical zones. In areas where irrigation is the main factor affecting the abundance of vector mosquitoes, transmission may occur year round. For these reasons, the periods of greatest risk for JE virus transmission to travellers are highly variable and depend on such factors as season, location, duration of stay and the type of activities undertaken. Crude estimates for North Americans travelling to Asia place the overall risk of JE illness at less than 1 per million. However, for travellers to rural areas during the transmission season, the risk per month of exposure can be as high as 1 per 5,000. Rare case reports suggest that even short-term, resort-based travellers can occasionally contract JE.

The risk of JE transmission to the traveller may be significantly reduced by the appropriate use of bednets, repellents and protective clothing.

Most JE infections do not result in obvious illness. Between 50 and 300 infections occur for each clinical case identified. However, when encephalitis does occur, it is usually severe, with 10% to 25% mortality rates and residual neuropsychiatric problems in 50% of survivors.

The disease usually affects children, but in countries where it has been recently introduced all age groups may be affected. In addition to children < 10 years of age, advanced age may be a risk factor for developing symptomatic illness.

Japanese encephalitis acquired during pregnancy carries the risk of intrauterine infection and miscarriage.

Preparations approved for use in Canada

This chapter will deal only with vaccines that are currently marketed in Canada

◆ JE-VAX® (Japanese encephalitis vaccine), Sanofi Pasteur Ltd. (distributor)

This vaccine is a highly purified, formalin-inactivated vaccine derived from mouse brain. The vaccine is based upon the Nakayama-INH strain; it is produced by the Research Institute of Osaka University (Biken) and distributed by Sanofi Pasteur Ltd. (Canada). The vaccine contains thimerosal as a preservative and other minor components.

Table 8. Areas where Japanese Encephalitis Has Been Recognized and Season of Epidemic Risk

Zone	Country
Temperate regions (Risk greatest July to October)	Bangladesh China Northern India Japan Kampuchea Korea Laos Myanmar Nepal Far Eastern Russia Northern Thailand Northern Vietnam
Tropical regions (Risk greatest during the rainy season. Note that the rainy season varies somewhat from region to region but is typically May to November)	Southern India Pakistan Indonesia Malaysia Philippines Sri Lanka Taiwan Southern Thailand Southern Vietnam

For a list of all approved products in Canada, please refer to Table 1 in the *General Considerations* chapter, page 7.

Efficacy and immunogenicity

The vaccine has been widely used in Asian countries such as Japan, where JE vaccine has been approved since 1954. In a study of children in Northern Thailand, JE vaccine was demonstrated to have an efficacy of 91% (95% confidence interval 70%-97%) after two doses of vaccine. Another field trial demonstrated that less than 80% of vaccinees developed neutralizing antibody after two doses of vaccine, as compared with 99% after three doses. Some studies have demonstrated higher geometric mean titres in Asian compared to non-Asian subjects after vaccination; this may reflect prior exposure to JE or other flaviviruses circulating in Asia. In summary, immunogenicity studies indicate that three doses of JE vaccine are needed to provide adequate protective levels of antibodies in non-immune vaccinees. As vaccine efficacy is never 100%, all travellers should be advised to take personal protective measures against mosquito bites.

Recommended usage

The vaccine is indicated for active immunization against JE for people ≥ 1 year of age who will spend 1 month or more in rural areas in endemic or epidemic areas during the transmission season or in urban areas if the urban area is part of the endemic or epidemic area, especially if travel will include rural areas. However, there have been several reports of JE in short-term travellers to endemic regions. Immunization should therefore be considered for some people spending < 30 days in endemic areas, e.g., travellers to areas where there is epidemic activity, travellers making repeated short trips, or those with extensive outdoor rural exposure.

Immunization is recommended for all laboratory personnel working with JE virus.

Schedule and dosage

A series of three 1.0 mL doses is given on days 0, 7 and 30. When time does not permit, these may be administered on days 0, 7 and 14, but the antibody response to this accelerated schedule is lower and may not be as durable. Two doses of vaccine 7 to 14 days apart can provide reasonable protection (80% efficacy) for short periods of time (< 1 year).

Route of administration

The vaccine should be administered subcutaneously.

Booster doses and re-immunization

No definitive recommendation can be made regarding the timing of booster doses in travellers. In a study of a small number of adults, protective titres of neutralizing antibodies persisted for 3 years after primary immunization. No pediatric data are currently available. Booster doses of 1.0 mL (0.5 mL for children < 3 years) are generally recommended at intervals of 3 years.

Serologic testing

There is no indication for pre- or post-immunization serology.

Storage requirements

The lyophilized preparation should be stored at +2° C to +8° C. After reconstitution, the vaccine should be stored at a temperature between +2° C and +8° C and used within 8 hours.

Simultaneous administration with other vaccines

There are only limited data on the safety and immunogenicity of JE vaccine when given concurrently with other vaccines, drugs, or biologics. As a general rule, given that JE is an inactivated vaccine, it can be given simultaneously with any other vaccine.

Adverse reactions

Serious adverse events are rare following immunization and, in most cases, data are insufficient to determine a causal association.

JE vaccine has been associated with injection site tenderness, redness and swelling. Other local effects have been reported in an average of 20% of vaccinees (range < 1% to 31%). Systemic side effects, principally fever, headache, malaise, rash and other reactions such as chills, dizziness, myalgia, nausea, vomiting and abdominal pain, are reported in 5% to 10% of vaccinees.

In an immunization program for US military personnel in Okinawa, an overall reaction rate of 62.4 per 10,000 vaccinees occurred, including reports of urticaria, angioedema, generalized itching and wheezing. These reactions were generally mild to moderate in severity. Nine out of 35,253 people who had been immunized were hospitalized, primarily to allow administration of intravenous steroids for refractory urticaria. None of these reactions was considered life-threatening. A more recent study of 14,249 U.S. military personnel (36-850 doses of vaccine) demonstrated overall reaction rates of 16/10,000 for the first two doses and only 2/10,000 for the third dose.

A Danish case control study in travellers suggests an overall risk of about 1/10,000 doses for allergic-type responses.

In the late 1980s and early 1990s, an apparent increase in the incidence of delayed systemic hypersensitivity reactions was reported in several developed countries. The reactions were characterized by urticaria, often in a generalized distribution, and/or angioedema of the extremities, face and oropharynx, especially of the lips. Distress or collapse due to hypotension or other causes led to hospitalization in several cases. Most of the reactions reported have been treated successfully with antihistamines and steroids given either orally or parenterally. Some individuals have complained of generalized itching without evidence of a rash. No deaths related to delayed hypersensitivity reactions to JE vaccine have been reported. An important feature of these reactions is the interval between immunization and onset of symptoms.

Delayed hypersensitivity reaction after a first dose of vaccine occurs a median of 12 hours after immunization; 88% of reactions occur within 3 days. The interval between a second dose and onset of symptoms is generally longer (median 3 days) and as long as 2 weeks. Reactions can occur after a second or third dose when preceding doses were received uneventfully.

Overall, the delay between vaccination and the onset of the delayed hypersensitivity reaction is less than 6 days in 80%-90% of cases. However, in a small minority of cases, a delay of 10-14 days has been reported.

Data on U.S. military personnel and Danish travellers suggest that the risk of developing a systemic allergic reaction is greater in younger subjects, women and those with a history of allergy (e.g., urticaria, allergic rhinitis, asthma), particularly to other immunizing agents. Post-marketing surveillance suggests that such late reactions continue to occur at a rate of approximately 6.3/100,000 doses in the United States. The vaccine constituents responsible for the late hypersensitivity syndrome have not been identified, although reactions to gelatin have been implicated in some cases.

Severe neurologic adverse effects such as encephalitis or encephalopathy have been reported after JE immunization but are very rare (approximately 0.2/100,000 doses in Japanese vaccine recipients and possibly fewer in North American vaccinees).

Contraindications and precautions

Allergic reactions (generalized urticaria or angioedema) to a previous dose of vaccine are contraindications to further doses. Possible allergic reactions exhibited as generalized urticaria and angioedema may occur after minutes or be delayed as long as 14 days after immunization. Most allergic reactions occur within 10 days, the majority occurring within 48 hours. Vaccinees should be observed for 30 minutes after immunization and warned against the possibility of delayed urticaria and angioedema of the face and airway. Ideally, vaccinees should not embark on international travel within 10 days of immunization because of the possibility of delayed allergic reactions. If travel must occur in less than 10 days from the time of vaccination, the benefits of vaccination must be weighed against the risk of a delayed allergic reaction.

JE vaccine is produced in mouse brains and therefore in individuals with known hypersensitivity to proteins of rodent or neural origin, a referral to an allergist is recommended to assess whether JE vaccine can safely be administered. JE vaccine should not be given to people with known hypersensitivity to any component of the vaccine.

A history of urticaria or angioedema particularly after other immunizing agents should be considered when weighing the risks and benefits of the vaccine for an individual patient.

Pregnancy and breastfeeding

There are no data that show whether JE vaccine can cause fetal harm when administered to a pregnant woman. Pregnant women who must travel to areas where the risk of JE infection is high should be immunized when the theoretic risks of immunization are outweighed by the risk of infection to the mother and developing fetus.

Although there are no data, breast-feeding is not considered a contraindication to JE vaccine.

Use in immunocompromised persons

People undergoing immunosuppressive therapy are likely to have a poor immune response to vaccines in general and killed vaccines in particular. JE immunization should be deferred, if possible, while patients are receiving such therapy. If travel must be undertaken, such patients may be immunized as already outlined, with the understanding that the antibody response may be suboptimal.

Selected references

Andersen MM, Ronne T. *Side-effects with Japanese encephalitis vaccine.* Lancet 1991;337(8748):1044.

Berg SW, Mitchell BS, Hanson RK et al. *Systemic reactions in US Marine Corps personnel who received Japanese encephalitis vaccine.* Clinical Infectious Diseases 1997;24(2):265-66.

Centers for Disease Control and Prevention. *Inactivated Japanese encephalitis virus vaccine: recommendations of the Immunization Practices Advisory Committee (ACIP).* Morbidity and Mortality Weekly Report 1993;42(RR- l):1-15.

Chambers TJ, Tsai TF, Pervikov Y et al. *Vaccine development against dengue and Japanese encephalitis: report of a World Health Organization meeting.* Vaccine 1997;15(14):1494-1502.

Defraites RF, Gambel JM, Hoke CH et al. *Japanese encephalitis vaccine (inactivated, Biken) in US soldiers: immunogenicity and safety of vaccine administered in two dosing regimens.* American Journal of Tropical Medicine and Hygiene 1999;61(2):288-93.

Gambel JM, DeFraites R, Hoke C Jr et al. *Japanese encephalitis vaccine: persistence of antibody up to 3 years after a three-dose series.* Journal of Infectious Diseases 1995;171(4):1074.

Hoke CH, Nisalak A, Sangawhipa N et al. *Protection against Japanese encephalitis by inactivated vaccines.* New England Journal of Medicine 1988;319(10):608-14.

Jelinek T, Nothdurft HD. *Japanese encephalitis vaccine in travellers. Is wider use prudent?* Drug Safety 1997;16(3):153-6.

Kurane I, Takasaki T. *Immunogenicity and protective efficacy of the current inactivated Japanese encephalitis vaccine against different Japanese encephalitis virus strains.* Vaccine 2000;18(S2):33-5.

Liu Z-L, Hennessy S, Strom BL et al. *Short-term safety of live attenuated Japanese encephalitis vaccine: results of a randomized trial with 26,239 subjects.* Journal of Infectious Diseases 1997;176(5):1366-69.

Plesner AM, Arlien-Soborg P, Herning M. *Neurological complications to vaccination against Japanese encephalitis.* European Journal of Neurology 1998;5(5):479-85.

Plesner A, Ronne T, Wachmann H. *Case-control study of allergic reactions to Japanese encephalitis vaccine.* Vaccine 2000;18(17):1830-36.

Poland JD, Cropp CB, Craven RB et al. *Evaluation of the potency and safety of inactivated Japanese encephalitis vaccine in U.S. inhabitants.* Journal of Infectious Diseases 1990;161(5):878-82.

Robinson HC, Russell ML, Csokonay WM. *Japanese encephalitis vaccine and adverse effects among travellers.* Canadian Disease Weekly Report 1991;17(32):173-77.

Ruff TA, Eisen D, Fuller A et al. *Adverse reactions to Japanese encephalitis vaccine.* Lancet 1991;338(8771):881-82.

Sakaguchi M, Yoshida M, Kuroda W et al. *Systemic immediate-type reactions to gelatin included in Japanese encephalitis vaccines.* Vaccine 1997;15(2):121-22.

Takahashi H, Pool V, Tsai TF et al. *Adverse events after Japanese encephalitis vaccination: review of post-marketing surveillance data from Japan and the United States.* Vaccine 2000;18(26):2963-69.

Tsai TF. *New initiatives for the control of Japanese encephalitis by vaccination: minutes of a WHO/CVI meeting, Bangkok, Thailand, 13-15 October 1998.* Vaccine 2000;18(S2):1-25.

Tsarev SA, Sanders ML, Vaughn DW et al. *Phylogenetic analysis suggests only one serotype of Japanese encephalitis virus.* Vaccine 2000;18(S2):36-43.

Measles Vaccine

Measles (rubeola) is a leading cause of vaccine-preventable deaths in children worldwide. There has been a marked reduction in incidence in countries where vaccine has been widely used, but measles remains a serious and common disease in many parts of the world. Complications such as otitis media and bronchopneumonia occur in about 10% of reported cases, even more commonly in those who are poorly nourished and chronically ill, and in infants < 1 year of age. Measles encephalitis occurs in approximately 1 of every 1,000 reported cases and may result in permanent brain damage. Measles infection causes subacute sclerosing panencephalitis (SSPE), a rare but fatal disease. In developed countries, including Canada, death is estimated to occur once in 3,000 cases. Measles during pregnancy results in a higher risk of premature labour, spontaneous abortion and low birth weight infants. Canada has made great progress in its goal of measles elimination, and endemic transmission of measles has been interrupted.

Since the publication of the 2002 *Canadian Immunization Guide* there have been some changes in the preparations approved for use in Canada.

Epidemiology

Before the introduction of the vaccine, measles occurred in cycles with an increasing incidence every 2 to 3 years. At that time, an estimated 300,000 to 400,000 cases occurred annually. Since the introduction of vaccine, the incidence has declined markedly in Canada (see Figure 8). Between 1989 and 1995, in spite of very high vaccine coverage, there were many large outbreaks involving mainly children who had received one dose of measles vaccine. It was estimated that 10% to 15% of immunized children remained unprotected after a single dose given at 12 months of age, a proportion large enough to allow circulation of the virus. These primary vaccine failures were mainly caused by the interference of persisting maternal antibody. The currently recommended second dose aims to achieve immunity in children who did not respond to their first dose.

In 1996/97, every province and territory added a second dose to its routine schedule, and most conducted catch-up programs in school-aged children with measles or measles/rubella vaccine. These interventions achieved vaccine coverage for the second dose in excess of 85%, reducing the proportion of vulnerable children to such a negligible level that viral transmission could not be sustained.

Measles elimination within a population should be possible, as an effective vaccine is available and there is no non-human reservoir or source of infection. During the XXIV Pan American Sanitary Conference in September 1994, representatives from Canada and other nations resolved to eliminate

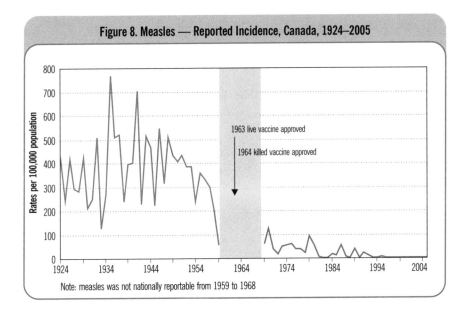

Figure 8. Measles — Reported Incidence, Canada, 1924–2005

1963 live vaccine approved

1964 killed vaccine approved

Rates per 100,000 population

Note: measles was not nationally reportable from 1959 to 1968

measles in the Americas by the year 2000. In Canada, sustained transmission has been eliminated by our current schedule and high vaccine coverage. However, as expected, imported cases continue to occur. Secondary spread from these imported cases is self-limited and involves the few Canadians who are still vulnerable. The largest outbreaks have occurred in isolated groups that are philosophically opposed to immunization. Nevertheless, there is very limited secondary transmission of measles in the general population. Between 2001 and 2005, the number of measles cases reported annually ranged from 6 (2005) to 34 (2001) with a yearly average of 14. All cases were imported or import-related.

Most other countries in North, Central and South America have also succeeded in eliminating sustained transmission. In 2005 fewer than 100 measles cases were reported in all of the Western Hemisphere. The situation in other regions is evolving at a slower pace, though measles deaths in Africa have been reduced by 60%, largely through the efforts of The Measles Initiative, a cooperative group led by the Red Cross, in partnership with UNICEF, the Centers for Disease Control and Prevention, the World Health Organization and the United Nations Foundation.

The greatest challenge for future years will be to continue achieving vaccine coverage rates of 95% or more as measles becomes increasingly unfamiliar to Canadian parents. Immunization against measles will continue to be necessary in Canada until global elimination of the disease has been achieved.

Preparations approved for use in Canada

This chapter will deal only with vaccines that are currently marketed in Canada.

◆ M-M-R® II (measles, mumps, and rubella vaccine, live, attenuated), Merck Frosst Canada Ltd.

◆ Priorix® (measles, mumps, and rubella vaccine, live, attenuated), GlaxoSmithKline Inc.

Measles vaccine is a live, attenuated virus vaccine and is available in combination with rubella and mumps vaccine. Measles vaccines are generally prepared in chick fibroblast cell cultures. All preparations may contain traces of antibiotics (e.g., neomycin) and stabilizer such as gelatin.

For a list of all approved products in Canada, please refer to Table 1 in the *General Considerations* chapter, page 7.

Efficacy and immunogenicity

The efficacy of the measles vaccine increases with age at immunization. The main mechanism explaining poor efficacy in children immunized at an early age is the interference by maternal antibody. These antibodies are transferred from the mother to the fetus in utero, and their levels slowly decrease after birth. Most infants have lost their maternal antibody by 12 months of age, but studies have shown that immunization at 15 months of age gives higher numbers of protected individuals. Maternal antibodies are not the only factor in vaccine failure, as the protection appears to reach a plateau after 15 months of age. The efficacy of a single dose given at 12 or 15 months is estimated to be 85% to 95%. With a second dose, almost 100% of children are protected.

Recommended usage

Infants and children

For routine immunization of all children, two doses of measles vaccine should be given. Infants should receive a first dose combined with mumps and rubella vaccines (MMR) on or shortly after their first birthday; the second dose should be given after 15 months of age but before school entry. It is convenient to link this dose with other routinely scheduled immunizations. Options include giving it with the scheduled immunization at 15 or 18 months of age, with school entry immunization at 4 to 6 years, or at any intervening age that is practicable (such as entry to day care).

Two doses of vaccine given at least 4 weeks apart are recommended for children who

- have missed MMR immunization on the routine schedule;
- are without an immunization record;
- are without reliable records of measles immunization (e.g., immigrants);
- were given live measles vaccine and immune globulin (Ig) separated by an inappropriate interval.

The recommended interval between Ig-containing products and MMR immunization varies from 3 to 11 months. Please refer to the *Recent Administration of Human Immune Globulin Products* chapter, page 53, for more information.

Vaccine may be recommended for children < 12 months of age during outbreaks or international travel to an area where measles is common. MMR may be given as early as 6 months of age. Under these circumstances, or if vaccine was inappropriately given before the child's first birthday, two doses of MMR should still be given after the first birthday.

Post-exposure use

Susceptible individuals > 12 months of age who are exposed to measles may be protected from disease if measles vaccine is given within 72 hours of the exposure. There are no known adverse effects of vaccine given to people incubating measles. Ig given within 6 days of the exposure can modify or prevent disease and may be used for this purpose in infants < 12 months of age, people for whom vaccine is contraindicated, or those for whom more than 72 hours but less than 1 week have elapsed since exposure. Please refer to the *Passive Immunizing Agents* chapter, page 353, for more information. Unless it is contraindicated, individuals who receive Ig should be given measles vaccine after the intervals specified in Table 4, page 54, see *Recent Administration of Human Immune Globulin Products* chapter for more information.

Adults

Adults born prior to 1970 can be assumed to have acquired natural immunity to measles. Adults born in 1970 or later who have not had a measles vaccine or have not had natural measles infection should receive a dose of MMR. A second dose of MMR should be offered only to adults born in 1970 or later who are at greatest risk of exposure. These people include

- travelers to a measles endemic area;
- health care workers;
- military recruits;
- students at post-secondary institutions.

Schedule and dosage

Two doses of MMR vaccine should be administered. The first dose should be given on or after the first birthday and the second dose given at least 1 month after the first and, in children, before school entry. The standard dosage is 0.5 mL.

For single vials, the entire contents of the vial should be injected promptly after reconstitution (0.5-0.7 mL).

Route of administration

The vaccine should be administered subcutaneously.

Booster doses and re-immunization

Re-immunization after the standard two-dose schedule is not thought to be necessary at this time.

Serologic testing

There are no routine indications for pre- or post-immunization serology. Persons can generally be presumed to be immune to measles if they were born before 1970, have documented evidence of vaccination with two doses of measles-containing vaccine after their first birthday, laboratory evidence of immunity, or a history of laboratory-confirmed measles disease.

Storage requirements

Measles-containing vaccine should be stored in the refrigerator at a temperature of +2° C to +8° C. Vaccine must be protected from light, which may inactivate the vaccine viruses. Once reconstituted, the vaccine should be administered promptly.

Simultaneous administration with other vaccines

Measles-containing vaccine can be given concurrently with other childhood vaccines. Vaccines should be administered using separate syringes and at separate sites. When administered with other live vaccines, like varicella vaccine, measles-containing vaccine should be given at the same time or separated by a minimum 4-week interval.

Adverse reactions

Serious adverse events are rare following immunization and, in most cases, data are insufficient to determine a causal association.

Measles vaccine produces a mild, non-transmissible and usually subclinical infection. The most frequent reaction (approximately 5% of immunized children) is malaise and fever with or without rash lasting up to 3 days and occurring 7 to 12 days after MMR immunization. One in 3,000 children with fever may have associated febrile convulsions. Rarely, transient thrombocytopenia occurs within 2 months after immunization, is usually benign and generally resolves within a month. Joint symptoms are associated with the rubella component of MMR. Adverse reactions are less frequent after the second dose of vaccine and tend to occur only in those not protected by the first dose.

Encephalitis has been reported in association with administration of live attenuated measles vaccine at a frequency of approximately 1 per million doses distributed in North America, which is so rare that it is uncertain whether the vaccine is the cause. Nevertheless, the reported incidence is much lower than that observed with the natural disease (approximately 1 per 1,000 cases). There has been a dramatic decline in the incidence of SSPE since the introduction of widespread measles immunization. No vaccine-strain viruses have been isolated from these patients.

In 1998, a group of researchers from the U.K. reported an association between MMR vaccine and autism and inflammatory bowel disease. There were claims that MMR can cause severe developmental problems and that separate injections of each component would be safer. Rigorous scientific studies have been done in countries all over the world, and there is strong scientific evidence to show that there is no association between measles vaccine and autism or inflammatory bowel disease. In 2004, 10 of the original 13 authors retracted the key interpretation concerning a potential association between MMR vaccine and autism and inflammatory bowel disease. Separate administration of the different components of MMR is strongly discouraged, as it will give no health benefit, will increase the proportion of children who fail to receive all three antigens and/or delay achieving complete protection against all three diseases, and will cause unnecessary pain and distress to children. Separate component vaccines are not currently available in Canada.

Contraindications and precautions

Since MMR vaccine contains trace amounts of neomycin and gelatin, people who have experienced anaphylactic reactions to neomycin or who have a documented gelatin allergy should not receive MMR vaccine. Anyone who has experienced anaphylaxis to a previous dose of MMR should not receive the vaccine again. Please refer to the *Anaphylaxis: Initial Management in Non-Hospital Settings* chapter, page 80, for more information.

As with other live vaccines, measles-containing vaccine should not be administered to people whose immune mechanism is impaired as a result of disease or therapy, except under special circumstances. The immune response in such individuals may be impaired. It is desirable to immunize close contacts of immunocompromised individuals in order to minimize the risk of exposure to measles. Please refer to the *Immunization of Immunocompromised Persons* chapter, page 117, for more information.

Infants infected with human immunodeficiency virus (HIV) who are asymptomatic should receive routine MMR vaccination. In addition, MMR is recommended for most symptomatic HIV-infected persons, including children who are symptomatic without evidence of severe immunosuppression. Please consult an infectious disease specialist/immunologist for more specific advice on MMR immunization for HIV-infected people. HIV-infected children should receive Ig after recognized exposures to measles because the response to prior immunization may be inadequate. When other susceptible people with immune deficiencies are exposed to measles, passive immunization with Ig should be given as soon as possible. Please refer to the *Passive Immunizing Agents* chapter, page 353, for more information.

Although there is no known risk from measles vaccine administered during pregnancy, it should not be given to pregnant women.

Clinical studies have demonstrated that egg allergy should no longer be considered a contraindication to immunization with MMR. In people who have a history of anaphylactic hypersensitivity to hens' eggs (urticaria, swelling of the mouth and throat, difficulty in breathing or hypotension), measles vaccine can be administered in the routine manner without prior skin testing. No special precautions are necessary for children with minor egg hypersensitivity who are able to ingest small quantities of egg uneventfully. No special measures are necessary for children who have never been fed eggs before MMR immunization. Prior egg ingestion should not be a prerequisite for MMR immunization. Please refer to the *Anaphylactic Hypersensitivity to Egg and Egg-Related Antigens* chapter, page 85.

Tuberculosis may be exacerbated by natural measles infection, but there is no evidence that measles vaccine has such an effect. The measles component in MMR vaccine can temporarily suppress tuberculin reactivity. However, tuberculin skin testing is not a prerequisite to the administration of MMR vaccine. If skin testing for tuberculosis is required, it should be done on the same day as immunization or delayed for 4-6 weeks.

Administration of MMR should be deferred if there is any severe acute illness. However, immunization should not be delayed because of minor acute illness, with or without fever.

Other considerations

Outbreak control

A full discussion of measles outbreak control is beyond the scope of this chapter. With the current childhood two-dose schedule for measles vaccine, large outbreaks of measles are not expected to recur. However, because many countries have lower immunization coverage, measles will continue to be imported into Canada. Imported cases will result in limited transmission of measles, usually among unvaccinated children and young adults who have not received two doses of vaccine.

Control interventions in schools or other facilities had little impact when Canada was using a single-dose program. With the two-dose strategy and high vaccine coverage, the benefits of control interventions are likely to be negligible except in settings where vaccine coverage is known to be low. Thus, before any intervention is started, suspected measles cases should be promptly confirmed by culture or serology. If cases are confirmed, contacts should be informed that measles is circulating and advised to update their immunization status if necessary. For practical purposes, all students attending the same school or facility should be considered contacts. Immunization within 72 hours of exposure will usually prevent measles. Should an individual already be immune or infected by measles virus, there is no increased risk of adverse reactions from immunization with live measles-containing vaccine.

Selected references

Advisory Committee on Epidemiology. *Guidelines for control of measles outbreaks in Canada.* Canada Communicable Disease Report 1995;21(21):189-95.

Bell A, King A, Pielak K et al. *Epidemiology of measles outbreak in British Columbia — February 1997.* Canada Communicable Disease Report 1997;23(7):49-51.

Bellini WJ, Rota JS, Lowe LE et al. *Subacute sclerosing panencephalitis: more cases of this fatal disease are prevented by measles immunization than was previously recognized.* Journal of Infectious Diseases 2005;192(10):1686-93.

De Serres G, Boulianne N, Meyer F et al. *Measles vaccine efficacy during an outbreak in a highly vaccinated population: incremental increase in protection with age at vaccination up to 18 months.* Epidemiology and Infection 1995;115(2):315-23.

De Serres G, Gay NJ, Farrington CP. *Epidemiology of transmissible diseases after elimination.* American Journal of Epidemiology 2000;151(11):1039-48.

De Serres G, Sciberras J, Naus M et al. *Protection after two doses of measles vaccine is independent of interval between doses.* Journal of Infectious Diseases 1999;180(1):187-90.

Gay NJ, De Serres G, Farrington CP et al. *Assessment of the status of measles elimination from reported outbreaks: United States, 1997-1999.* Journal of Infectious Diseases 2004;189(Suppl 1):S36-42.

Halsey NA, Hyman SL. *Measles-mumps-rubella vaccine and autistic spectrum disorder: report from the New Challenges in Childhood Immunizations Conference convened in Oak Brook, Illinois, June 12-13, 2000.* Pediatrics 2001;107(5):E84.

Institute of Medicine, Immunization Safety Review Committee (Stratton K, Gable A, Shetty P et al, eds.). *Measles-mumps-rubella vaccine and autism.* Washington DC: National Academy Press, 2001.

Jadavji T, Scheifele D, Halperin S. *Thrombocytopenia after immunization of Canadian children, 1992 to 2001.* Pediatric Infectious Disease Journal 2003;22(2):119-22.

King A, Varughese P, De Serres G et al. *Measles elimination in Canada.* Journal of Infectious Diseases 2004;189(Suppl 1):S236-42.

Madsen KM, Hviid A, Vestergaard M et al. *A population-based study of measles, mumps, and rubella vaccination and autism.* New England Journal of Medicine 2002;347(19):1477-82.

Markowitz L, Albrecht P, Orenstein WA et al. *Persistence of measles antibody after revaccination.* Journal of Infectious Diseases 1992;166(1):205-8.

Measles Initiative. *Together we can save a life.* URL: <http://www.measlesinitiative.org/index3.asp.>.

Miller E, Andrews N, Grant A et al. *No evidence of an association between MMR vaccine and gait disturbance.* Archives of Disease in Childhood 2005;90(3):292-96.

Murch SH, Anthony A, Casson DH et al. *Retraction of an interpretation.* Lancet 2004;363(9411):750.

Ratnam S, Chandra R, Gadag V. *Maternal measles and rubella antibody levels and serologic response in infants immunized with MMRII vaccine at 12 months of age.* Journal of Infectious Diseases 1993;168(6):1596-98.

Ratnam S, West R, Gadag V et al. *Immunity against measles in school-aged children: implications for measles revaccination strategies.* Canadian Journal of Public Health 1996;87(6):407-10.

Strauss B, Bigham M. Does measles-mumps-rubella (MMR) vaccination cause inflammatory bowel disease and autism? Canada Communicable Disease Report 2001;27(8):65-72.

Taylor B, Miller E, Lingam R et al. *Measles, mumps and rubella vaccination and bowel problems or developmental regression in children with autism: population study.* British Medical Journal 2002;324(7334):393-96.

Meningococcal Vaccine

Since the publication of the 2002 *Canadian Immunization Guide*, a third meningococcal C conjugate vaccine has been approved for use, guidelines for the prevention and control of meningococcal disease have been published and further information concerning the duration of protection provided by meningococcal C conjugate vaccines in infancy has been published.

Epidemiology

Invasive meningococcal disease (IMD) is endemic in Canada, showing periods of increased activity roughly every 10 to 15 years with no consistent pattern. The incidence rate varies considerably with different serogroups, age groups, geographic locations and time. Implementation of universal meningococcal C immunization programs will also affect disease epidemiology.

Since 1985, the overall incidence of IMD has remained at or below 2 per 100,000 per year (range 0.5 to 2.1). Overall, the incidence rate has been highest among children < 1 year of age and then declines as age increases, except for a smaller peak in the 15 to 19 year age group. An average of 298 cases of meningococcal disease have been reported annually. Disease occurs year round, but there is seasonal variation with the majority of cases occurring in the winter months.

Serogroups A and C *Neisseria meningitidis* were the groups most frequently identified from 1971 to 1974. From 1975 to 1989, serogroup B predominated. Since 1993, serogroups B and C have been responsible for most of the cases of endemic disease in Canada (incidence rates ranging between 0.13 to 0.65 per 100,000 population and 0.2 to 0.44 per 100,000 population for C and B respectively). However, there has been less fluctuation in the incidence of serogroup B than of serogroup C disease over time. Between the years 2000 and 2003, the average number of serogroup C cases per year in children < 1 year was 4 (range 1-8). In those aged 1-4 the average was 9 (range 4-14). During the same time period, the average number of cases in the 15-19 and 20-24 age groups was 25 (range 12-40) and 13 (range 5-18) respectively. Meningococcal outbreaks are almost exclusively due to serogroup C. There were sporadic localized outbreaks and periods of elevated incidence of serogroup C disease during 1989-1993 and 1999-2001. Immunization campaigns using serogroup C polysaccharide and conjugate vaccines were implemented in some regions during the 1999-2001 outbreak period. Recent data suggest that incidence rates of serogroup C are decreasing; however, more data are needed.

An increasing trend in the incidence of serogroup Y disease has been observed in the United States during the past decade, although no such trends have been observed in Canada over this time. In this country, from 1993 to 2003, serogroup Y incidence has remained relatively stable at 0.06 to 0.13 per 100,000 population per year (average 28 confirmed cases per year, range 17 to 41). Serogroup Y disease has tended to affect older adults (median age 45 years, range 0-94).

Incidence rates for serogroup W135 have remained below 0.05 per 100,000 population. Cases of serogroup A disease remain rare in Canada (< 10 cases reported between 1993 and 2005).

The epidemiology of meningococcal disease varies throughout the world. International travellers should be aware of the risk of IMD at their destination of choice. IMD occurs sporadically worldwide and in focal epidemics. The traditional endemic or hyperendemic areas of the world (the "meningitis belt") include the savannah areas of sub-Saharan Africa extending from Gambia and Senegal in the west to Ethiopia and Western Eritrea in the east. Health care providers advising Canadian travellers should remain current with global meningococcal activity. The Committee to Advise on Tropical Medicine and Travel (CATMAT) provides guidelines for health care providers counselling Canadian international travellers on meningococcal vaccination. In deciding on the need for immunization, there should be particular consideration of the destination to be visited, the nature and duration of exposure, and the age and health of the traveller. Current meningococcal outbreak information can be obtained through the Public Health Agency of Canada, Travel Medicine Program (http://www.travel-health.gc.ca) and the World Health Organization (WHO) (http://www.who.int/csr/don/archive/disease/meningococcal_disease/en/)

Preparations approved for use in Canada

This chapter will deal only with vaccines that are currently marketed in Canada.

Two different types of meningococcal vaccine are available: purified capsular polysaccharide vaccines and protein-polysaccharide conjugate C vaccines.

Conjugate vaccines (Men-C-C)

◆ Meningitec™ (composed of *N. meningitidis* group C oligosaccharides conjugated to cross reacting material 197 [CRM197]), Wyeth Canada (distributor)

◆ Menjugate™ (meningococcal group C oligosaccharides conjugated to a purified non-toxic variant of diphtheria toxin CRM197), Chiron Corporation

◆ NeisVac-C™ (contains meningococcal group C polysaccharide conjugated to tetanus toxoids), GlaxoSmithKline Inc. (distributor)

Polysaccharide vaccines

Bivalent vaccines (Men-P-AC)

- Menomune® A/C (meningococcal polysaccharide vaccine, groups A and C combined), Sanofi Pasteur Ltd.

Quadrivalent vaccine (Men-P-ACW135Y)

- Menomune® A/C/Y/W-135 (containing capsular polysaccharide from serogroups A, C, Y and W135 meningococci), Sanofi Pasteur Ltd.

Efficacy and immunogenicity

Conjugate vaccines

A high level of protection produced by immunization with meningococcal C conjugate vaccine has been predicted from immunogenicity data. In addition, data related to the effectiveness of the meningococcal C conjugate vaccine program after its introduction in England in November 1999 are available. Children received three doses of the vaccine at ages 2, 3 and 4 months. Children from 5 months to 18 years of age were provided vaccination as part of a catch-up campaign. This involved two doses at least 4 weeks apart for children aged 5 months to 1 year and a single dose for children > 1 year of age. Assessment of the immunization program in its first year showed that vaccine effectiveness ranged from 87% to 98%. There was no significant difference in effectiveness between age groups. However, after 4 years of follow-up, the vaccine effectiveness among children who had received the routine infant immunization declined significantly to 66% and was lower than in the catch-up cohorts, in whom effectiveness remained high, ranging from 83% to 100%.

Polysaccharide vaccines

The immunogenicity and clinical efficacy of the serogroups A and C polysaccharide vaccines have been well established. The serogroup A polysaccharide induces antibody response among certain children as young as 3 months of age, although a response comparable with that occurring in adults is not achieved until 4-5 years of age; the serogroup C component is poorly immunogenic among recipients aged < 2 years. The serogroups A and C polysaccharide vaccines have demonstrated estimated clinical efficacies of 85% to 100% among older children and adults, and are useful in controlling epidemics. Serogroups Y and W-135 polysaccharides are safe and immunogenic in adults and in children > 2 years of age. Although clinical protection has not been documented, vaccination with these polysaccharides induces bactericidal antibody. The antibody responses to each of the four polysaccharides in the vaccine are serogroup-specific and independent.

Part 4 — Active Immunizing Agents – Meningococcal Vaccine

Polysaccharide vaccines have been widely used to control outbreaks of serogroup A and C meningococcal disease in Canada and throughout the world. Vaccine efficacy within the year of immunization is between 87% and 94%. Lower efficacy (0% to 67%) has generally been observed in young children, especially those < 2 years of age. In Quebec, where 1.7 million doses of polysaccharide vaccine were given during an outbreak of serogroup C disease in the early 1990s, efficacy after 5 years was estimated at 79% among children and young adults. After further follow-up in Quebec, protection from serogroup C meningococcal disease was observed in the first 2 years after vaccine administration (vaccine efficacy 65%) but not in the next 3 years (vaccine efficacy 0%). Vaccine efficacy was strongly related to age at immunization: 83% for ages 15 to 20 years, 75% for ages 10 to 14 years, and 41% for ages 2 to 9 years. There was no evidence of protection in children < 2 years.

During a serogroup A epidemic in Africa, the efficacy of polysaccharide vaccines against serogroup A was estimated as 87%. Although protection against serogroup A after use of polysaccharide vaccines may persist in school-aged children and adults for at least 3 years, the efficacy in children aged < 5 years may decrease markedly within this period.

Measurable levels of antibodies against the group A and C polysaccharides decrease markedly during the first 3 years after a single dose of vaccine. This decrease in antibody occurs more rapidly in children < 5 years of age than in adults.

Recommended usage

The meningococcal C conjugate vaccines have been approved for use in infants, children and adults, and the National Advisory Committee on Immunization (NACI) recommends that they be used as follows.

Infants

Meningococcal C conjugate vaccines are recommended for routine immunization of infants. The recommended schedule differs depending upon the vaccine used. Three doses of either Meningitec™ or Menjugate™ are recommended to be given to infants beginning no earlier than 2 months of age and separated by at least 1 month. Two doses of NeisVac-C™ should be administered at least 2 months apart, with the first dose not to be administered before 2 months of age. At least one dose of the primary immunization series should be given after 5 months of age. Infants 4 to 11 months of age who have not previously received the vaccine should be immunized with two doses given at least 4 weeks apart. Infants born prematurely should receive the vaccine at the same chronological age as term infants.

Polysaccharide vaccine is not recommended for routine infant immunization.

Individuals ≥ 1 year of age

Meningococcal C conjugate vaccines are recommended for immunization of children aged 1-4 years and for adolescents and young adults to prevent the increased risk of serogroup C meningococcal disease in these age groups. For children ≥ 5 years of age who have not reached adolescence, immunization with a single dose of MenC-conjugate vaccine may also be considered. A single dose is required for any person ≥ 1 year of age.

Polysaccharide vaccine is not recommended for routine childhood immunization.

Contacts of cases

Close contacts of individuals with meningococcal infections are at increased risk of IMD; this risk is greatest for household contacts. The vaccination status of close contacts, including the type of meningococcal vaccine, the number of doses and age at vaccine administration, should be determined. Vaccination of susceptible close contacts, in addition to chemoprophylaxis, should be considered when the serogroup is vaccine preventable, as it may further reduce the risk of subsequent meningococcal disease; vaccination should be carried out as soon as possible. The increased risk of disease for household contacts persists for up to 1 year after disease in the index case and beyond any protection from antibiotic chemoprophylaxis. In general, this prolonged risk is not seen among other contacts who do not have ongoing exposure.

Thus, the following individuals are considered close contacts for whom immunoprophylaxis and chemoprophylaxis (as detailed in Table 9), should be given:

- Household contacts of a case
- Persons who share sleeping arrangements with the case
- Persons who have direct contaminations of their nose or mouth with oral/nasal secretions of a case (e.g., kissing on the mouth, shared cigarettes, shared drinking bottles)
- Children and staff in child care and nursery school facilities

The following individuals are close contacts who should receive only chemoprophylaxis (not immunoprophylaxis):

- Health care workers (HCWs) who have had **intensive unprotected contact** (without wearing a mask) with infected patients (i.e., intubating, resuscitating or closely examining the oropharynx)
- Airline passengers sitting immediately on either side of the case (but not across the aisle) when the total time spent aboard the aircraft was at least 8 hours

Part 4 — Active Immunizing Agents – Meningococcal Vaccine

Table 9. Chemoprophylaxis* for Close Contacts of Individuals with Meningococcal Infection

Drug	Dosage**	Comments
Ciprofloxacin	Adults ≥ 18 years of age: PO 500 mg x 1 dose	Contraindicated during pregnancy and lactation. Only approved for persons > 18 years of age. Not recommended for prepubertal children.
Rifampin	Adults: 600 mg PO q 12 h x 4 doses Children ≥ 1 month of age: 10 mg/kg (maximum 600 mg) per dose PO q 12 h x 4 doses Infants < 1 month of age: 5 mg/kg per dose PO q 12 h x 4 doses	Contraindicated in pregnancy. Urine and tears may be stained red. Advise against wear of soft contact lenses as they can also be stained. Can reduce effectiveness of oral contraceptives. Advise use of alternative/additional contraceptive measures.
Ceftriaxone	Adults and adolescents ≥ 12 years: 250 mg IM x 1 dose Children < 12 years: 125 mg IM x 1 dose	Recommended drug for pregnant women. Alternative for persons who cannot tolerate oral medication. Dilute in 1% lidocaine to reduce pain at injection site.

* Chemoprophylaxis should be offered to all persons having close contact with an IMD case during the infectious period (the 7 days before onset of symptoms in the case to 24 hrs after onset of effective treatment), regardless of their immunization status. If antibiotics such as penicillin, which do not reliably eliminate nasopharyngeal carriage, have been used for treatment the index case should also receive antibiotics that clear nasal carriage before discharge.

** PO, orally; IM, intramuscularly

For susceptible close contacts of known serogroup C disease, meningococcal C conjugate vaccine is preferred because of longer duration of protection and induction of immunologic memory; however, polysaccharide vaccines will provide protection in older children and adults during the 1-year period of increased risk. Polysaccharide vaccines are ineffective against serogroup C disease in children < 2 years of age, and meningococcal C conjugate vaccine should be given to children in that age group. Bivalent (A, C) or quadrivalent (A, C, Y, W135) polysaccharide vaccine should be considered for susceptible close contacts of cases with IMD known to be caused by serogroup A; quadrivalent polysaccharide vaccine should be considered for susceptible close contacts of cases of serogroup Y or W135 disease. No vaccine is currently available for contacts of individuals with serogroup B disease, and vaccine is not recommended for contacts of cases of disease in which the serogroup has not been determined. For decisions regarding persons previously immunized, please refer to the section on *Booster Doses and Re-Immunization*.

High-risk groups

Routine immunization with meningococcal vaccine is recommended for certain groups at increased risk of meningococcal disease. Such individuals include those with functional or anatomic asplenia (vaccines should be given at least 2 weeks before splenectomy) and people with complement, properdin or factor D deficiency. More durable protection against serogroup C meningococcal disease may be achieved by giving meningococcal C conjugate vaccine to these individuals in addition to polysaccharide vaccine. If the conjugate C vaccine is given first, a period of at least 2 weeks before immunization with polysaccharide vaccine is recommended to allow time for generation of an antibody response, as it is possible that a shorter interval may interfere with this response. If the polysaccharide vaccine is given first, an adequate response to conjugate vaccine has been observed after a delay of 6 months in adults. This is the recommended interval until further data are available. Children < 2 years of age with these immunodeficiencies should be immunized with conjugate vaccine as described in the routine infant schedule above, and should then receive polysaccharide vaccine at 2 years of age. Please refer to the *Immunization of Immunocompromised Persons* chapter, page 117, for further information.

Routine immunization with the quadrivalent polysaccharide vaccine is recommended for military recruits and may be considered for other groups or institutions where there is an increased risk of disease. The choice between conjugate or polysaccharide meningococcal vaccine would depend on whether the individual is staying in Canada (conjugate C preferred as this strain is currently the most prevalent one circulating) or traveling to or working in areas where additional serogroups are prevalent (quadrivalent polysaccharide preferred).

Although there are no data to suggest an increased risk of meningococcal disease among students in Canada living in residential accommodation, an elevation in risk has been observed in the United States among freshmen living in dormitory accommodation and in the United Kingdom among university students in catered hall accommodation. Clusters of cases of meningococcal disease in students have been reported in a number of countries, and carriage rates increase rapidly among freshmen during the first week of term in the U.K. In this age group in Canada, there is an increase in the rate of meningococcal disease; the risk is mainly from serogroup C disease. NACI recommends that all Canadian adolescents and young adults be immunized with meningococcal C conjugate vaccine. As students attending colleges and universities are included in this recommendation by virtue of their age, there is no need to make special recommendations for this group of people.

Laboratory and health care workers

Nosocomial transmission of IMD is very uncommon, especially when routine practices and droplet (large) and contact precautions are followed to prevent the transmission of IMD. In rare instances, direct contact with respiratory secretions of infected persons (e.g., during mouth-to-mouth resuscitation) has resulted in transmission to HCWs. Therefore, HCWs are considered as close contacts only if they have had intensive, unprotected contact (without wearing a mask) with infected patients (e.g., intubating, resuscitating or closely examining the oropharynx). It is recommended that HCWs use barrier precautions to avoid direct contact with respiratory secretions of patients with meningococcal disease during the first 24 hours after commencement of antibiotic therapy. Routine immunization of HCWs is not recommended.

Laboratory-acquired meningococcal infection is believed to be rare. However, the rate of disease in a U.S. survey conducted by the Centers for Disease Control and Prevention (CDC), Atlanta, was higher than expected among microbiology laboratory workers dealing with N. meningitidis cultures in the absence of any breaches in laboratory safety practices. Research, industrial and clinical laboratory personnel who are routinely exposed to N. meningitidis should be offered immunization with quadrivalent polysaccharide vaccine and may be additionally offered conjugate C vaccine to provide enhanced protection against serogroup C meningococcal infection (see *Booster Doses and Re-immunization*).

Outbreaks of meningococcal disease

Consultation with public health officials and/or experts in communicable disease is important in the assessment and control of meningococcal disease outbreaks in various settings, and reference to published guidelines should be made. Most recent outbreaks of meningococcal disease in Canada have involved teenagers and young adults suffering from serogroup C disease. Such outbreaks may be controlled by the use of conjugate C vaccine or polysaccharide (either bivalent or quadrivalent) vaccine. The use of conjugate C vaccine may be preferable because of induction of immunologic memory and prolonged duration of protection. In those previously immunized with a polysaccharide vaccine for whom re-vaccination is considered, conjugate C vaccine is preferred (see *Booster Doses and Re-immunization*), as further immunization with polysaccharide vaccine may induce immunologic hyporesponsiveness, although the clinical significance of this phenomenon is unknown. In younger children (< 10 years) conjugate C vaccine is recommended for control of outbreaks in view of its superior immunogenicity and efficacy in this age group.

For the control of outbreaks of serogroup A meningococcal disease, which are exceedingly rare in Canada, bivalent or quadrivalent polysaccharide vaccine is recommended as a single dose for people ≥ 2 years of age. Children aged 3 to 23 months should receive two doses of vaccine given 2 to 3 months apart. For the control of outbreaks associated with serogroup Y or W135 meningococci, one dose of quadrivalent polysaccharide vaccine is recommended for people ≥ 2 years of age.

International travel

Quadrivalent polysaccharide vaccine is recommended for Canadian international travellers when meningococcal vaccine is indicated or required. Conjugate C vaccine alone is not appropriate for protection of travellers, as it does not protect against serogroup A, which is endemic in selected regions of the world, or serogroup W135 disease. Pilgrims making the annual Hajj pilgrimage to Mecca should receive a single dose of quadrivalent vaccine at least 2 weeks before departure. Despite the frequency of travel to regions where meningococcal epidemics occur, disease in travellers appears to be very unusual.

Schedule and dosage

Meningococcal C conjugate vaccine is given as a 0.5 mL dose. The recommended schedule differs depending upon the vaccine used and the age at vaccination (see *Recommended Usage*).

Bivalent and quadrivalent polysaccharide vaccines are given as a 0.5 mL dose to people aged ≥ 2 years. For specific protection against serogroup A meningococcal disease these vaccines may be given from 3 months of age, but two doses are required 2 to 3 months apart in infants 3-23 months of age.

There are no published data related to the interchangeability of the three conjugated meningococcal C vaccines, but the vaccines have been used safely in this manner in the U.K. without a noticeable decrease in efficacy. When possible, the infant series should be completed with the same vaccine.

Route of administration

Meningococcal C conjugate vaccine is to be given by intramuscular injection at a separate anatomic site from that of other co-administered vaccines.

Bivalent and quadrivalent polysaccharide vaccines are to be given by subcutaneous injection to people aged ≥ 2 years at a separate anatomic site from that of other co-administered vaccines.

Booster doses and re-immunization

Re-immunization with meningococcal C conjugate vaccines is not thought to be necessary at present, although there are insufficient data to predict persistence of immunologic memory (and presumed protection).

The need for, or effectiveness of, re-immunization with meningococcal polysaccharide vaccine has not been fully established. Repeated immunization may induce immunologic hyporesponsiveness to polysaccharide vaccines, although the clinical significance of this phenomenon is unknown. Re-immunization should be considered, according to Table 10, for those continuously or repeatedly exposed to serogroup A disease who have been previously immunized with bivalent or quadrivalent vaccine, particularly for children initially immunized at < 5 years of age. Children or adults with immunodeficiencies resulting in increased risk of meningococcal disease caused by serogroup A, Y or W135 meningococci may be re-immunized with quadrivalent polysaccharide vaccine according to Table 10.

Individuals who have previously received polysaccharide vaccine may receive conjugate C vaccine for continued protection against serogroup C disease. Since an adequate response to conjugate vaccine has been observed with a delay of 6 months after immunization with purified polysaccharide vaccine in adults, this remains the recommended interval until further data are available. In other circumstances, when conjugate C vaccine has already been administered and protection against serogroup A, Y or W135 meningococci is required, a period of 2 weeks should elapse before immunization with polysaccharide vaccine to allow time for generation of an antibody response and avoid possible interference with this response by the polysaccharide vaccine.

Serologic testing

There is no indication for pre- or post-immunization serology.

Storage requirements

All of the available products should be stored at a temperature between +2° C and +8° C and must not be frozen. The vaccines that need to be reconstituted should be done so immediately before use according to the manufacturer's instructions.

Table 10. Recommended Interval Between Repeat Doses of Meningococcal Polysaccharide Vaccines in Individuals Repeatedly or Continuously Exposed to Serogroup A, Y, W135 Disease

Age when first immunized	No. of primary doses	Interval since last dose as indication for repeat dose
3-12 months	2 doses: 2-3 months apart	6-12 months
13-23 months	2 doses: 2-3 months apart	1-2 years
2-5 years	1	2-3 years
≥ 6 years	1	≥ 5 years

Simultaneous administration with other vaccines

If necessary or convenient, meningococcal C conjugate vaccine may be administered at the same time as IPV, DTaP, Td, Tdap, Hib, hepatitis B, MMR, varicella or pneumococcal conjugate vaccines, at separate sites and with a separate needle and syringe. The meningococcal polysaccharide vaccine may also be given simultaneously with other vaccines, except the meningococcal conjugate vaccine, at a separate location and using a separate needle and syringe.

When used after administration of the meningococcal C conjugate vaccine, a delay of at least 2 weeks is recommended before immunization with meningococcal polysaccharide vaccine to allow time for generation of an antibody response, as it is possible that a shorter interval may interfere with this response. If the meningococcal polysaccharide vaccine has been administered first, an adequate response to conjugate vaccine has been observed after a delay of 6 months in adults. This is the recommended interval until further data are available.

Adverse reactions

Conjugate vaccines

Mild reactions, including local reactions (redness, tenderness, and swelling at the injection site), occur in up to 50% of vaccinees, irritability in up to 80% of infants and fever of > 38° C in up to 9% when other vaccines were administered. Headaches and malaise occur in up to 10% of older children and adults. Severe reactions are very uncommon and include systemic allergic reactions in < 0.01%.

Purified polysaccharide vaccines

Both bivalent and quadrivalent polysaccharide vaccines have been used extensively in many countries for mass immunization programs and to immunize military recruits, people who are immunocompromised and travellers. Mild reactions to the vaccines include pain and redness at the injection site in up to 50% and transient fever in 5%, particularly infants. Severe reactions to these vaccines are very unusual but include systemic allergic reactions (urticaria, wheezing and rash) at a rate of ≤ 0.1/100,000 doses, anaphylaxis in < 1 per million doses and occasional neurologic reactions. These vaccines have an established safety record. No adverse events have been documented during pregnancy or in newborn infants of immunized mothers.

Part 4 — Active Immunizing Agents – Meningococcal Vaccine

Contraindications and precautions

Contraindications

Conjugate vaccines and polysaccharide vaccines are contraindicated in people with a known hypersensitivity to any component of the vaccine and in those who have shown signs of hypersensitivity after previous administration of the vaccine.

Precautions

Meningococcal C conjugate vaccine will not protect against meningococcal diseases caused by any of the other types of meningococcal bacteria (A, B, 29e, H, I, K, L, W135, X, Y or Z, including non-typed). Complete protection against meningococcal serogroup C infection cannot be guaranteed. Conjugate vaccines containing CRM197 or tetanus toxoid should not be considered as immunizing agents against diphtheria or tetanus, and no changes in the schedule for administering vaccines containing diphtheria or tetanus toxoids are recommended. Conjugate C vaccine has not been studied in pregnant women; however, in specific circumstances in which the benefits outweigh the risks, its use can be considered.

Other considerations

The effect of meningococcal C conjugate vaccine on meningococcal population biology is unknown. With the use of widespread meningococcal immunization, close epidemiologic and laboratory-based surveillance is necessary to monitor changes in meningococcal biology and epidemiology.

New quadrivalent protein-polysaccharide conjugate vaccines are in development. At the time of publication of this edition of the *Guide*, Menactra™ (quadrivalent meningococcal conjugate vaccine, Sanofi Pasteur Ltd) had just been approved for use in Canada. Please see future NACI statements for recommendations. These vaccines might provide broad protection against the vaccine serogroups after introduction of an infant immunization program; they could presumably replace the currently used polysaccharide vaccines. None of these vaccines offers protection against serogroup B meningococci, a feature that limits the impact that any meningococcal vaccine can have on the invasive meningococcal disease burden, especially in children.

Selected references

Anderson EL, Bowers T, Mink CM et al. *Safety and immunogenicity of meningococcal A and C polysaccharide conjugate vaccine in adults.* Infection and Immunity 1994;62(8):3391-95.

Borrow R, Fox AJ, Richmond PC et al. *Induction of immunological memory in UK infants by a meningococcal A/C conjugate vaccine.* Epidemiology and Infection 2000;124(3):427-32.

Borrow R, Southern J, Andrews N et al. *Comparison of antibody kinetics following meningococcal serogroup C conjugate vaccine between healthy adults previously vaccinated with meningococcal A/C polysaccharide vaccine and vaccine-naive controls.* Vaccine 2001;19(23-24):3043-50.

Centers for Disease Control and Prevention. *Laboratory-acquired meningococcemia – California and Massachusetts.* Morbidity and Mortality Weekly Report 1991;40(3):46-7, 55.

Centers for Disease Control and Prevention. *Prevention and control of meningococcal disease: recommendations of the Advisory Committee on Immunization Practices (ACIP).* Morbidity and Mortality Weekly Report 2005;54(RR-7):1-21.

Choo S, Zuckerman J, Goilav C et al. *Immunogenicity and reactogenicity of a group C meningococcal conjugate vaccine compared with a group A+C meningococcal polysaccharide vaccine in adolescents in a randomised observer-blind controlled trial.* Vaccine 2000;18(24):2686-92.

Committee to Advise on Tropical Medicine and Travel (CATMAT). *Statement on meningococcal vaccination for travellers.* Canada Communicable Disease Report 1999;25(ASC5):1-12.

Cooke RP, Riordan T, Jones DM et al. *Secondary cases of meningococcal infection among close family and household contacts in England and Wales, 1984-7.* British Medical Journal 1989;298(6673):555-58.

De Wals P, De Serres G, Niyonsenga T. *Effectiveness of a mass immunization campaign against serogroup C meningococcal disease in Quebec.* Journal of the American Medical Association 2001;285(2):177-81.

English M, MacLennan JM, Bowen-Morris JM et al. *A randomised, double-blind, controlled trial of the immunogenicity and tolerability of a meningococcal group C conjugate vaccine in young British infants.* Vaccine 2000;19(9-10):1232-38.

Erickson L, De Wals P. *Complications and sequelae of meningococcal disease in Quebec, Canada, 1990-1994.* Clinical Infectious Diseases 1998;26(5):1159-64.

Fairley CK, Begg N, Borrow R et al. *Conjugate meningococcal serogroup A and C vaccine: reactogenicity and immunogenicity in United Kingdom infants.* Journal of Infectious Diseases 1996;174:1360-63.

Gilmore A, Stuart J, Andrews N. *Risk of secondary meningococcal disease in health-care workers.* Lancet 2000;356(9242):1654-55.

Gold R, Lepow ML, Goldschneider I et al. *Immune response of human infants of polysaccharide vaccines of group A and C Neisseria meningitidis.* Journal of Infectious Diseases 1977;136:S31-5.

Hastings L, Stuart J, Andrews N. *A retrospective survey of clusters of meningococcal disease in England and Wales, 1993 to 1995: estimated risks of further cases in household and educational settings.* Communicable Disease Report 1997;7(13):R195-200.

MacDonald NE, Halperin SA, Law BJ et al. *Induction of immunologic memory by conjugated vs plain meningococcal C polysaccharide vaccine in toddlers: a randomized controlled trial.* Journal of the American Medical Association 1998;280(19):1685-89.

MacLennan J, Obaro S, Deeks J et al. *Immune response to revaccination with meningococcal A and C polysaccharides in Gambian children following repeated immunisation during early childhood.* Vaccine 1999;17(23-24):3086-93.

MacLennan J, Obaro S, Deeks J et al. *Immunologic memory 5 years after meningococcal A/C conjugate vaccination in infancy.* Journal of Infectious Diseases 2001;183(1):97-104.

MacLennan JM, Shackley F, Heath PT et al. *Safety, immunogenicity, and induction of immunologic memory by a serogroup C meningococcal conjugate vaccine in infants: a randomized controlled trial* [see comments]. Journal of the American Medical Association 2000;283(21):2795-801.

National Advisory Committee on Immunization. *Statement on recommended use of meningococcal vaccines.* Canada Communicable Disease Report 2001;27(ACS-6).

Neal KR, Nguyen-Van-Tam J, Monk P et al. *Invasive meningococcal disease among university undergraduates: association with universities providing relatively large amounts of catered hall accommodation.* Epidemiololgy and Infection 1999;122(3):351-57.

PHLS Meningococcal Infections Working Group and Public Health Medicine Environmental Group. *Control of meningococcal disease: guidance for consultants in communicable disease control.* Communicable Disease Report 1995;5(13):R189-95.

Public Health Agency of Canada. *Guidelines for the prevention and control of meningococcal disease.* Canada Communicable Disease Report 2005;31(S1):1-26.

Ramsay ME, Andrews N, Kaczmarski EB et al. *Efficacy of meningococcal serogroup C conjugate vaccine in teenagers and toddlers in England.* Lancet 2001;357(9251):195-96.

Richmond P, Borrow R, Goldblatt D et al. *Ability of 3 different meningococcal C conjugate vaccines to induce immunologic memory after a single dose in UK toddlers.* Journal of Infectious Diseases 2001;183(1):160-63.

Richmond P, Borrow R, Miller E et al. *Meningococcal serogroup C conjugate vaccine is immunogenic in infancy and primes for memory.* Journal of Infectious Diseases 1999;179(6):1569-72.

Richmond P, Goldblatt D, Fusco PC et al. *Safety and immunogenicity of a new Neisseria meningitidis serogroup C-tetanus toxoid conjugate vaccine in healthy adults.* Vaccine 1999;18(7-8):641-46.

Richmond P, Kaczmarski E, Borrow R et al. *Meningococcal C polysaccharide vaccine induces immunologic hyporesponsiveness in adults that is overcome by meningococcal C conjugate vaccine.* Journal of Infectious Diseases 2000;181(2):761-64.

Trotter CL, Andrews NJ, Kaczmarski EB et al. *Effectiveness of meningococcal serogroup C conjugate vaccine 4 years after introduction.* Lancet 2004;364(9431):365-67.

Mumps Vaccine

Mumps is an acute infectious disease caused by mumps virus. About 40% of those infected develop acute parotitis, which is unilateral in about 25% of cases. Nonspecific or primarily respiratory symptoms occur in about half of those who acquire infection. Subclinical infection is common. Although complications are relatively frequent, permanent sequelae are rare. Before the widespread use of mumps vaccine, mumps was a major cause of viral meningitis. Mumps meningoencephalitis can, rarely, result in permanent neurologic sequelae, including paralysis, seizures, cranial nerve palsies and hydrocephalus. Transient but occasionally permanent deafness may occur, at an estimated rate of 0.5 to 5.0 per 100,000 reported mumps cases. Orchitis occurs in 20% to 30% of post-pubertal male cases and oophoritis in 5% of post-pubertal female cases. Involvement of the reproductive organs is commonly unilateral; therefore, sterility as a result of mumps is rare. Mumps infection in pregnancy has not been associated with congenital malformations, but mumps infection during the first trimester of pregnancy may increase the rate of spontaneous abortion.

Since the publication of the 2002 *Canadian Immunization Guide* there have been some changes in the preparations approved for use in Canada.

Epidemiology

Since the approval of vaccine in 1969, the number of reported mumps cases has decreased by greater than 99% from an average of 34,000 cases reported per year in the early 1950s to under 400 cases per year in the early 1990s. A further reduction in incidence was observed following the introduction of the routine second dose of MMR. The annual number of reported cases has continued to drop; during the period 2000-2004, an average of 87 cases were reported annually, ranging from 32 (2004) to 205 cases (2002).

In Canada, large outbreaks have been rare in recent years, but three localized outbreaks occurred between 2001 and 2005. The first outbreak, of 193 cases, occurred between September 2001 and March 2002 and involved an under-vaccinated community in northern Alberta following importation of the disease from Bolivia. Most members of the community were philosophically opposed to vaccination. Immunization rates in the affected community were greatly below the provincial average. The majority of cases (80%) occurred in unimmunized individuals, spreading through area schools and to a lesser extent the surrounding community. Two small outbreaks involving 13 and 19 cases occurred in Nova Scotia in the spring and fall of 2005 respectively. The cases ranged in age from 13 to 19 years (average age 14) for the former and 20 to 27 years in a university community (average age 23 years) for the latter. Four of the 13 cases in the first Nova Scotia outbreak and all of the cases in the second outbreak reported receiving only one dose of MMR. The latter outbreak resulted in three secondary cases in other provinces.

Globally there has been an ongoing outbreak in the United Kingdom from 2004 to 2006, which has involved > 70,000 cases. Most of the cases have occurred among unvaccinated young adults. The circulating genotype has been identified as genotype G. The G genotype is not an unusual or rare genotype and, like the rest of known genotypes of mumps, it has been circulating globally for decades or longer. In 2005-2006, multi-state outbreaks of mumps involving several hundred individuals, mostly young adults, many of whom had been vaccinated (with one dose of mumps vaccine), have occurred in the United States. These outbreaks have also been identified as associated with genotype G. Mumps remains endemic in many countries throughout the world, and mumps vaccine is used in only 57% of World Health Organization member countries, predominantly in countries with more developed economies.

Preparations approved for use in Canada

This chapter will deal only with vaccines that are currently marketed in Canada.

- ◆ M-M-R® II (measles, mumps, and rubella vaccine, live, attenuated), Merck Frosst Canada Ltd.

- ◆ Priorix® (measles, mumps, and rubella vaccine, live, attenuated), GlaxoSmithKline Inc.

Mumps virus vaccine is a live, attenuated virus vaccine and is only available in the combined form as measles, mumps and rubella (MMR) vaccine.

For a list of all approved products in Canada, please refer to Table 1 in the *General Considerations* chapter, page 7.

Efficacy and immunogenicity

A single dose of mumps vaccine produces an antibody response in over 95% of susceptible individuals. In controlled clinical trials, one dose of mumps vaccine was 95% efficacious in preventing mumps disease. However, field studies have demonstrated lower estimates of vaccine efficacy, usually around 80% with single-dose regimens. Antibody levels are lower than those that follow natural disease. The duration of vaccine-induced immunity is unknown, but serologic and epidemiologic data show the persistence of antibody, suggesting continuing protection against infection for at least 20 years. Although no data are currently available correlating specific antibody titres with susceptibility to mumps, outbreaks have been reported in highly vaccinated populations. A two-dose measles, mumps, and rubella immunization schedule used in Finland resulted in higher mumps-specific antibody levels, a higher seropositivity rate and slower decay of antibody levels.

Recommended usage

Administration of live attenuated mumps vaccine in combination with measles and rubella vaccines (MMR) is recommended for all children 12 months of age. The combined vaccine should be used even in individuals who may have prior immunity to components of the vaccine, and it can be used to immunize susceptible adults against mumps.

Although mumps immunization after exposure to mumps may not prevent the disease, it is not harmful. Should the exposure not result in an infection, the vaccine should confer protection against future exposures.

Schedule and dosage

One dose of MMR vaccine should be administered for mumps protection, with the second dose given for measles protection. The first dose should be given on or after the first birthday and the second dose given at least 1 month after the first and before school entry. The standard dose is 0.5 mL. See the *Measles Vaccine* chapter on page 228 for details of indications for a second dose.

For single vials, the entire contents of the vial should be injected promptly after reconstitution (0.5-0.7 mL).

Route of administration

MMR vaccine should be administered subcutaneously.

Booster doses and re-immunization

Re-immunization after the standard two-dose schedule is not thought to be necessary at this time.

Serologic testing

There is no indication to routinely check pre- or post-vaccination serology. Persons can generally be presumed to be immune to mumps if they have documented evidence of vaccination on or after their first birthday, laboratory evidence of immunity, a history of laboratory-confirmed mumps disease, or if they were born before 1970.

Part 4 — Active Immunizing Agents – Mumps Vaccine

Storage requirements

MMR vaccine should be stored in the refrigerator at a temperature of +2° C to +8° C. Vaccine must be protected from light, which may inactivate the vaccine viruses. Once reconstituted, the vaccine should be administered promptly.

Simultaneous administration with other vaccines

MMR can be administered simultaneously with other vaccines, at separate anatomic sites and in separate syringes. When administered with other live vaccines, such as varicella vaccine, MMR should be given at the same time or separated by a minimum 4-week interval.

Adverse reactions

Serious adverse events are rare following immunization and, in most cases, data are insufficient to determine a causal association.

The most frequent reaction (approximately 5% of immunized children) is malaise and fever with or without rash lasting up to 3 days and occurring 7 to 12 days after MMR immunization. One in 3,000 children with fever may have associated febrile convulsions. Historically, parotitis has occasionally occurred after immunization. Thrombocytopenia has been reported within 2 months after vaccination and is thought to be associated with the measles component of MMR. Joint symptoms are associated with the rubella component of MMR. Refer to the *Measles Vaccine* chapter on page 228 and the *Rubella Vaccine* chapter on page 298 for additional details.

Contraindications and precautions

Since MMR vaccine contains trace amounts of neomycin and gelatin, people who have experienced anaphylactic reactions to neomycin or who have a documented gelatin allergy should not receive MMR vaccine. Anyone who has experienced anaphylaxis to a previous dose of MMR should not receive the vaccine again. Please refer to the *Anaphylaxis: Initial Management in Non-Hospital Settings* chapter, page 80, for more information.

As with other live vaccines, mumps-containing vaccine should not be administered to people whose immune mechanism is impaired as a result of disease or therapy, except under special circumstances. The immune response in such individuals may be impaired. Please refer to the *Immunization of Immunocompromised Persons* chapter, page 117, for more information

Infants infected with human immunodeficiency virus (HIV) who are asymptomatic should receive routine MMR vaccination. In addition, MMR is recommended for most symptomatic HIV-infected persons, including children who are symptomatic without evidence of severe immunosuppression. Please consult an infectious disease specialist/immunologist for more specific advice on MMR immunization for HIV-infected people.

Although there is no known risk from mumps vaccine administered during pregnancy, it should not be given to pregnant women.

The recommended interval between immune globulin-containing products and MMR immunization varies from 3 to 11 months. Please refer to Table 4 in the *Recent Administration of Human Immune Globulin Products* chapter, page 54, for more information.

Convincing evidence supports the safety of routine administration of MMR vaccines to all children who have allergy to eggs. Fewer than 2 per 1,000 vaccinated egg-allergic children have been found to be at risk of anaphylactic reaction to MMR. Please refer to the *Anaphylactic Hypersensitivity to Egg and Egg-Related Antigens* chapter, page 85, for more information.

Selected references

Boulianne N, De Serres G, Ratnam S et al. *Measles, mumps and rubella antibodies in children 5-6 years after immunization: effect of vaccine type and age at vaccination.* Vaccine 1995; 13(16):1611-16.

Buxton J, Craig C, Daly P et al. *An outbreak of mumps among young adults in Vancouver, British Columbia, associated with "rave parties".* Canadian Journal of Public Health 1999;90(3):160-63.

Caplan CE. *Mumps in the era of vaccines.* Canadian Medical Association Journal 1999;160(6):865-66.

Cheek JE, Baron R, Atlas H et al. *Mumps outbreak in a highly vaccinated school population.* Archives of Pediatrics and Adolescent Medicine 1995;149(7):774-78.

Cooney MK, Fox JP, Hall CE. *The Seattle Virus Watch, VI. Observations of infections with and illness due to parainfluenza, mumps, and respiratory syncytial viruses and Mycoplasma pneumoniae.* American Journal of Epidemiology 1975;101(6):532-51.

Davidkin I, Valle M, Julkunen I. *Persistence of anti-mumps virus antibodies after a two-dose MMR vaccination at nine-year follow-up.* Vaccine 1995;13(16):1617-22.

Duclos P, Ward BJ. *Measles vaccines: a review of adverse events.* Drug Safety 1998;19(6):435-54.

Falk WA, Buchan K, Dow M et al. *The epidemiology of mumps in Southern Alberta, 1980-1982.* American Journal of Epidemiology 1989;130(4):736-49.

Griffin MR, Ray WA, Mortimer EA et al. *Risk of seizures after measles-mumps-rubella immunization.* Pediatrics 1991;88(5):881-85.

Health Protection Agency, U.K. *Confirmed cases of mumps by age and region: 1996-2005.* URL:<www.hpa.org.uk/infections/topics_az/mumps/data_reg_age.htm>.

Jadavji T, Scheifele D, Halperin S. *Thrombocytopenia after immunization of Canadian children, 1992 to 2001.* Pediatric Infectious Disease Journal 2003;22(2):119-22.

James JM, Burks AW, Roberson PK et al. *Safe administration of the measles vaccine to children allergic to eggs.* New England Journal of Medicine 1995;332(19):1262-66.

Miller E, Goldacre M, Pugh S et al. *Risk of aseptic meningitis after measles, mumps and rubella vaccine in U.K. children.* Lancet 1993;341(8851):979-82.

Peltola H, Heinonen OP, Valle M et al. *The elimination of indigenous measles, mumps and rubella from Finland by a 12 year two-dose vaccination program.* New England Journal of Medicine 1994;331(21):1397-1402.

West R, Roberts PM. *Measles, mumps and rubella vaccine: current safety issues.* BioDrugs 1999;12(6):423-29.

Pertussis Vaccine

Pertussis (whooping cough) is a highly communicable infection of the respiratory tract caused by *Bordetella pertussis*. The disease can affect individuals of any age; however, severity is greatest among young infants. One to three deaths occur each year in Canada, particularly in infants too young to have begun their immunization and in partially immunized infants (e.g., one or two doses). The number of affected adolescents and adults has steadily increased, and the morbidity in these cases is not insignificant. The goal of pertussis control is to decrease the morbidity and mortality of pertussis across the entire lifespan. Protection of adolescents and adults is a worthy goal for the benefit of these individuals themselves, notwithstanding the added indirect protection that it may provide to infants.

Pertussis has been partially controlled in Canada through immunization, and during the last 50 years its incidence has decreased by > 90% (see Figure 9), although outbreaks continue to occur.

Since the publication of the 2002 *Canadian Immunization Guide*, a statement about prevention of pertussis in adolescents and adults has been published, as has information about the interval between administration of vaccines against diphtheria, tetanus and pertussis. Information related to these issues is included in the chapter.

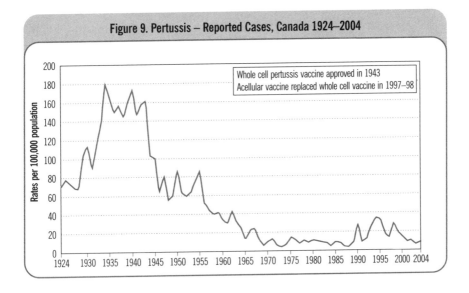

Figure 9. Pertussis – Reported Cases, Canada 1924–2004

Epidemiology

The whole-cell pertussis vaccine was introduced in Canada in the 1940s. It was replaced by the adsorbed whole-cell vaccine in the 1980s and by acellular vaccine in 1997-98. Since the introduction of pertussis vaccination, the number of reported cases has dropped dramatically, from 160 cases per 100,000 just before the introduction of the vaccine to < 20 cases per 100,000 in the 1980s. The incidence of pertussis in Canada was low during the 1980s but has increased since 1990. Between 1990 and 2004, the annual number of reported cases has ranged from 2,165 to 10,151, although this likely under-represents the true burden because of incomplete diagnosis and reporting. The resurgence of pertussis was likely due to a combination of factors, including the low efficacy of the combined adsorbed diphtheria-tetanus-pertussis whole-cell vaccine used in children in Canada between 1980 and 1997, waning immunity among adolescents and adults, as well as increased physician awareness and improved diagnosis and reporting of pertussis disease. A cohort of children immunized solely with the vaccine used between 1980 and 1997 was poorly protected and constitutes the population that has been most affected by pertussis since 1990. The increasing age of cases parallels that of children belonging to the vulnerable cohort.

The proportion of pertussis cases in adolescents (≥ 15 years) and adults increased from 9.6% in 1995 to 16.4%, 21.2%, and 31.3% in 1998, 2001 and 2004 respectively. In addition to a greater incidence, part of this increase may be attributable to better recognition, diagnosis and reporting of pertussis in adolescents and adults, as well as waning immunity. The increased incidence among adolescents has also been observed in the United States, France and other countries. Waning of vaccine-induced protection is a

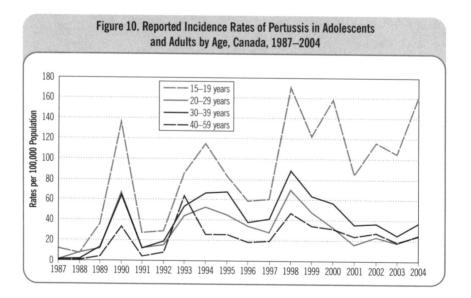

Figure 10. Reported Incidence Rates of Pertussis in Adolescents and Adults by Age, Canada, 1987–2004

universal phenomenon affecting adolescents and adults worldwide. These persons constitute a major reservoir of the disease and are an important source of transmission to infants.

Pertussis is a common cause of prolonged cough illness in adolescents and adults. Active surveillance for pertussis in Canada using a combination of laboratory methods has documented pertussis infection in 10% to 20% of adolescents and adults with a cough illness lasting 7 days or more without improvement. In a placebo-controlled clinical trial of acellular pertussis vaccine conducted in the United States involving 2,781 adults, nine participants from the placebo group developed pertussis in the 2-year follow-up period for an estimated annual rate of 3 per 1,000 person-years. This result was observed during non-epidemic years and would correspond to 60,000 adult cases in Canada annually.

Preparations approved for use in Canada

This chapter will deal only with vaccines that are currently marketed in Canada

- Adacel® (tetanus and diphtheria toxoids adsorbed combined with component pertussis vaccine, [Tdap]), Sanofi Pasteur Ltd.

- Pentacel® (Act-HIB® [*Haemophilus influenzae* b conjugate vaccine (tetanus protein conjugate)] reconstituted with Quadracel®), Sanofi Pasteur Ltd.

- Quadracel® (component pertussis vaccine and diphtheria and tetanus toxoids adsorbed combined with inactivated poliomyelitis vaccine, [DTaP-IPV]), Sanofi Pasteur Ltd.

- Tripacel® (component pertussis vaccine combined with diphtheria and tetanus toxoids adsorbed [classic formulation and hybrid formulation], [DTaP]), Sanofi Pasteur Ltd.

Only acellular vaccines made from purified antigens of *B. pertussis* are now available in Canada; whole-cell preparations are no longer in use. Acellular vaccines have decreased the frequency and severity of both local and systemic adverse reactions compared with whole-cell pertussis vaccines. In Canada, there is no monovalent acellular pertussis vaccine. Pertussis vaccine is only available in combined form with other agents such as diphtheria (D) and tetanus (T) toxoids with or without inactivated polio vaccine (IPV) and/or Hib conjugate vaccine (Hib).

There are two formulations of acellular pertussis vaccine, the infant/pediatric formulation (aP) and the adolescent/adult formulation (ap). The latter contains a lower concentration of pertussis antigens than the former. For the combination vaccines, the diphtheria toxoid is also present in a lower concentration in the adolescent/adult formulation compared with the infant/pediatric formulation. Therefore, Tdap refers to the adolescent/adult

259

formulation, whereas DTaP refers to the infant/pediatric formulation. The infant/pediatric formulation is approved for use in children from 2 months of age until their seventh birthday. The adolescent/adult formulation is approved for use in persons aged 11 to 54 years.

For a list of all approved products in Canada, please refer to Table 1 in the *General Considerations* chapter, page 7.

Efficacy and immunogenicity

Immunologic correlates of protection against pertussis are still not well-defined. In general, all of the acellular pertussis combination vaccines currently approved for use have demonstrated good immunogenicity of their component antigens and decreased reactogenicity when compared with the whole-cell products. It is likely that antibodies to the different component antigens all play a role in protection against clinical disease, pertussis toxoid being a major contributor. All acellular pertussis vaccines approved for use in Canada have an estimated efficacy of approximately 85%. In adults, one clinical trial has shown an efficacy of 92% over the 2.5 years following immunization.

The duration of protection afforded by acellular pertussis vaccines is not known, but the data seem to indicate that protection does not decline during the first 4 years of follow-up. Long-term follow-up will continue for several of the cohorts that participated in the efficacy studies and will guide future recommendations.

Recommended usage

Acellular pertussis vaccine is recommended for all children ≥ 2 months of age for whom there are no contraindications. All adolescents should receive a single booster dose of the adolescent/adult formulation. All adults who have not previously received a dose of acellular vaccine should receive a single dose of Tdap. The prevention of pertussis in adults, particularly if they are in regular contact with infants (health care workers, parents and grandparents of young children), is desirable. The infant/pediatric formulation of acellular pertussis should be used in children < 7 years and the adolescent/adult formulation should be used thereafter. In children ≥ 7 years of age who have not had a primary immunization series or for whom the immunization status is unknown (e.g., immigrant children), the adolescent/adult pertussis-containing formulation should be used.

Persons who have had natural pertussis infection should continue to receive pertussis-containing vaccines. This practice is preferred because the duration of protection induced by pertussis infection is unknown (waning may begin as early as 7 years after infection) and because the diagnosis of pertussis can be difficult to confirm, particularly with test results other than positive culture for *B. pertussis*. There are no data to suggest that administering pertussis vaccines to persons with a history of pertussis is unsafe. As well, continuation of immunization with acellular pertussis vaccine may confer additional benefit to infants < 6 months of age, who often have a suboptimal antibody response to natural pertussis infection.

The primary immunization series should, whenever possible, be completed with the same combination product. However, if the original vaccine is not known or not available, it is recommended that an alternative combination DTaP-IPV/Hib product be used to complete the primary immunization series. The National Advisory Committee on Immunization (NACI) recommends that the DTaP-IPV/Hib and DTaP-IPV combination vaccines currently approved for sale in Canada may be used interchangeably for the 18 month and 4-6 year booster, respectively. Since there is no monovalent acellular pertussis vaccine currently available in Canada, a combination product, Tdap, must be used whenever there is a need for a pertussis booster in adolescents and adults who have recently received Td vaccine. NACI has concluded that there is no evidence of increased risk of severe adverse events for Canadian adolescents after receiving diphtheria and tetanus toxoid-containing vaccines at intervals of < 5 years. In the context of catch-up programs, given the vulnerability of this group to pertussis, the pertussis booster (Tdap) should not be delayed for fear of adverse events related to the diphtheria or tetanus toxoid component. Since the evidence is still limited, post-marketing studies remain a priority.

Outbreak control

Acellular pertussis vaccine has been used safely for the control of pertussis outbreaks in defined populations, such as in schools or hospitals, although data supporting its effectiveness are lacking. If Tdap is considered for people ≥ 7 years to achieve outbreak control, this should be undertaken with evaluation of its effectiveness. Ensuring that all children and adolescents are completely immunized remains the most important preventive measure in maximizing control of pertussis. Establishing that the immunizations of daycare, school and community contacts are up to date should be undertaken by public health authorities.

Contacts

Children exposed to a case should have their immunization status reviewed. If immunization is incomplete and in the absence of contraindications, any necessary doses should be given (see *Schedule and Dosage*).

The role of chemoprophylaxis in the management of contacts is not discussed here. Readers are referred to the proceedings of the 2002 *National Consensus Conference on Pertussis* for further information.

Schedule and dosage

Primary immunization against pertussis with the infant/pediatric formulation (aP) consists of three doses given at 2, 4 and 6 months of age. Booster doses with the infant/pediatric formulation (aP) should be administered at 18 months of age and 4 to 6 years of age. A booster dose with the adolescent/adult formulation (ap) should be administered at 14-16 years of age. It is very important that immunization against pertussis begin at 2 months and be completed on time to ensure that the greatest possible protection is provided to young infants, in whom the disease can be very serious.

Children < 7 years of age not immunized in early infancy should receive three doses of the infant/pediatric formulation (aP) with an interval of 2 months between doses, followed by a fourth dose administered 6-12 months after the third. A booster dose of infant/pediatric formulation (aP) should be administered between 4 and 6 years. This dose is unnecessary if the fourth dose was administered after the fourth birthday. A booster dose with the adolescent/adult formulation (ap) should be given at 14-16 years of age.

When more rapid protection is preferred, the first three doses may be administered at intervals of 4 weeks and the fourth dose given as soon as 6 months after the third dose. The dose to be administered is that recommended by the manufacturer.

For children 7 to 17 years of age who have not been immunized, including immigrants with unknown status, three doses of adolescent/adult formulation of acellular pertussis vaccine (Tdap) should be administered using a 3-dose schedule: at 0 months, 2 months and 6-12 months later. Adults ≥ 18 years of age who have not been immunized, including immigrants with unknown status, should receive a single dose of the adolescent/adult formulation (Tdap) and receive two more doses of Td using the appropriate schedule. After 17 years of age, it is considered unnecessary to give three doses of pertussis vaccine as the probability of having been in contact with pertussis is quite high, in Canada and elsewhere in the world. This recommendation is based on expert opinion since there is a lack of available evidence; further research may modify this.

For adults who have not previously received a dose of acellular pertussis vaccine, it is recommended that the diphtheria-tetanus (Td) booster dose be replaced by the combined Tdap vaccine. The duration of protection induced by acellular pertussis vaccine is unknown, and therefore at this time there is no recommendation for more booster doses. Further research may modify this recommendation.

Please refer to the *Immunization of Immunocompromised Persons* chapter, page 117, for recommendations on hematopoietic stem cell and solid organ transplant recipients.

Route of administration

All combined acellular pertussis vaccines are adsorbed vaccines and must be given intramuscularly.

Booster doses and re-immunization

The recommendations for booster doses vary with age. See *Schedule and Dosage* section.

Serologic testing

There is no indication for pre- or post-immunization serology.

Storage requirements

Pertussis-containing vaccines should be stored at a temperature between +2° and +8° C and should not be frozen. As with all adsorbed vaccines, pertussis-containing vaccines that have been frozen should not be used.

Simultaneous administration with other vaccines

Vaccines that combine antigens against multiple diseases enhance immunization compliance by decreasing the necessary number of injections and visits, and therefore should be encouraged. Acellular pertussis vaccines are available in combination with diphtheria and tetanus toxoids, as well as with inactivated polio vaccine and Hib conjugate vaccine.

If necessary or convenient, vaccines containing acellular pertussis may be administered simultaneously with other inactivated and live vaccines at separate sites and with separate syringes. Not to do so is a missed opportunity and is likely to result in under-immunization. None of the products should be mixed in the same syringe with any other vaccines, unless specifically approved and described in the package insert.

Adverse reactions

Serious adverse events are rare following immunization and, in most cases, data are insufficient to determine a causal association.

The rate of reactions to acellular pertussis vaccines is less than that reported with whole-cell preparations. In clinical trials, the incidence rates of local adverse reactions, including tenderness, erythema, swelling and general reactions of fever, irritability and drowsiness, were significantly lower after immunization with acellular than with whole-cell pertussis vaccines. Less common adverse reactions, such as persistent crying and hypotonic-hypo-responsive episodes, were also less frequent after administration of acellular pertussis vaccines and were reported with a frequency similar to that among recipients of vaccines not containing pertussis. Convulsions were unusual and were reported less often after immunization with acellular pertussis vaccines in some of the efficacy studies but not in others.

The size and frequency of local reactions increase with the number of doses administered. These local reactions produce large swelling, but pain is generally limited. The presence of a large, local reaction to a previous dose should not be considered a contraindication to continuing the recommended schedule.

Contraindications and precautions

Pertussis vaccine should not be given to individuals who have had an anaphylactic reaction to a previous dose or to any constituent of the vaccine. Because these events are so rare, it is not known which component of the combined DTaP-IPV-Hib, DTaP-IPV, DTaP or Tdap is responsible for allergic reactions. Therefore, no further doses of any of the vaccine components should be given unless an assessment by an allergist can determine the responsible antigen or other vaccine component. In order to maximize the child's benefit, an assessment should be done rapidly.

Inactivated vaccines and toxoids are usually considered safe for the fetus, but the effect of administration of Tdap on the development of the embryo and the fetus has not been assessed. Maternal antibody might provide passive protection to the infant in early life; however, the effect of interference by passive maternal antibody on the ability of the infant to mount an adequate response to pediatric DTaP during infancy is unknown. Immunization of a pregnant woman may be warranted when the risk of disease outweighs the risk of vaccine both for the mother and the fetus. If this condition is not met, vaccination should be deferred until after delivery. Health care providers who choose to administer Tdap should discuss with the pregnant woman the lack of data confirming the safety and immunogenicity of Tdap in pregnant women, and the potential benefits and possible adverse effect on the infant.

Although a causal association has not been established between tetanus and Guillain- Barré syndrome (GBS), at the present time it is prudent to withhold subsequent vaccinations in children and adults who develop GBS within 8 weeks of a previous tetanus vaccine dose. Those who develop GBS outside this interval or have an alternative cause identified (e.g., *Campylobacter jejuni* infection) may receive subsequent tetanus vaccinations. As pertussis is given in combination with tetanus vaccine, withholding tetanus would necessitate withholding the pertussis component as well.

Conditions not considered contraindications to pertussis vaccine

Certain other events temporally associated with whole-cell pertussis immunization were at one time considered contraindications or precautions to further pertussis immunization. With the use of acellular vaccine, they are no longer considered contraindications.

◆ High fever within 48 hours of vaccination, attributed to immunization and not to intercurrent illness, indicates the likelihood of recurrence of fever with subsequent doses. Febrile convulsions may be more likely in a susceptible child who develops high fever. However, there are no long-term sequelae from these convulsions, and pertussis immunization can continue.

◆ Afebrile convulsions have not been shown to be caused by pertussis vaccine and are not a contraindication to immunization.

◆ Persistent, inconsolable crying and an unusual, high-pitched cry after pertussis vaccination are not associated with any sequelae and are likely to be pain responses at the site of injection in young infants. These reactions do not preclude further pertussis immunization. Acetaminophen prophylaxis may reduce discomfort with subsequent doses.

◆ Hypotonic-hyporesponsive episodes are not a contraindication to the use of acellular pertussis vaccine. Because these episodes occur after both DTaP and DT, it is difficult to attribute causation to the pertussis components of DTaP; continued immunization with all antigens is recommended.

◆ Onset of encephalopathy temporally related to pertussis immunization does not indicate that the vaccine was the cause. Encephalopathy itself, from whatever cause, is not a contraindication to pertussis immunization. For further information see the *Immunization of Persons with Neurologic Disorders* chapter, page 131.

Selected references

David ST, Hemsley C, Pasquali PE et al. *Enhanced surveillance for vaccine-associated adverse events: dTap catch-up of high school students in Yukon.* Canada Communicable Disease Report 2005;31(11):117-26.

Decker MD, Edwards KM, Steinhoff MC et al. *Comparison of 13 acellular pertussis vaccines: adverse reactions.* Pediatrics 1995;96(3 Pt 2):557-66.

De Serres G, Shadmani R, Boulianne N et al. *Effectiveness of a single dose of acellular pertussis vaccine to prevent pertussis in children primed with pertussis whole cell vaccine.* Vaccine 2001;19(20-22):3004-8.

Edwards KM, Decker MD. *Acellular pertussis vaccines for infants.* New England Journal of Medicine 1996;334(6):391-92.

Edwards KM, Meade BD, Decker MD et al. *Comparison of 13 acellular pertussis vaccines: overview and serologic response.* Pediatrics 1995;96(3 Pt 2):548-57.

Part 4 — Active Immunizing Agents – Pertussis Vaccine

Greco D, Salmaso S, Mastrantonio P et al. *A controlled trial of two acellular vaccines and one whole-cell vaccine against pertussis.* New England Journal of Medicine 1996;334(6):341-48.

Gustafsson L, Hallander HO, Olin P et al. *A controlled trial of a two-component acellular, a five-component acellular, and a whole-cell pertussis vaccine.* New England Journal of Medicine 1996;334(6):349-55.

Halperin SA, Smith B, Russell M et al. *An adult formulation of a five component acellular pertussis vaccine combined with diphtheria and tetanus toxoids is safe and immunogenic in adolescents and adults.* Pediatric Infectious Disease Journal 2000;19(4):276-83.

Health Canada. *National Consensus Conference on Pertussis.* Canada Communicable Disease Report 2003;29(S3):1-39.

Mikelova LK, Halperin SA, Scheifele D et al. *Predictors of death in infants hospitalized with pertussis : a case-control study of 16 pertussis deaths in Canada.* Journal of Pediatrics 2003;143:576-81.

National Advisory Committee on Immunization. *Prevention of pertussis in adolescents and adults.* Canada Communicable Disease Report 2003;29(ACS-5):1-9.

National Advisory Committee on Immunization. *Statement on adult/adolescent formulation of combined acellular pertussis, tetanus, and diphtheria vaccine.* Canada Communicable Disease Report 2000;26(ACS-1):1-8.

National Advisory Committee on Immunization. *Statement on pertussis vaccine.* Canada Communicable Disease Report 1997;23(ACS-3):1-16.

Ntezayabo B, De Serres G, Duval B. *Pertussis resurgence in Canada largely caused by a cohort effect.* Pediatric Infectious Disease Journal 2003;22(1):22-7.

Schmitt HJ, von Konig CH, Neiss A et al. *Efficacy of acellular pertussis vaccine in early childhood after household exposure.* Journal of the American Medical Association 1996;275(1):37-41.

Stehr K, Cherry JD, Heininger U et al. *A comparative efficacy trial in Germany in infants who received either the Lederle-Takeda acellular pertussis component DTP (DTap) vaccine, the Lederle whole-cell component DTP vaccine, or DT vaccine.* Pediatrics 1998;101(1 Pt 1):1-11.

Trollfors B, Taranger J, Lagergard T et al. *A placebo-controlled trial of a pertussis-toxoid vaccine.* New England Journal of Medicine 1995;333(16):1045-50.

Ward JI, Cherry JD, Chang S et al. *Efficacy of an acellular pertussis vaccine among adolescents and adults.* New England Journal of Medicine 2005;353(15):1555-63.

Pneumococcal Vaccine

Streptococcus pneumoniae (pneumococcus) is the leading cause of bacteremia, meningitis, bacterial pneumonia and acute otitis media (AOM) in children. Invasive pneumococcal disease (IPD) is most common in the very young, the elderly and certain specific groups at high risk, such as individuals with functional or anatomic asplenia and congenital or acquired immune deficiency, including those with acquired immune deficiency syndrome (AIDS).

Since the publication of the 2002 *Canadian Immunization Guide*, the pneumococcal conjugate vaccine has been incorporated into the publicly funded immunization programs of all provinces and territories in Canada, and information has become available about the effect of its use on the epidemiology of this infection. The chapter has been updated to reflect this. It also includes specific recommendations for children whose immunization schedule is interrupted and information concerning the utilization of a three-dose infant immunization schedule. Finally, recommendations for re-immunization have been clarified.

Epidemiology

IPD has been nationally notifiable since 2000. Age-specific incidence rates (per 100,000 population per year) during the period 2000 to 2004 were 39.8 among infants < 1 year of age, 24.6 among children 1 to 4 years, and 13.3 among adults ≥ 60 years. Children < 1 year of age accounted for 7% of cases (mean 130 cases per year), those aged 1 to 4 years accounted for 18% (mean 345 cases per year), and adults ≥ 60 years accounted for 37% (mean 711 cases per year) of Canadian IPD cases.

The serotypes contained in the 7-valent vaccine consist of serotypes circulating during the pre-vaccine era in Canada, as follows: > 80% of serotypes isolated from the blood or cerebrospinal fluid (CSF) of children, 95% of serotypes isolated with high level penicillin resistance, and 73% of those isolated with intermediate level resistance. There may be populations or communities, such as Aboriginal children in northern communities, with a different distribution of serotypes.

In northern Canadian regions participating in the International Circumpolar Surveillance project between 1999 and 2004 (i.e., Yukon, Northwest Territories, Nunavut and northern regions of Quebec and Labrador), 62.5% of IPD isolates from children < 2 years of age were serotypes contained in the 7-valent vaccine. Among persons ≥ 65 years of age, 86.4% of isolates obtained were serotypes contained in the 23-valent vaccine. In Nunavut and Northern Quebec, the two regions with universal conjugate programs in place during 2002, there were 19 cases of preventable IPD (i.e., caused by the seven serotypes in the vaccine) among children < 2 years before program implementation (1999-2002) and none after (2003-2004).

The introduction of universal pneumococcal conjugate immunization for infants in the Calgary region of Alberta, in September 2002 led to a prompt and large decline in the incidence of IPD among children < 2 years of age (Figure 11). There has also been a decline in the incidence of IPD caused by the seven serotypes contained in the conjugate vaccine among adults ≥ 65 years (See Figure 12). As in the United States, the magnitude of the decline among older people is likely due to the indirect effect of conjugate vaccine rather than a direct effect of polysaccharide vaccine, because the reduction among adults ≥ 65 years was only for infections caused by serotypes contained in the conjugate vaccine and was larger than any reduction expected from the use of polysaccharide vaccine.

Preparations approved for use in Canada

This chapter will deal only with vaccines that are currently marketed in Canada.

Conjugate vaccine

♦ Prevnar® (pneumococcal 7-valent conjugate vaccine), Wyeth Canada

This pneumococcal conjugate vaccine is approved for use in Canada for children from 6 weeks to 9 years of age and is composed of the purified polysaccharides of the capsular antigens of seven *S. pneumoniae* serotypes,

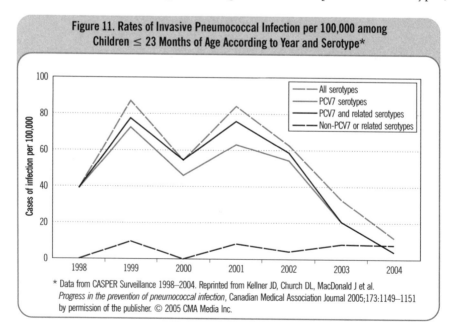

Figure 11. Rates of Invasive Pneumococcal Infection per 100,000 among Children ≤ 23 Months of Age According to Year and Serotype*

* Data from CASPER Surveillance 1998–2004. Reprinted from Kellner JD, Church DL, MacDonald J et al. *Progress in the prevention of pneumococcal infection*, Canadian Medical Association Journal 2005;173:1149–1151 by permission of the publisher. © 2005 CMA Media Inc.

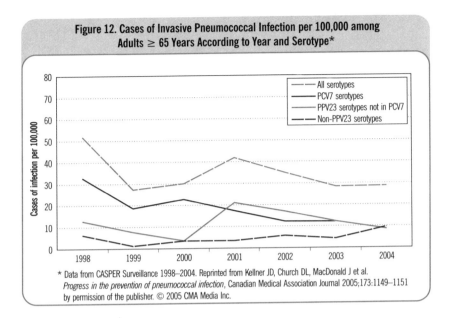

Figure 12. Cases of Invasive Pneumococcal Infection per 100,000 among Adults ≥ 65 Years According to Year and Serotype*

* Data from CASPER Surveillance 1998–2004. Reprinted from Kellner JD, Church DL, MacDonald J et al. *Progress in the prevention of pneumococcal infection*, Canadian Medical Association Journal 2005;173:1149–1151 by permission of the publisher. © 2005 CMA Media Inc.

individually conjugated to CRM197 (cross-reacting material 197), a purified non-toxic variant of diphtheria toxin. The vaccine is manufactured as a liquid suspension. Each 0.5 mL dose of vaccine is formulated to contain 2 μg of each polysaccharide for serotypes 4, 9V, 14, 18C, 19F and 23F, and 4 μg of serotype 6B per dose (16 μg total of polysaccharide); approximately 20 μg of CRM197 carrier protein; and 0.125 mg of aluminum as aluminum phosphate adjuvant. The vaccine contains no thimerosal or other preservatives.

Polysaccharide vaccine

* Pneumovax® 23 (pneumococcal vaccine, 23-valent), Merck Frosst Canada Ltd.

* Pneumo 23® (pneumococcal polysaccharide vaccine), Sanofi Pasteur Ltd.

Both of the two pneumococcal polysaccharide vaccines currently available in Canada contain 25 μg of capsular polysaccharide from each of 23 types of pneumococci: 1, 2, 3, 4, 5, 6B, 7F, 8, 9N, 9V, 10A, 11A, 12F, 14, 15B, 17F, 18C, 19A, 19F, 20, 22F, 23F and 33F (Danish nomenclature). Approximately 90% of cases of pneumococcal bacteremia and meningitis are caused by these 23 types. The six serotypes that are most often found to be resistant to one or more antibiotics are included in this vaccine.

For a list of all approved products in Canada, please refer to Table 1 in the *General Considerations* chapter, page 7.

Efficacy and immunogenicity

Conjugate vaccine

Infants immunized with a three-dose primary series beginning at 2 months of age, with doses separated by 4 to 8 weeks, develop a 3.4- to 20-fold increase in serum antibodies for the vaccine serotypes. The minimum serum antibody concentration necessary for protection against pneumococcal disease has not been determined for any serotype. Functional antibodies are induced in infants together with strong and rapid anamnestic responses upon boosting with either conjugate or polysaccharide vaccines in the 6 to 12 months after the primary series. The observed protective efficacy against invasive disease due to vaccine serotypes is 89% to 97%. Protection against development of AOM ranges from 6% against an episode from any cause to a 34% reduction in pneumococcal-associated AOM and a 54% reduction in AOM due to the serotypes included in the vaccine. A 20% reduction in tympanostomy tube placement has also been observed with the use of the vaccine. The immunogenicity of conjugate pneumococcal vaccine has been demonstrated in children with sickle cell disease and human immunodeficiency virus (HIV) infection.

The long-term efficacy of the conjugate pneumococcal vaccines is not known, but immunologic memory has been demonstrated 18 months after two to three doses in infancy and up to 20 months after one dose in children 2 to 3 years of age.

Polysaccharide vaccine

In healthy young adults, a single dose of polysaccharide vaccine stimulates an antibody response to each of the compound capsular polysaccharides. The immunity conferred is type specific. Efficacy, as measured by serotype-specific protection against IPD, can surpass 80% among healthy young adults. It is in the range of 50% to 80% among the elderly and in specific patient groups, such as those with diabetes mellitus, anatomic or physiologic asplenia, congestive heart failure or chronic pulmonary disease. Antibody response and clinical protection are decreased in certain groups at particularly high risk of pneumococcal infection. These include patients with renal failure, sickle-cell anemia or impaired immune responsiveness, including HIV infection. In general, children < 2 years of age respond poorly to polysaccharide vaccine; safety and effectiveness in children < 2 years have not been established. Following polysaccharide pneumococcal immunization, serotype-specific antibody levels decline after 5 to 10 years and decrease more rapidly in some groups than others. The duration of immunity is not precisely known.

Recommended usage

Conjugate pneumococcal vaccine is recommended for routine administration to all children ≤ 23 months of age. It is also recommended for children 24-59 months of age at higher risk of IPD. High-risk children include those who attend child care centres, are Aboriginal, have sickle cell disease and other sickle cell hemoglobinopathies, have other types of functional or anatomic asplenia, HIV infection, immunocompromising conditions (e.g., primary immunodeficiencies; malignancies; conditions resulting from immunosuppressive therapy, solid organ transplantation, or use of long-term systemic corticosteroids; nephrotic syndrome), chronic medical conditions (e.g., chronic cardiac and pulmonary disease such as bronchopulmonary dysplasia, diabetes mellitus, chronic renal disease or CSF leak) and children with cochlear implants or those receiving cochlear implants. The conjugate vaccine should be considered for all other children in this age group.

Polysaccharide vaccine is not recommended for children < 2 years of age, as it is relatively ineffective, and the conjugate vaccine is superior. Children aged 2 years to < 5 years of age who are at increased risk of IPD (defined earlier) should receive the conjugate vaccine, the polysaccharide vaccine being used as a booster dose in this age group to increase the serotype coverage (see *Schedule and Dosage* below).

Polysaccharide vaccine should be given to all individuals ≥ 5 years of age who have not received the vaccine previously and who are at higher risk of IPD. This includes the conditions defined earlier, as well as cirrhosis and alcoholism. Polysaccharide vaccine should also be given to those who smoke, since they are also at increased risk. When circumstances permit, some experts suggest that the conjugate vaccine may be given as the initial dose followed by the polysaccharide vaccine, as this may theoretically improve antibody response and immunologic memory. However, the polysaccharide vaccine is the vaccine of choice for these individuals, and if only one vaccine can be provided it should be the polysaccharide vaccine.

Polysaccharide pneumococcal vaccine is recommended for all individuals ≥ 65 years of age. Individuals with unknown immunization histories should receive the vaccine.

Immunologic abnormalities may decrease both the antibody response to and protection by either type of vaccine. When possible, vaccine should be given at least 2 weeks before splenectomy or initiation of immunosuppressive therapy and early in the course of HIV infection. Because of the variable vaccine efficacy in certain age groups, those at highest risk (and their families) should be counseled regarding the risk of fulminant pneumococcal sepsis, which may occur despite immunization.

Part 4 — Active Immunizing Agents – Pneumococcal Vaccine

Schedule and dosage

The dose of both the conjugate and the polysaccharide vaccine for all age groups is 0.5 mL.

The recommended optimal schedule for infants is four doses of the conjugate vaccine administered at 2, 4, 6, and 12-15 months of age (Table 11). Children ≤ 6 months should receive the first dose at 2 months of age (minimum age is 6 weeks) and at intervals of approximately 2 months (minimum interval 4 weeks). The fourth dose should be administered after 12 months of age and at least 2 months after the third dose. Infants of very low birth weight (< 1500 grams) should be given their first dose according to their chronological age and not their calculated gestational age. Children 7 to 11 months old who have not been previously immunized against IPD should receive two doses at least 4 weeks apart followed by a third dose after 12 months of age and at least 2 months after the second dose. Children 12 to 23 months of age not previously immunized should receive two doses at least 2 months apart. For children 2 to 5 years old, one dose is sufficient for healthy children, but two doses given 2 months apart is recommended for children with chronic conditions that place them at higher risk of IPD.

Children who present for pneumococcal conjugate immunization after an interruption of their schedule should be assessed to determine the number of doses required to complete the series. This is because the schedule varies by the age of the child. Children who are < 12 months of age when they re-present should complete their immunization schedule as if no interruption had occurred. Children who present at 12 to 23 months of age who have not received a complete primary series (i.e., three doses) require two doses, 2 months apart. Children who present at 12 to 23 months of age who have received the complete primary series (i.e., three doses) only require one dose (i.e., the booster dose). Healthy children who present at ≥ 2 years of age require only one dose.

Table 11. Summary Schedule for Pneumococcal Conjugate Vaccine in Previously Unvaccinated Children

Age at first dose	Primary series	Booster*
2-6 months**	3 doses, 2 months† apart	1 dose at 12 to 15 months of age
7 to 11 months	2 doses, at least 4 weeks apart	1 dose after 12 months of age
12 to 23 months	2 doses, 2 months apart	None
24-59 months		
Healthy children	1 dose	None
High-risk children	2 doses, 2 months apart	

* Booster doses to be given at least 2 months after the final dose of the primary series.

** Minimum age of 6 weeks

† Minimum interval of 4 weeks

When used after administration of the conjugate vaccine, pneumococcal polysaccharide vaccine should be given only after a delay of at least 8 weeks. Polysaccharide vaccine should be administered as a single dose.

Some jurisdictions are considering or have already implemented a three-dose conjugate vaccine schedule at 2, 4 and 12-15 months of age. At this time, the available data do not allow for a direct comparison of the efficacy of the three-dose and the four-dose schedule. The available data indicate that the short-term efficacy of the three-dose schedule after the third dose is comparable. The long-term efficacy of a three-dose schedule has not been determined, but this is generally not known for most vaccines at the time of approval. As the studies evaluating a three-dose schedule were not conducted among children at high risk of IPD, the National Advisory Committee on Immunization (NACI) emphasizes that such children should continue to receive the recommended four-dose schedule in jurisdictions that have implemented a routine three-dose schedule.

Route of administration

The conjugate vaccine is given as an intramuscular injection. The polysaccharide vaccine may be given by either intramuscular or subcutaneous injection.

Booster doses and re-immunization

Conjugate vaccine

Data are not yet available on any decrease in immunity over time following the use of conjugate vaccine in infancy and early childhood, and further booster doses are not thought to be necessary at this time.

Polysaccharide vaccine

Results from serologic and case studies indicate that immunity induced by polysaccharide vaccine decreases over time. At present, routine re-immunization for those who have been vaccinated with polysaccharide vaccine is not recommended. However re-immunization should be considered for those of any age at highest risk of invasive infection, including those with functional or anatomic asplenia or sickle cell disease; hepatic cirrhosis, chronic renal failure or nephrotic syndrome; HIV infection; and immuno-suppression related to disease or therapy. Experience with re-immunization is limited. If re-immunization is carried out, only a single re-immunization is recommended after 5 years in those aged > 10 years at the time of initial immunization with polysaccharide vaccine and after 3 years for those who received the initial vaccine when they were ≤ 10 years of age. See chapter on *Immunization of Immunocompromised Persons*, page 117, for considerations for persons undergoing hematopoietic stem cell transplantation.

Serologic testing

There is no indication for routine pre- or post-immunization serology.

Storage requirements

These vaccines should both be stored, refrigerated, at a temperature of +2° C to +8° C as per the manufacturers' package inserts. Freezing must be avoided.

Simultaneous administration with other vaccines

If necessary or convenient, pneumococcal conjugate vaccine may be administered at the same time as diphtheria, tetanus, acellular pertussis (DTaP), polio (IPV), *Haemophilus influenzae* type b (Hib), hepatitis B, measles, mumps and rubella (MMR), varicella or meningococcal conjugate vaccines, at separate sites and with separate syringes. The pneumococcal polysaccharide vaccine may also be given simultaneously with other vaccines (except the pneumococcal conjugate vaccine) at a separate location and using a separate needle and syringe. When used after administration of the pneumococcal conjugate vaccine, pneumococcal polysaccharide vaccine should be administered only after a delay of at least 8 weeks. Similarly, when used after administration of pneumococcal polysaccharide vaccine, pneumococcal conjugate vaccine should be delayed by at least 8 weeks. Providers should be aware that minimal safety or efficacy data are available regarding these sequences.

Adverse reactions

Conjugate vaccine

The pneumococcal conjugate vaccine is generally well tolerated when administered at the same time as other childhood vaccines. Fever has been reported more frequently among children receiving their primary immunization series when conjugate vaccine was included. Few serious side effects have been reported. Redness, swelling and tenderness at the injection site may occur; this might be more commonly reported in recipients of multiple injections. The severity or frequency of these reactions has not been found to increase with subsequent doses in the primary series or with booster doses.

Polysaccharide vaccine

Reactions to the pneumococcal polysaccharide vaccine are usually mild. Local soreness and erythema are quite common. Occasionally, slight fever may occur. Re-immunization of healthy adults < 2 years after the initial dose is associated with increased local and systemic reactions. Subsequent studies have suggested that revaccination after intervals of $\geq$ 4 years is not associated with an increased incidence of adverse side effects. Severe local reactions are rare.

Contraindications and precautions

Anaphylactic reaction to pneumococcal conjugate vaccine or pneumococcal polysaccharide vaccine is a contraindication to re-immunization with that product.

Neither pregnancy nor breast-feeding is a contraindication to pneumococcal polysaccharide vaccine.

Conjugate vaccines containing CRM197 should not be considered as immunizing agents against diphtheria, and no changes in the schedule for administering vaccines containing diphtheria toxoid are recommended.

Other considerations: strategies to improve vaccine utilization

Immunization is a safe and effective means of preventing IPD among individuals at increased risk of serious illness or death. It offers a partial solution to the emerging problem of disease caused by strains resistant to antibiotics. In general, immunization recommendations for young children are well followed. However, surveys show that less than 5% of the population > 2 years of age at increased risk have received the polysaccharide vaccine. Several provinces and territories have initiated programs to make the polysaccharide pneumococcal vaccine more readily available to target populations.

Recommended strategies for delivering pneumococcal vaccine to individuals at higher risk of invasive disease include the following:

♦ Ensuring that all recipients of influenza vaccine are also immunized with pneumococcal vaccine, if appropriate. Providers should have both vaccines available to facilitate concurrent administration.

♦ Implementing standing orders for pneumococcal immunization of residents on admission to long-term care facilities, if indicated.

♦ Implementing standing orders in hospitals for pneumococcal immunization of patients in high-risk groups to be immunized on discharge or during ambulatory visits.

♦ Delivering pneumococcal vaccine in adult day care and community centres to people at risk.

♦ Promoting pneumococcal and influenza immunization programs concurrently to both consumers and providers.

Selected references

American Academy of Pediatrics. Committee on Infectious Diseases. *Policy statement: recommendations for the prevention of pneumococcal infections, including the use of pneumococcal conjugate vaccine (Prevnar), pneumococcal polysaccharide vaccine, and antibiotic prophylaxis.* Pediatrics 2000;106:362-66.

American Academy of Pediatrics. Committee on Infectious Diseases. *Technical report: prevention of pneumococcal infections, including the use of pneumococcal conjugate and polysaccharide vaccines and antibiotic prophylaxis.* Pediatrics 2000;106(2 Pt1):367-76.

Black S, Shinefield H, Fireman B et al. *Efficacy, safety and immunogenicity of heptavalent pneumococcal conjugate vaccine in children.* Pediatric Infectious Disease Journal 2000;19(3):187-95.

Butler JC, Breiman RF, Campbell JF et al. *Pneumococcal polysaccharide vaccine efficacy: an evaluation of current recommendations.* Journal of the American Medical Association 1993;270(15):1826-31.

Centers for Disease Control and Prevention. *Direct and indirect effects of routine vaccination of children with 7-valent pneumococcal conjugate vaccine on incidence of invasive pneumococcal disease – United States, 1998-2003.* Morbidity and Mortality Weekly Report 2005;54(36):893-97.

Eskola J, Anttila M. *Pneumococcal conjugate vaccines.* Pediatric Infectious Disease Journal 1999;18(6):543-51.

Eskola J, Kilpi T, Palmu A et al. *Efficacy of a pneumococcal conjugate vaccine against acute otitis media.* New England Journal of Medicine 2001;334(6):403-09.

Fine MJ, Smith MA, Carson CA et al. *Efficacy of pneumococcal vaccination in adults: a meta-analysis of randomized clinical trials.* Archives of Internal Medicine 1994;154(23):2666-77.

Kellner JD, Church DL, MacDonald J et al. *Progress in the prevention of pneumococcal infection.* Canadian Medical Association Journal 2005;173(10):1149-51.

National Advisory Committee on Immunization. *Statement on recommended use of pneumococcal conjugate vaccine.* Canada Communicable Disease Report 2002;28(ACS-2):1-32.

National Advisory Committee on Immunization. *Statement on the recommended use of pneumococcal conjugate vaccine: addendum.* Canada Communicable Disease Report 2003; 29(ACS-8):14-5.

Rodriguez R, Dyer PD. *Safety of pneumococcal revaccination.* Journal of General Internal Medicine 1995;10(9):511-12.

Scheifele D, Halperin S, Pelletier L et al. *Invasive pneumococcal infections in Canadian children 1991-1998: implications for new vaccination strategies.* Clinical Infectious Diseases 2000;31(1):58-64.

Shapiro ED, Berg AT, Austrain R et al. *The protective efficacy of polyvalent pneumococcal polysaccharide vaccine.* New England Journal of Medicine 1991;325(21):1453-60.

Shinefield HR, Black S, Ray P et al. *Safety and immunogenicity of heptavalent pneumococcal CRM197 conjugate vaccine in infants and toddlers.* Pediatric Infectious Disease Journal 1999;18(9):757-63.

Poliomyelitis Vaccine

Poliomyelitis is a disease that may cause irreversible paralysis in less than 1% of infected individuals. It is a highly infectious disease caused by three serotypes of poliovirus. It is spread from person to person principally through the fecal-oral route. The virus is extremely stable and can remain viable in the environment for long periods of time. Following the introduction of inactivated poliovirus vaccines (IPV) in Canada in 1955 and of trivalent oral poliovirus vaccine (OPV) in 1962, indigenously acquired disease has been eliminated (see Figure 13).

Changes since the publication of the 2002 *Canadian Immunization Guide* include 1) information on the global polio eradication initiative, 2) removal of OPV from the market in Canada but continued use in developing countries, and 3) a change in the guidelines for IPV use in outbreaks and in travellers.

Epidemiology

In Canada

Canada was certified polio-free in 1994. The last major Canadian epidemic of wild poliovirus occurred in 1959, with 1,887 paralytic cases reported. Smaller clusters occurred after that time. In 1978-79, there were 11 paralytic cases among unimmunized individuals in religious groups in Ontario, Alberta and British Columbia, who had contact with imported cases. In 1993, 22 asymptomatic persons with imported wild polio infection were found in the same religious group in Alberta, and in 1996 an asymptomatic person was reported in Ontario. In none of these instances was spread of the virus seen outside the unimmunized groups, presumably because of high levels of immunization in the rest of the population, nor did cases of clinical illness occur in the affected communities in Canada.

More recent cases of paralytic poliomyelitis in Canada have been associated with OPV use. Eleven of 12 paralytic cases in Canada reported between 1980 and 1995 were vaccine associated paralytic poliomyelitis (VAPP). Eight occurred in the contacts of vaccinated persons (three confirmed and five possible), and one was a confirmed vaccine recipient. The remaining two cases were not reviewed but occurred in known contacts of OPV-vaccinated children. Vaccine programs in Canada switched from OPV to IPV in 1995/1996; the last VAPP case occurred in 1995.

In 1985, the Pan American Health Organization (PAHO) adopted a goal of elimination of poliomyelitis from the Americas, and this goal was achieved in 1994. To ensure that Canada remains polio-free, the Public Health Agency of Canada reviews surveillance data for acute flaccid paralysis (AFP) col-

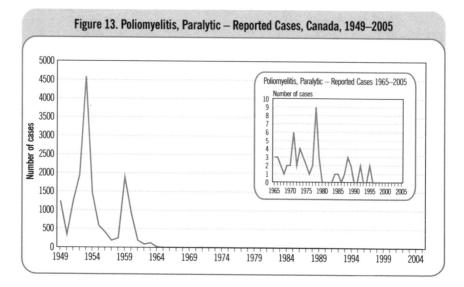

Figure 13. Poliomyelitis, Paralytic – Reported Cases, Canada, 1949–2005

lected by the Immunization Monitoring Program ACTive (IMPACT) system and the Canadian Paediatric Surveillance Program (CPSP), operated by the Canadian Paediatric Society. From 1996 to 2004, between 30 and 63 cases of AFP in children < 15 years of age were reported to the CPSP each year, none attributed to wild or vaccine-derived poliovirus.

The global polio eradication initiative

The World Health Organization (WHO) initially established a goal for the global eradication of polio by 2000. This was amended to 2005 and subsequently to 2008, because polio cases continued to occur in south Asia and west/central Africa. The temporary suspension of OPV vaccination in northern Nigeria in 2003-04 resulted in an outbreak that spread to 14 previously polio-free countries, and wild poliovirus transmission was re-established in six previously polio-free countries. In 2005, three out of six WHO regions have achieved polio eradication: the Americas, the Western Pacific and the European regions.

The WHO's eradication strategy for 2004-08 consists of the following steps: (a) interrupting poliovirus transmission in 2004-05 by increasing OPV coverage in epidemic areas using national immunization days and "mop-up" campaigns, (b) ensuring that there is access to WHO-accredited laboratories for AFP surveillance, (c) achieving certification of global polio eradication in all regions by 2006-08, (d) cessation of OPV use by 2006-08 to prevent circulation of vaccine-derived poliovirus, and (e) ensuring that all regions conduct proper laboratory containment of wild and vaccine-derived polioviruses.

To manage unforeseen outbreaks, WHO may develop a stockpile of the current trivalent OPV or monovalent OPV (mOPV) for each of the three serotypes of poliovirus. The advantage of mOPV is that it would induce mucosal immunity to the specific outbreak strain and would not result in the ongoing circulation of the remaining two vaccine strains in the community. However, mOPV is not available in North America. The alternative is to establish an adequate supply of IPV to vaccinate susceptible individuals.

Preparations approved for use in Canada

This chapter will deal only with vaccines that are currently marketed in Canada.

◆ DT Polio Adsorbed (diphtheria and tetanus toxoids adsorbed and polio-myelitis vaccine), Sanofi Pasteur Ltd.

◆ Inactived Poliomyelitis Vaccine [IPV], Sanofi Pasteur Ltd.

◆ Pentacel® (Act-HIB® [*Haemophilus influenzae* b conjugate vaccine (teta-nus protein conjugate)] reconstituted with Quadracel®), Sanofi Pasteur Ltd.

◆ Quadracel® (component pertussis vaccine and diphtheria and tetanus toxoids adsorbed combined with inactivated poliomyelitis vaccine, [DTaP-IPV]), Sanofi Pasteur Ltd.

◆ Td Polio Adsorbed (tetanus and diphtheria toxoids and inactivated polio-myelitis vaccine adsorbed), Sanofi Pasteur Ltd.

Only IPV is currently marketed in Canada and recommended for routine use. All provinces and territories use IPV in routine immunization programs. OPV is no longer recommended because most cases of paralytic polio from 1980 to 1995 were associated with OPV. Furthermore, OPV is no longer marketed in Canada.

IPV preparations are produced either in Vero cells or in human diploid (MRC-5) cells. All are formalin-inactivated products with enhanced potency and are significantly more immunogenic than the first-generation IPV. They each contain the three types of wild poliovirus: type 1 (Mahoney), type 2 (MEF-1) and type 3 (Saukett). Streptomycin, polymyxin B and neomycin may be present as preservatives.

For a list of all approved products in Canada, please refer to Table 1 in the *General Considerations* chapter, page 7.

Efficacy and immunogenicity

IPV produces immunity to all three types of poliovirus in over 90% of people following two doses of vaccine given at least 4-8 weeks apart, and in close to 100% following a booster given 6 to 12 months later.

Recommended usage

Infants and children

To avoid the risk of VAPP, the exclusive use of IPV for routine immunization is recommended in Canada.

Adults

Routine polio immunization is not considered necessary for previously unimmunized adults in Canada who do not intend to travel to areas in which polio outbreaks occur, as there is a negligible risk of exposure to wild polioviruses in the Americas.

Exposure to wild polioviruses

Immunization with IPV is recommended for previously unimmunized adults and children who may be or are exposed to wild polioviruses. These include

- travellers to areas of countries where these viruses are circulating;
- residents of communities in which a visitor or new refugee/immigrant may be excreting the viruses;
- health care workers in close contact with individuals who may be excreting the viruses;
- laboratory workers handling specimens that may contain the viruses.

Schedule and dosage

Children (< 18 years of age)

For routine immunization beginning in infancy, four doses of IPV are recommended, in combination with other routinely administered vaccines (diphtheria, tetanus, acellular pertussis (DTaP) and *Haemophilus influenzae* type b (Hib)) at 2 months, 4 months, 18 months and 4 to 6 years of age (pre-school booster). The fourth dose is not needed if the third dose is given on or after the fourth birthday. It is acceptable to give an additional dose of IPV at 6 months of age for convenience of administration in combination with DTaP and Hib.

For unimmunized children > 4 years of age, two doses of IPV plus a third dose constitute a complete series. The first two doses of IPV are recommended 4 to 8 weeks apart, followed by a third dose 6 to 12 months later. For children who began their polio immunization series in a country where OPV was used, immunization may be completed in Canada using IPV, and there is no need to re-start the series.

No additional doses of IPV are recommended for traveling children whose primary series of IPV is complete. Previously unimmunized children exposed to imported wild polio or traveling to areas with polio outbreaks should start the primary series of IPV, with due consideration given to a more accelerated schedule (i.e. three doses with only 4 to 6 weeks between each dose). If IPV cannot be secured, children traveling in a region where OPV is available may receive the necessary doses of OPV to complete their series. These parents should be informed that there is a small risk of VAPP with OPV (see *Adverse Reactions*, below).

Adults (≥ 18 years of age)

Adults who completed the primary series of IPV or OPV during childhood and are traveling to developed countries (e.g., North America, Europe, Mediterranean, Japan, Australia, New Zealand) do not require a booster of IPV. However, those traveling to areas that have wild polio or vaccine-derived poliovirus outbreaks should receive a single booster of IPV.

Unimmunized adults or those with unknown polio immunization history who may be exposed to imported wild polio cases in Canada or who are traveling to areas where there are polio outbreaks should receive two doses of IPV, given 4 to 8 weeks apart, with a third dose 6-12 months later. Travelers departing in less than 4 weeks should receive the first dose of IPV and the remaining doses later, at the recommended intervals. Incompletely immunized adults who have previously received less than a full primary course of IPV or OPV should receive the remaining dose(s) of poliovirus vaccine as IPV, regardless of the interval since the last dose.

Route of administration

IPV is injected subcutaneously according to the dose specified in the manufacturer's package insert. Combination vaccines must be administered intramuscularly because of the presence of adsorbed tetanus and diphtheria toxoids.

Booster doses and re-immunization

The need for booster doses of poliovirus vaccine in fully immunized adults has not been demonstrated. Hence, booster doses of vaccine are not *routinely* recommended for adults who have completed the primary series during childhood. For those at high risk of exposure to polio (e.g., military personnel, workers in refugee camps in endemic areas, travelers to areas where there are epidemics), a single booster dose of IPV is recommended.

Children and adults who undergo hematopoietic stem cell or bone marrow transplantation will lose any previously acquired immunity to poliovirus after the transplantation. These patients require three doses of IPV to reconstitute their immunity to poliovirus, starting 12 months after the transplantation. Please refer to the *Immunization of Immunocompromised Persons* chapter, page 117, for the recommended intervals.

Serologic testing

There is no indication for pre- or post-immunization serology.

Storage requirements

IPV-containing vaccines should be stored in the refrigerator at a temperature of +2° C to +8° C. The vaccine should not be frozen.

Simultaneous administration with other vaccines

IPV vaccine, usually given in combination as DTaP-IPV or DTaP-IPV-Hib, may be given at the same time as measles, mumps and rubella (MMR), varicella, pneumococcal conjugate, meningococcal C conjugate, hepatitis B vaccines and influenza vaccines at separate sites and with a separate needle and syringes. IPV may be simultaneously given with the adolescent Tdap vaccine, but at separate sites and with separate syringes.

Adverse reactions

Serious adverse events are rare following immunization and, in most cases, the data are insufficient to determine a causal association.

The side effects of currently available IPV are normally limited to minor local reactions. As with all vaccines, anaphylaxis has been reported rarely. OPV may cause paralytic disease in recipients and incompletely immunized contacts at a rate of approximately 1 per 2.4 million doses distributed. Individuals travelling or living abroad whose children may be exposed to OPV should be made aware of this risk.

Contraindications and precautions

IPV should not be administered to people who have experienced an anaphylactic reaction to a previous dose of IPV, streptomycin, polymyxin B or neomycin. IPV can be given without risk to those who are immunodeficient or immunosuppressed and to people who will have household or close contact with such people. Less than optimal protection may be induced in those who are immunocompromised.

There are no contraindications to the use of IPV in susceptible women who are either pregnant or lactating. However, there is no reason to use IPV during pregnancy (a primary series or a booster dose), unless there is significant risk of exposure to poliovirus (e.g., travel to a country experiencing wild polio cases, or exposure to an imported polio case within Canada).

Selected references

American Academy of Pediatrics, Committee on Infectious Diseases. *Prevention of poliomyelitis: recommendations for use of only inactivated poliovirus vaccine for routine immunization.* Pediatrics 1999;104(6):1404-6.

Caceres VM, Sutter RW. *Sabin monovalent oral polio vaccines: review of past experiences and their potential use after polio eradication.* Clinical Infectious Diseases 2001;33(4):531-41.

Carlson J, Bell A, Cashman N et al. Health Canada Working Group on Polio Eradication. *Protocol for the investigation of acute flaccid paralysis and suspected paralytic poliomyelitis.* Canada Communicable Disease Report 1998;24(4):25-30.

Centers for Disease Control and Prevention. *Isolation of wild poliovirus type 3 among members of a religious community objecting to vaccination – Alberta, Canada, 1993.* Morbidity and Mortality Weekly Report 1993;42(17):337-39.

Centers for Disease Control and Prevention. *Epidemiologic notes and reports follow-up on poliomyelitis – United States, Canada, Netherlands.* Morbidity and Mortality Weekly Report 1997;46(50):1195-99.

Centers for Disease Control and Prevention. *Poliomyelitis prevention in the United States: updated recommendations of the Advisory Committee on Immunization Practices (ACIP).* Morbidity and Mortality Weekly Report 2000;49(RR-5):1-22.

Committee to Advise on Tropical Medicine and Travel (CATMAT). *Poliomyelitis vaccination for international travellers.* Canada Communicable Disease Report 2003;29(ACS-10):1-7.

Modlin JF, Halsey NA, Thomas ML et al. *Humoral and mucosal immunity in infants induced by three sequential inactivated poliovirus vaccine-live attenuated oral poliovirus vaccine immunization schedules.* Journal of Infectious Diseases 1997;175(Suppl 1):S228-34.

NVAC-ACIP Joint Working Group and Centers for Disease Control and Prevention. *Ensuring preparedness for potential poliomyelitis outbreaks: recommendations for the US poliovirus vaccine stockpile from the National Vaccine Advisory Committee and the Advisory Committee on Immunization Practices.* Archives of Pediatrics and Adolescent Medicine 2004;158(12):1106-12.

Patriarca PA, Sutter RW, Oostvogel PM. *Outbreaks of paralytic poliomyelitis, 1976-1995.* Journal of Infectious Diseases 1997;175(Suppl 1):S165-72.

Plotkin SA, Orenstein WA. *Vaccines.* 3rd edition. Philadelphia: W.B. Saunders Company, 1999.

Part 4 — Active Immunizing Agents – Poliomyelitis Vaccine

Rutty CJ, Barreto L, Van Exan R et al. *Conquering the crippler: Canada and the eradication of polio.* Canadian Journal of Public Health 2005;96(2):I2-24.

Varughese PV and Canadian Paediatric Society. Acute flaccid paralysis. In: *Canadian Paediatric Surveillance Program (CPSP): 2003 results.* Ottawa: CPS, 2003.

Varughese PV, Carter AO, Acres SE et al. *Eradication of indigenous poliomyelitis in Canada: impact of immunization strategies.* Canadian Journal of Public Health 1989;80(5):363-68.

Vidor E, Meschievitz C, Plotkin S. *Fifteen years of experience with Vero-produced enhanced potency inactivated poliovirus vaccine.* Pediatric Infectious Disease Journal 1997;16(3):312-22.

World Health Organization. *Acute flaccid paralysis surveillance: a global platform for detecting and responding to priority infectious diseases.* Weekly Epidemiological Record 2004;79(48):425-32.

World Health Organization. *Global polio eradication initiative, strategic plan 2004-2008.* Weekly Epidemiological Record 2004;79(6):55-7.

World Health Organization. *Progress towards global eradication of poliomyelitis, 2003 and January-April 2004.* Weekly Epidemiological Record 2004;79(25):229-34.

Rabies Vaccine

Rabies is a neurotropic viral infection that has two clinical presentations and is a fatal disease. After infection, the usual incubation period is 20 to 60 days, although it may vary from several days to years. The more common, agitated (furious) form presents with the classic symptoms of hydrophobia or aerophobia with a rapidly progressing encephalitis and death. The paralytic form of the disease manifests as progressive flaccid paralysis, has a more protracted course and is more difficult to diagnose.

Since the publication of the 2002 *Canadian Immunization Guide*, a new rabies vaccine product has become available, and new recommendations have been made regarding the intradermal administration of rabies vaccine in certain pre-exposure situations.

Epidemiology

Human rabies

In 2000 and 2003, two people in Canada died of rabies infection, one in Quebec (2000) and one in British Columbia (2003). These were the first cases of human rabies in Canada since 1985. The most likely sources of infection for both of these people were unrecognized bat exposures. Since 1924, a total of 23 people in six provinces have died of rabies in Canada (Figure 14): Quebec (12), Ontario (6), Saskatchewan (2) and Alberta, British Columbia and Nova Scotia (1 case each). In 2004, the US Centers for Disease Control and Prevention confirmed the first reported case of rabies following solid organ transplantation.

Animal rabies

The rabies virus can infect any mammal. In North America, it occurs mainly in certain wild terrestrial carnivore species and can spread to domestic livestock and pets. Over the past few years the overall number of animal rabies cases in Canada has been steadily decreasing. There remain regional differences in the prevalence of animal rabies across the country, and the specific species infected in each region vary over time. For up-to-date details on animal rabies activity in Canada, please see the Canadian Food Inspection Agency (CFIA) Web site (http://www.inspection.gc.ca/english/anima/heasan/disemala/rabrag/statse.shtml).

During the past 6 years (2000-2005) a total of 2,238 cases of confirmed animal rabies were reported in Canada (average: 373 per year). Skunks accounted for 40% of the total cases, followed by bats (26%), foxes (11%) and raccoons (8%). Bat rabies was detected in most regions across Canada, except the three territories and Prince Edward Island (PEI). Three provinces accounted for the majority of cases: Ontario (43%), Manitoba (24%) and Saskatchewan (14%). The species most affected, by region, during the 6-year period were as follows: skunks in Manitoba (434/540 or 80%) and Saskatchewan (243/316 or 77%); bats in British Columbia (91/95 or 96%), Alberta (20/21 or 95%) and Quebec (66/118 or 56%); foxes in the Northwest Territories/Nunavut (57/74 or 77%) and Newfoundland/Labrador (33/44 or 75%); and raccoons in New Brunswick (55/70 or 79%). In Ontario the most affected species were bats (356/956 or 37%) and skunks (226/956 or 24%). Over the past 6 years, PEI reported one case of animal rabies (cat), and Nova Scotia reported three. Yukon had no reported cases of animal rabies. Spread to domestic species of animals, such as pets (e.g., cats and dogs) and livestock (horses and cows) has occurred. Dogs and cats accounted for 4.5% of animal rabies cases.

Bat rabies has accounted for 58% of the human rabies cases in the United States since 1980 and appears to be increasing in frequency. The increased incidence is due, in part, to the failure to recognize the small wound inflicted by a biting bat and thus omission of post-exposure prophylaxis. In most of the recently reported cases, there has not been a history of a bat bite although there has been contact, either recognized or unrecognized at the onset of the illness, with infected colonies. In the past, four cases were thought to have been acquired through aerosolized virus across mucous membranes.

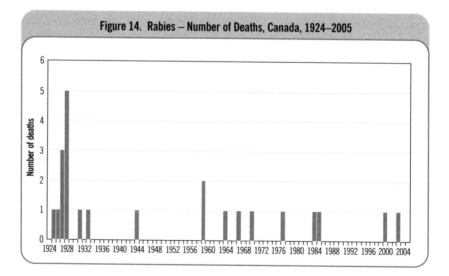

Figure 14. Rabies – Number of Deaths, Canada, 1924–2005

Preparations approved for use in Canada

This chapter will deal only with vaccines that are currently marketed in Canada.

Two rabies vaccines are currently marketed for active immunization of humans in Canada:

◆ Imovax® Rabies, Sanofi Pasteur Ltd

◆ RabAvert®, Merck Frosst (distributor)

Both products may be used for pre-exposure and post-exposure prophylaxis. Imovax® Rabies is prepared from rabies virus grown in human diploid cell culture (HDCV), concentrated by ultrafiltration and then inactivated with beta-propiolactone. Sterile diluent is supplied for reconstitution into a single 1.0 mL dose. RabAvert is a purified chick embryo cell vaccine (PCECV) produced by growing the fixed-virus strain Flury low egg passage in primary cultures of chicken fibroblasts. The virus is inactivated with beta-propiolactone and processed by zonal centrifugation. The vaccine has no preservative. Sterile diluent is supplied for reconstitution into a single 1.0 mL dose.

Two human rabies immune globulin (RabIg) products are approved in Canada for passive immunization. RabIg is concentrated by cold ethanol fractionation from the plasma of hyperimmunized donors and undergoes multiple procedures for human viral pathogen clearance during preparation. It is supplied at a standardized concentration of 150 IU per mL. Please refer to the *Passive Immunizing Agents* chapter, page 353, for more information on immune globulin products.

For a list of all approved products in Canada, please refer to Table 1 in the *General Considerations* chapter, page 7.

Pre-exposure management

Pre-exposure rabies immunization with either HDCV or PCECV should be offered to people at potentially high risk of contact with rabid animals, e.g., certain laboratory workers, veterinarians, animal control and wildlife workers, spelunkers, and persons hunting and trapping in high-risk areas. Travellers to endemic areas where there is poor access to adequate and safe post-exposure management should consider pre-travel immunization. As well, children who are too young to understand either the need to avoid animals or to report a traumatic contact are considered at greater risk of rabid animal exposure and should be offered pre-exposure immunization when travelling to endemic areas (please refer to the *Immunization of Travellers* chapter, page 136, for more information).

Part 4 — Active Immunizing Agents – Rabies Vaccine

Post-exposure management

HDCV or PCECV together with RabIg and local treatment are highly effective in preventing rabies in exposed individuals. No post-exposure failures have occurred in Canada or the United States. The few reported failures elsewhere in the world have been attributed to delay in treatment, lack of appropriate cleansing of wounds, suboptimal methods of immunization or omission of passive immunization. Responses to vaccines received in other countries may be less predictable.

Rabies prophylaxis must be considered in every incident in which potential animal exposure to rabies virus has occurred, unless rabies is known to be absent from the local animal population. In evaluating each case, local public health officials should be consulted. If there has been no exposure, as described below, post-exposure treatment is not indicated.

1. Species of animal

The animals in Canada most often proven rabid are wild terrestrial carnivores (skunks, foxes and raccoons), bats, cattle, and stray dogs and cats. As the distribution of animal rabies and the species involved vary considerably across Canada it is important to consult the local medical officer of health or government veterinarian in cases of possible exposure. Human exposures to livestock are usually confined to salivary contamination, with the exception of horses and swine, from which bites have been reported. The risk of infection after exposure to rabid cattle is low. Squirrels, hamsters, guinea-pigs, gerbils, chipmunks, rats, mice or other rodents, rabbits and hares are only rarely found to be infected with rabies and are not known to have caused human rabies in North America; post-exposure prophylaxis should be considered only if the animal's behaviour was highly unusual.

The manifestations of rabies and the incubation periods vary in different species. The length of time virus may be excreted in saliva before the development of symptoms has not been determined for the purpose of defining rabies exposure except in domestic dogs, cats and ferrets. In these animals, rabies virus excretion does not generally precede symptom development beyond 10 days. It remains unclear as to whether asymptomatic carriage of rabies virus in wild animals is possible.

2. Type of exposure

Rabies is transmitted when the virus is inoculated into tissues. This occurs most commonly through bites, although when cuts or wounds are contaminated by rabies virus from saliva or infected tissue, transmission is possible. Rarely, transmission has been recorded when virus was inhaled, or infected grafts/organs were transplanted into patients. Thus, three broad categories of exposure are recognized as warranting post-exposure prophylaxis: bite, non-bite and bat exposures.

Bite: This is defined as any penetration of the skin by teeth. Bites inflicted by most animals are readily apparent with the exception of bats (see below). Wild or stray animals, or any domestic animal behaving unusually should never be handled by untrained individuals. Children should be taught this.

Non-bite: This category includes contamination of scratches, abrasions or cuts of the skin or mucous membranes by saliva or other potentially infectious material, such as the brain tissue of a rabid animal. Petting a rabid animal or handling its blood, urine or feces is not considered to be an exposure, but such contact should be avoided. Being sprayed by a skunk is also not considered an exposure. These incidents do not warrant post-exposure prophylaxis.

Exposures incurred in the course of caring for humans with rabies could theoretically transmit the infection. No case of rabies acquired in this way has been documented, but post-exposure prophylaxis should be considered for exposed individuals.

Bat exposures: Recently, the majority of individuals who have died in North America from bat rabies have not had a bite history or even, in several situations, a known bat exposure history. In addition, bites inflicted by bats to a sleeping person may not be felt, and may leave no visible bite marks. Hence, when people are sleeping unattended in a room where a bat is found, when there has been close contact with bats or when the possibility of a bite cannot be reasonably excluded – e.g., if a bat is discovered in proximity to an individual who is cognitively impaired or near a young child – post-exposure prophylaxis should be initiated. Bats should never be handled with bare hands.

Four cases of rabies were thought to have been acquired through aerosolized virus across mucous membranes. However, each of these likely had exposure to large quantities of aerosolized virus, as two were spelunkers and two laboratory workers. Post-exposure prophylaxis is therefore warranted and recommended in rare instances of non-bite exposure, such as inhalation of aerosolized virus by spelunkers exploring caves inhabited by infected bats or by laboratory technicians homogenizing tissues infected with rabies virus; however, the efficacy of prophylaxis after such exposures is unknown.

3. Investigation of the incident

Each incident of possible exposure requires a full investigation. This should include an assessment of the risk of rabies in the animal species involved and, in a low prevalence area such as Canada, the behaviour of the particular domestic animal implicated. An unprovoked attack is more likely to indicate that the animal is rabid. Nevertheless, rabid cats and dogs may become uncharacteristically quiet. Bites inflicted on a person attempting to feed or handle an apparently healthy animal should generally be regarded as provoked.

Domestic pets with up-to-date rabies vaccination are unlikely to become infected with rabies. If vaccinated animals exhibit signs suggestive of rabies they must be carefully evaluated by a veterinarian.

Any animal that has bitten a human and/or is suspected of being rabid should be reported to the local medical officer of health and to the nearest CFIA veterinarian. These veterinarians are familiar with the regulations concerning rabies and, if necessary, will collect and ship appropriate specimens to a federal laboratory for diagnosis. Further information and advice is obtainable from the CFIA regional offices or local district office on the CFIA Web site (www.inspection.gc.ca/english/anima/heasan/offbure.shtml) or by consulting the blue pages of the local telephone directory.

Signs of rabies cannot be reliably interpreted in wild animals. These animals, as well as stray or unwanted dogs or cats and other biting animals, should immediately be humanely killed in a way that does as little damage as possible to the head, which should be submitted for laboratory examination. For advice regarding appropriate killing of animals please call your local public health office. A domestic dog, cat or ferret that is evaluated by a veterinarian and determined to be normal should be kept under secure observation for 10 days even if it has a history of vaccination. If the animal is still clinically well after that time, it can be concluded that it was not shedding rabies virus at the time of the exposure and was therefore non-infectious. If illness suggestive of rabies develops during the holding period, the animal should be humanely killed and the head submitted for examination. Rabies virus is only readily demonstrable in brains of animals that have neurologic symptoms.

If the animal escapes during the 10-day observation period, the need for post-exposure prophylaxis should be carefully re-assessed. Exotic pets (other than ferrets) should be treated as wild animals because the incubation period and period of rabies virus shedding in these animals are unknown. Recent information regarding the pathogenesis of rabies in domestic ferrets has prompted them to be considered in the same category as domestic dogs and cats rather than wild carnivores.

Management of people after possible exposure to rabies

Table 12 outlines the recommendations for the management of people after possible exposure to rabies. These recommendations are intended as a guide and may need to be modified in accordance with the specific circumstances of the exposure.

Immediate washing and flushing of the wound with soap and water is imperative and is probably the most effective procedure in the prevention of rabies. Suturing the wound should be avoided if possible. Tetanus prophylaxis and antibacterial drugs should be given as required.

If a rabies exposure is considered likely then post-exposure prophylaxis should never be delayed. If an observed animal such as a cat, dog or domestic ferret remains asymptomatic over a 10-day period or the animal is tested and there is no pathologic evidence of rabies, the course can be discontinued.

Table 12. Post-exposure Prophylaxis for Persons Not Previously Immunized Against Rabies

Animal species	Condition of animal at time of exposure	Management of exposed person
Dog, cat or ferret	Healthy and available for 10 days' observation	1. Local treatment of wound 2. At first sign of rabies in animal, give RabIg (local and intramuscular) and start HDCV or PCECV, unless bite wound to the head or neck (begin immediately)
	Rabid or suspected to be rabid*. Unknown or escaped	1. Local treatment of wound 2. RabIg (local and intramuscular) and HDCV or PCECV
Skunk, bat, fox, coyote, raccoon and other carnivores. Includes bat found in room when a person was sleeping unattended.	Regard as rabid* unless geographic area is known to be rabies free	1. Local treatment of wound 2. RabIg (local and intramuscular) and HDCV or PCECV**
Livestock, rodents or lagomorphs (hares and rabbits)	Consider individually. Consult appropriate public health and CFIA officials. Bites of squirrels, chipmunks, rats, mice, hamsters, gerbils, other rodents, rabbits and hares may warrant post-exposure rabies prophylaxis if the behaviour of the biting animal was highly unusual.	

RabIg = (human) rabies immune globulin, HDCV = human diploid cell vaccine, PCECV= purified chick embryo cell culture vaccine

* If possible, the animal should be humanely killed and the brain tested for rabies as soon as possible; holding for observation is not recommended. Discontinue vaccine if fluorescent antibody test of animal brain is negative.

** See text for potential bat exposure.

Schedule and dosage

Pre-exposure immunization

Three doses of HDCV or PCECV are required and should be given on days 0, 7 and 21. The vaccine is given as a 1.0 mL dose intramuscularly into the deltoid muscle or the thigh in infants. See discussion on intradermal administration below.

Post-exposure prophylaxis of previously unimmunized individuals

Five doses of 1.0 mL of HDCV or PCECV should be given, the first dose (on day 0) as soon as possible after exposure and additional doses on each of days 3, 7, 14 and 28 after the first dose. Vaccine should be administered intramuscularly into the deltoid muscle (never in the gluteal region) or the anterolateral upper thigh in infants. An appropriate dose of RabIg, as described below, should also be given on day 0.

Post-exposure prophylaxis should be started as soon as possible after exposure and should be offered to exposed individuals regardless of the elapsed interval. If the suspect animal is domestic and is available for quarantine, then immunization may be withheld pending the animal's status after the 10-day observation period. However, if the bite wound is to the head and neck region, prophylaxis should begin immediately and not be delayed until after the 10-day period. When notification of an exposure is delayed, prophylaxis may be started as late as 6 or more months after exposure.

The vaccine series may be discontinued after consultation with public health/infectious disease experts if the direct fluorescent antibody test of the brain of an animal killed at the time of attack is negative. However, if suspicion of rabies in the animal remains high, even in the presence of a negative test, the immunization series should be continued.

The recommended dose of human RabIg is 20 IU/kg body weight. This formula is applicable to all age groups, including children. Preferably, the full dose of RabIg should be thoroughly infiltrated into the wound and surrounding area. If not anatomically feasible, any remaining volume should be injected intramuscularly at a site distant from vaccine administration. When more than one wound exists, each should be locally infiltrated with a portion of the RabIg using a separate needle and syringe if possible. In such instances, the RabIg may be diluted 2- to 3-fold in a solution of 0.9% sodium chloride in order to provide the full amount of human RabIg required for good infiltration of sites at risk of rabies. If the site of the wound is unknown, the entire dose should be administered intramuscularly. Because of interference with active antibody production, the recommended dose should not be exceeded. Since vaccine-induced antibodies begin to appear within 1 week, there is no value in administering RabIg more than 8 days after initiating an approved vaccine course.

Vaccine and RabIg should be used concurrently for optimum post-exposure prophylaxis against rabies, except in certain previously immunized people, as indicated below. **Under no circumstances should vaccine be administered in the same syringe or at the same site as RabIg.**

Post-exposure prophylaxis of previously immunized individuals

Post-exposure prophylaxis for people who have previously received rabies vaccine differs according to which preparation of vaccine was received.

1. Two doses of HDCV or PCECV, one injected immediately and the other 3 days later, without RabIg, are recommended for exposed individuals with the following rabies immunization history:

   - completion of an approved course of pre-or post-exposure prophylaxis with HDCV or PCECV within the previous 2 years;

   - completion of immunization with other types of rabies vaccine or with HDCV or PCECV according to unapproved schedules as long as neutralizing rabies antibody has been demonstrated in serum (see serologic testing below).

2. A complete course of HDCV or PCECV plus RabIg is recommended for those who may have received rabies vaccines in the past but do not fulfill the criteria listed in A above. A serum sample may be collected before vaccine is given, and if protective antibody (> 0.5 IU/mL) is demonstrated the course may be discontinued, provided at least two doses of vaccine have been given. If in doubt, consultation with an infectious diseases or public health physician is recommended.

Route of administration

RabIg is always given intramuscularly and preferably directly into the edges surrounding the wound.

Rabies vaccine for post-exposure prophylaxis must be administered intramuscularly. Both HDCV and PCECV are approved in Canada for intramuscular (IM) use.

For pre-exposure prophylaxis, the intradermal (ID) route may be considered in some circumstances: while IM administration of rabies vaccine is the gold standard, the World Health Organization (WHO) considers the ID regimen an acceptable alternative as it uses less vaccine to produce a comparable degree of protection against rabies. The ID route should not be used in all individuals. The immune response to ID vaccination in persons who are immunocompromised or taking steroids or chloroquine has been unreliable. In these individuals vaccine should be administered by the IM route only. It is also important to note that improper administration may cause the vaccine to be injected subcutaneously. In addition, a suboptimal dose of vaccine may be administered. The proper syringe and needle are imperative to ensure that the correct route and dose are used. ID vaccines should therefore only be given by well-trained staff and in situations in which there is a well-established cold chain and preferably when a large group of individuals is being vaccinated at the same time. Post-immunization antibody titres should be determined to ensure that an acceptable level of protection has been achieved at least 1 month after completion.

For pre-exposure vaccination three 0.1 mL doses of HDCV or PCECV can be given on days 0, 7 and 21 or 28 intradermally (on the upper arm, over the deltoid). The WHO recommends that the vaccine should contain at least 2.5 IU per IM dose.

If a decision is made to give pre-exposure prophylaxis by the ID route, then ample time must be available to allow for choloroquine use to be delayed for at least 1 month after vaccination.

Booster doses and re-immunization

Some individuals with ongoing high-risk exposure to rabies may require pre-exposure booster doses if their antibody titres fall below 0.5 IU/mL (see *Serologic Testing*). People with continuing high risk of exposure, such as certain veterinarians, should have their serum tested for rabies antibodies every 2 years; others working with live rabies virus in laboratories or vaccine-production facilities who are at risk of inapparent exposure should be tested every 6 months. Those with inadequate titres should be given a booster dose of either HDCV or PCECV. People previously immunized with other vaccines should also be tested for evidence of protective antibody, and those with inadequate titres should be given a booster dose of HDCV or PCECV.

Previously immunized individuals must still receive two additional immunizations at 0 and 3 days following a rabies exposure. An incompletely or inadequately immunized individual requires the complete series of active and passive immunization following rabies exposure.

Both RabAvert® and Imovax® Rabies have been shown to be effective in boosting immunity in previously immunized individuals in both the pre-exposure booster and post-exposure prophylaxis settings. A rapid anamnestic response is obtained regardless of whether the primary vaccine was PCECV or HDCV.

Serologic testing

Three doses of either HDCV or PCECV given intramuscularly over 21 to 28 days have produced protective antibodies in 100% of individuals in all age groups. Numerous studies comparing the pre-exposure immunogenic responses to PCECV and HDCV have shown both vaccines to be comparable in terms of antibody induction, and the height and persistence of antibody response. Therefore, healthy people immunized with an appropriate regimen do not require routine post-immunization antibody determinations unless vaccinated by the ID route.

Neutralizing antibodies develop 7 days after immunization and persist for at least 2 years. The Canadian national rabies reference laboratory is the Ontario Provincial Public Health Laboratory, which considers an acceptable antibody response to be a titre of > 0.5 IU/mL by the rapid fluorescent-focus inhibition test. Determination of post-immunization antibody titre may be advisable for those whose immune response may be reduced by illness, medication or advanced age.

Corticosteroids, immunosuppressive agents and immunosuppressive illnesses may interfere with the antibody response. Upon completion of a post-exposure course of vaccine in these populations, antibody titres should be determined to ensure that an acceptable level has been achieved. Antibody titre determination may also be advisable after pre-exposure immunization in these populations.

Protective antibodies are present immediately after passive vaccination with RabIg, but they have a half-life of only approximately 21 days.

Storage requirements

Both HDCV and PCECV must be stored protected from light at +2° to +8° C.

Simultaneous administration with other vaccines

No clinical trial data are available regarding the concurrent administration of rabies vaccines with other vaccines. Other essential inactivated vaccines may be given at the same time as rabies vaccines but at separate sites using a separate needle and syringe.

Adverse reactions

Serious adverse events are rare following immunization and, in most cases, data are insufficient to determine a causal association.

HDCV: Local reactions such as pain, erythema, swelling and itching at the injection site may occur in 30% to 74% of recipients; mild systemic reactions such as headache, nausea, abdominal pain, muscle aches and dizziness may occur in about 5% to 40%. Systemic allergic reactions characterized by generalized urticaria and accompanied in some cases by arthralgia, angio-edema, fever, nausea and vomiting have been reported. These reactions are uncommon in people receiving primary immunization but have occurred in up to 7% of those receiving a booster dose, with onset after 2 to 21 days. Such reactions have been shown to follow the development of IgE antibodies to beta propiolactone-altered human serum albumin in the vaccine. Immediate anaphylactic reactions have occurred in 1 in 10,000 people given HDCV. Neurologic complications are rare, but three cases of neurologic illness resembling Guillain-Barré syndrome, which resolved without sequelae within 12 weeks, were reported in the early 1980s.

PCECV: Local reactions commonly reported (i.e., > 10% of recipients) with RabAvert® consist of pain, tenderness and induration at the injection site, which lasts for 2-3 days. Other local reactions, including erythema, itching and swelling, have also been reported. Systemic reactions are generally less common (i.e., 1%-10% of recipients) and may consist of malaise, myalgia, arthralgia, headache and fever. Lymphadenopathy, nausea and rash have been reported occasionally. Temporally associated neurologic and anaphylactic events have been very rarely reported following the administration of RabAvert®.

RabIg: Local pain and low-grade fever may follow administration of RabIg.

Contraindications and precautions

Contraindications

There are no definite contraindications to the use of rabies vaccine after significant exposure to a proven rabid animal.

Precautions

Persons with egg allergies are not necessarily at increased risk of a hypersensitivity reaction to RabAvert®. However, for pre-exposure vaccination, an alternative vaccine (HDCV) should be given to persons with a history of severe hypersensitivity reactions to egg or egg products. If an alternative vaccine is not available, post-exposure prophylaxis should be administered with strict medical monitoring. Facilities for emergency treatment of anaphylactic reactions should be available. Persons with a history of hypersensitivity to the vaccine or any of its components should not be given the vaccine for pre-exposure immunization if possible. For more specific advice please consult an allergy specialist.

Serious allergic or neuroparalytic reactions occurring during the administration of rabies vaccine in the post-exposure situation pose a serious dilemma. The risk of rabies developing must be carefully considered before a decision is made to discontinue immunization. The use of corticosteroids as a possible treatment may inhibit the immune response. The patient's blood should be tested for rabies antibodies and expert opinion should be sought in the management of these individuals.

Pregnancy is not a contraindication to post-exposure prophylaxis, but it would be prudent to delay pre-exposure immunization of pregnant women unless there is a substantial risk of exposure.

Other considerations

Vaccine interchangeability: wherever possible, an immunization series should be completed with the same product. However, if this is not feasible, RabAvert® and Imovax® Rabies are considered interchangeable in terms of indications for use, immunogenicity, efficacy and safety.

Selected references

Centers for Disease Control and Prevention. *Compendium of animal rabies prevention and control, 2005.* Morbidity and Mortality Weekly Report 2005;54(RR-3):1-8.

Centers for Disease Control and Prevention. *Human rabies prevention — United States, 1999: recommendations of the Advisory Committee on Immunization Practices (ACIP).* Morbidity and Mortality Weekly Report 1999;48(RR-1):1-21.

National Association of State Public Health Veterinarians. *Compendium of animal rabies control, 1998.* Morbidity and Mortality Weekly Report 1998;47(RR-9):1-9.

Parker R, McKay D, Hawes C et al. *Human rabies, British Columbia – January, 2003.* Canada Communicable Disease Report 2003;29(16):137-38.

Plotkin SA. *Rabies.* Clinical Infectious Diseases 2000;30(1):4-12.

Turgeon N, Tucci M, Deshaies D et al. *A case report: human rabies in Montreal, Quebec, October 2000.* Canada Communicable Disease Report 2000;26(24):209-10.

Varughese P. *Human rabies in Canada — 1924-2000.* Canada Communicable Disease Report 2000:26(24):210-11.

World Health Organization. *WHO recommendations on rabies post-exposure treatment and the correct technique of intradermal immunization against rabies.* Geneva: World Health Organization, 1997. WHO/EMC/Zoo.96.6.

World Health Organization. *World survey of rabies —1997.* Canada Communicable Disease Report 2000;26(2):13-6.

Part 4 — Active Immunizing Agents – Rabies Vaccine

Rubella Vaccine

Rubella is a viral disease that results in a transient erythematous rash, post-auricular or suboccipital lymphadenopathy, arthralgia and low-grade fever. As symptoms are non-specific, it may be mistaken for infection due to parvovirus, adenoviruses or enteroviruses. Adult infection is frequently accompanied by transient polyarthralgia or polyarthritis. Serious complications are rare, and up to 50% of infections are subclinical.

The main goal of immunization is the prevention of rubella infection in pregnancy, which may give rise to congenital rubella syndrome (CRS). This syndrome can result in miscarriage, stillbirth and fetal malformations, including congenital heart disease, cataracts, deafness and mental retardation. Fetal infection can occur at any stage of pregnancy, but the risk of fetal damage following maternal infection is particularly high in the earliest months after conception (85% in the first trimester) with progressive diminution of risk thereafter, and it is very uncommon after the 20th week of pregnancy. Infected infants who appear normal at birth may later show eye, ear or brain damage. Congenital infection may give rise to such problems as diabetes mellitus and panencephalitis later in life. Congenitally infected infants may shed the virus in the urine and in nasopharyngeal secretions for 1 year or more.

The changes since the previous edition of the *Canadian Immunization Guide* include 1) discontinuation of the marketing of monovalent rubella (R) and measles and rubella (MR) vaccines in Canada, and 2) the development of newer diagnostic methods (specifically polymerase chain reaction and IgG avidity tests) to detect or confirm rubella infection.

Epidemiology

An MMR immunization program for all infants was introduced in Canada in April 1983. The average number of rubella cases reported decreased from approximately 5,300 (1971-1982) to fewer than 30 cases per year (1998-2004). The average annual incidence decreased from 0.08 per 100,000 in 1998 to 0.03 per 100,000 in 2004 (range: 0.02-0.09 per 100,000 per year).

In the two decades following the introduction of routine infant immunization, epidemics of rubella continued to occur every 3 to 10 years with incidence peaking both in the spring and winter months. Many of these outbreaks, including one involving over 3,900 cases in Manitoba in 1997, differentially affected males aged 15-24 years of age who had not been immunized because of previous (before 1983) selective rubella immunization of pre-pubertal girls in some jurisdictions. Since the late 1990s, outbreaks have largely been restricted to isolated clusters of unimmunized people, including those who decline immunization for religious or philosophical reasons.

From 2000 to 2004, fewer than 30 sporadic cases of rubella and 0 to 3 cases of CRS were reported each year in Canada. However, in 2005, in addition to sporadic cases reported in several provinces and territories, there was a rubella outbreak involving over 300 cases in an unimmunized southwestern Ontario community which was philosophically opposed to immunization. These outbreak-related cases accounted for the vast majority of rubella cases in 2005 and primarily involved unimmunized children < 19 years old (median age 11, range 0.3-34 years). Ten cases involved pregnant women, but no cases of CRS have been reported as of March 14, 2006. As a result of immunization rates in excess of 95% in the general population, the outbreak did not spread to the surrounding community.

In Canada, routine infant immunization programs have resulted in sustained high rates of immunity in the general population. In addition, measles elimination strategies since the mid 90s have indirectly resulted in a reduction in the proportion of the susceptible population with the use of rubella-containing vaccines (MR and MMR) for the two-dose routine program and measles elimination catch-up campaigns.

Canada is making progress towards elimination of indigenous rubella infection in pregnancy through routine immunization programs, together with CRS-specific policies to screen 100% of pregnant women for rubella and to offer immunization to all women who are susceptible post-partum. Yet while the rarity of CRS in Canada is a reflection of the impact of these rubella elimination strategies, the risk of cases resulting from importation and limited transmission still exists, both for immigrants arriving from areas of low rubella coverage as well as for Canadian communities and individuals who decline immunization for religious or philosophical reasons. CRS has also been reported in infants of Canadian women who developed rubella infection in pregnancy during travel abroad. Travel-related risk of exposure to rubella may change as more countries initiate childhood rubella immunization programs. By 2003, the majority of Caribbean and South and Central American countries had included rubella in their childhood immunization schedule to comply with the Pan American Health Organization's rubella elimination goals.

Preparations approved for use in Canada

This chapter will deal only with products currently marketed in Canada.

- ◆ M-M-R®II (measles, mumps and rubella vaccine, live, attenuated), Merck Frosst Canada Ltd.

- ◆ Priorix® (measles, mumps, rubella vaccine, live, attenuated), GlaxoSmithKline Inc.

The rubella virus vaccine currently marketed in Canada incorporates live attenuated virus strain RA 27/3. The RA 27/3 strain replaced other vaccine strains that were less immunogenic. It was introduced in 1980 and is prepared in human diploid cell culture. Rubella vaccine is only available in combination with measles and mumps vaccines (MMR). Consequently, the term "rubella-containing vaccine" is synonymous with MMR. The vaccine is lyophilized and should be reconstituted just before administration with the diluent provided.

For a list of all approved products in Canada, please refer to Table 1 in the *General Considerations* chapter, page 7.

Efficacy and immunogenicity

Rubella-containing vaccine stimulates the formation of antibody to rubella virus in over 97% of susceptible individuals. Titres are generally lower than those observed in response to natural rubella infection. Asymptomatic re-infection, manifest by a rise in antibody, has been observed in some vaccinees. Asymptomatic re-infection has also been observed in women with naturally acquired immunity associated with very low antibody titres. Rarely, transient viremia can occur in people who have had natural disease or prior immunization, but transmission to the fetus in this circumstance is believed to be rare.

Recommended usage

Infants and children

One dose of rubella-containing vaccine (MMR) is recommended routinely for all children on or as soon as practical after their first birthday. The second dose, given for measles protection, should be given after 15 months of age and before school entry. The acceptable minimum interval between the first and second dose is at least 1 month. Although a second dose of the rubella component is not believed to be necessary for achieving elimination of CRS, it is not harmful and may benefit those who do not respond to primary immunization (1% to 3% of people).

Adolescents and adults

Rubella-containing vaccine (MMR) should be given to all adolescents and adults unless they have proof of immunity, which is either a record of prior immunization, a documented history of laboratory-confirmed rubella disease or serologic proof of immunity. A *clinical* history of rubella without laboratory confirmation is not a reliable indicator of immunity. If there is no documentation of prior immunization, one dose of MMR should be given to ensure that these individuals will be protected against rubella and also protected against measles. Refer to the *Measles Vaccine* chapter on page 228 for information on indications for receipt of two doses of MMR vaccine.

A priority is to immunize non-pregnant, foreign-born adolescents and women from countries where rubella vaccine is not in use as soon as possible after entry to Canada (see *Epidemiology* section). Similarly, the rubella immune status of people planning to travel to rubella-endemic countries should be reviewed. Immunization with a single dose of rubella-containing vaccine is recommended if they do not have proof of immunity.

Since up to one-third of cases of CRS occur in second and subsequent pregnancies, it is essential that all women found to be susceptible during pregnancy receive one dose of rubella-containing vaccine in the immediate post-partum period, before hospital discharge. Canadian, U.S. and U.K. studies show that a large proportion of rubella-susceptible women are not immunized post-partum. Hospital standing order policies have been shown to be effective in increasing post-partum immunization rates.

In educational institutions, such as schools, colleges and universities, particular emphasis should be placed on immunization of susceptible female staff and female students of childbearing age because of their relatively high risk of exposure.

In health care settings, the rubella immune status of female employees of childbearing age should be carefully reviewed. Those without documented immunity should be immunized with MMR vaccine. In addition, it is also important that health care workers of either sex be actively immunized against rubella because they may, through frequent face-to face contact, expose pregnant women to rubella.

Schedule and dosage

One dose of MMR vaccine should be administered for rubella protection, with the second dose given for measles protection. The first dose should be given on or after the first birthday and the second dose given at least 1 month after the first and, in children, before school entry. The standard dosage is 0.5 mL. See the *Measles Vaccine* chapter on page 228 for details of indications for a second dose.

For single vials, the entire contents of the vial should be injected promptly after reconstitution (0.5-0.7 mL).

Route of administration

Rubella-containing vaccine (MMR) should be administered subcutaneously.

Booster doses and re-immunization

Antibody levels developed in response to earlier generation rubella vaccines declined over time, but this may not have clinical significance since any detectable antibody generally protects against viremic infection. The duration of protection is not yet known, but studies indicate that the duration of both cellular and humoral immunity exceeds 20 years. Booster doses are not considered necessary. However, if a booster dose is given, it is not harmful and may provide protection to the small proportion of individuals left unprotected by the first dose.

Serologic testing

Pre-immunization

A documented history of immunization is evidence of immunity. For those without documented immunization, serologic screening is neither necessary nor recommended before vaccination. Performing serologic tests may cause undue delay and result in a missed opportunity to immunize.

Post-immunization

Serologic testing after immunization is unnecessary. It is not necessary to repeat immunization even if subsequent serologic tests are also negative.

Prenatally

Serologic testing for rubella antibody is not necessary during prenatal care for those with documented evidence of serologic immunity or prior immunization. Women without a prior record of immunization who are tested and found to be non-immune serologically should be vaccinated with one dose of rubella-containing vaccine (MMR) in the immediate post-partum period and before discharge from hospital. They need not be screened for rubella antibodies either after immunization or in subsequent pregnancies, since they are likely protected against CRS.

Storage requirements

Rubella-containing vaccine (MMR) should be stored in the refrigerator at a temperature of +2° C to +8° C. The vaccine must be protected from light, which may inactivate the vaccine viruses. Once reconstituted, the vaccine should be administered promptly.

Simultaneous administration with other vaccines

Rubella-containing vaccine (MMR) may be administered at the same time but at a separate injection site as hepatitis B, pneumococcal conjugate, meningococcal conjugate C, *Haemophilus influenzae* type b, DTaP-IPV and the adolescent/adult Tdap vaccines. Other live vaccines such as varicella may be administered at the same time as MMR vaccine but at separate injection sites. If not administered at the same visit, other live vaccines must be separated by at least a 4-week interval.

Adverse reactions

Serious adverse events are rare following immunization and, in most cases, data are insufficient to determine a causal association.

Rash and lymphadenopathy occur occasionally. Acute transient arthritis or arthralgia may occur 1 to 3 weeks after immunization, persisting for approximately 1 to 3 weeks and rarely recurring. These reactions are uncommon in children, but the frequency and severity increase with age. They are more common in post-pubertal females, among whom arthralgia develops in 25% and arthritis-like signs and symptoms in 10% after immunization with rubella vaccine. The frequency of adverse reactions in seronegative women is higher in those who have never been vaccinated than in revaccinated seronegative women.

Published studies indicate no evidence of increased risk of new onset, chronic arthropathies or neurologic conditions in women receiving rubella vaccine. There is some evidence to suggest a genetic predisposition to joint manifestations following rubella immunization. Paresthesia or pain in the extremities lasting 1 week to 3 months has been reported rarely. Both the frequency and severity of adverse reactions are less than those associated with natural disease, and serious adverse reactions are rare.

Contraindications and precautions

Rubella-containing vaccine (MMR) should not be administered to people known to have anaphylaxis to the vaccine components, such as neomycin. There is evidence that it is safe to immunize children who have allergy to eggs with MMR, since fewer than 2 per 1,000 immunized egg-allergic children were found to be at risk of anaphylactic reaction to MMR vaccine. Please refer to the *Anaphylactic Hypersensitivity to Egg and Egg-Related Antigens* chapter, page 85, for more information.

As with other live vaccines, rubella-containing vaccine should not be administered to people whose immune mechanism is impaired as a result of disease or therapy, except under special circumstances. The immune response in such individuals may be impaired. Please refer to the *Immunization of Immunocompromised Persons* chapter, page 117, for more information.

Infants infected with human immunodeficiency virus (HIV) who are asymptomatic should receive routine MMR vaccination. In addition, MMR is recommended for most symptomatic HIV-infected persons, including children who are symptomatic without evidence of severe immunosuppression. Please consult an infectious disease specialist/immunologist for more specific advice on MMR immunization for HIV-infected people.

Administration of live rubella-containing vaccine during pregnancy should be avoided because of the theoretical risk of CRS in the fetus. Women of childbearing age should be advised to avoid pregnancy for 1 month after immunization. This recommendation is based on the expected duration of viremia after natural infection and the record of vaccine safety. Rubella-containing vaccine has occasionally been administered to women who were unknowingly pregnant at the time or who became pregnant shortly after immunization. Reassurance can be given that no fetal damage has been observed in the babies of over 1,000 susceptible women who received vaccine during their pregnancy and carried to term. The theoretical risk of teratogenicity, if any, is very small. Therefore, receipt of rubella-containing vaccine in pregnancy or conception within 1 month after receipt is not a reason to consider termination of pregnancy.

Breast-feeding is not a contraindication to rubella immunization. Although vaccine virus has been detected in breast milk and transmission can occur, no illness has been reported in the infants.

Small quantities of vaccine-strain virus may be detected in the nasopharynx of some vaccinees 7 to 28 days after immunization, but the risk of transmission to contacts seems to be very low. After many years of vaccine use, only a few cases of possible transmission have been documented. Therefore, it is safe to administer vaccine to those (including health care workers) who are in contact with susceptible pregnant women and with immunocompromised people.

Rh immune globulin (RhIg) may theoretically interfere with the response to rubella-containing vaccine. Rubella-susceptible women who receive RhIg post-partum should be vaccinated with rubella-containing vaccine (MMR) at a separate site, tested 2 months later for rubella immunity and revaccinated if the result is negative.

Rubella-containing vaccine (MMR) must be administered at least 2 weeks before an immune globulin injection. The recommended interval between immune globulin-containing products and MMR immunization varies from 3 to 11 months. Please refer to the *Recent Administration of Human Immune Globulin Products* chapter, page 53, for more information. It has been shown that simultaneous red blood transfusion does not interfere with the antibody response to MMR immunization. In such cases, however, it is recommended that a serologic test be done 6 to 8 weeks after immunization to assess the individual's immune status. If the individual is seronegative, a second dose of vaccine should be administered.

Other considerations

Passive immunization

Immune globulin given soon after exposure to rubella may modify or suppress symptoms but is not certain to prevent infection, including congenital infection. Therefore, the routine use of immune globulin in susceptible women exposed to rubella early in pregnancy is not recommended.

Management of outbreaks

During rubella outbreaks, people who have not been immunized or do not have serologic proof of immunity should be given rubella-containing vaccine (MMR) promptly without prior serologic testing. As previously stated, a history of rubella illness is not a reliable indicator of immunity. Although immunization is ineffective after exposure to wild-type rubella, it is not harmful and will provide future protection if the current exposure does not result in infection. It will also provide protection against measles and mumps.

Surveillance and diagnosis

All suspected and confirmed cases of rubella and CRS must be reported to the appropriate local or provincial/territorial public health authority. Laboratory confirmation of rubella is carried out by serologic tests, viral culture and/or reverse transcriptase polymerase chain reaction (RT-PCR). Confirming the diagnosis is particularly important in pregnant women (especially during the first trimester), suspected cases who have contact with pregnant women, suspected cases of CRS and during outbreaks.

Rapid confirmation may be obtained by testing for rubella-specific IgM antibody in a serum sample. The sensitivity of commercial rubella IgM enzyme immunoassays has been found to be approximately 50% for samples collected ≤ 5 days after rash onset and > 90% for samples collected 1 week to 4 weeks afterwards. There may be false-negative IgM results if the serum sample is taken too early or too late after the clinical illness.

A limitation of the IgM test is that some people may have prolonged positive results (> 1 year), and the test has a low positive predictive value outside an outbreak setting. Consequently, when rubella is suspected in pregnant women, positive rubella IgM results should be confirmed using IgG avidity testing, available through the National Microbiology Laboratory in Winnipeg. The presence of low IgG avidity implies a recent infection and confirms the IgM result. In contrast, high IgG avidity implies that the IgM result is false positive (prolonged positive result or re-infection) and therefore does not indicate recent rubella infection; there is thus minimal risk of CRS.

Seroconversion, defined as a greater than four-fold rise in rubella IgG antibody titre between samples obtained at the acute and the convalescent stages, is also confirmatory, the first sample being taken within the first 7 days after illness onset and the second 10 days after the first.

Sporadic cases are those with no epidemiologic link to a laboratory-confirmed case or with no travel history to an area with known rubella activity. These cases must be laboratory-confirmed either by rubella virus isolation or seroconversion. A false-positive IgM result may occur in a sporadic case, even with highly specific IgM assays, because of the very low incidence of disease in Canada (in non-outbreak situations). Therefore, IgM serology is not a reliable test to diagnose sporadic cases.

In addition to serum collection for serologic confirmation, all suspected rubella cases should have a nasopharyngeal sample collected for viral culture and genotyping. Genotyping or molecular epidemiology is necessary to track transmission pathways, link cases in outbreaks and document the elimination of a rubella virus strain from a geographic region. Rubella virus genotyping is done at the National Microbiology Laboratory in Winnipeg.

Consultation with an obstetrician is advised when attempting to diagnose fetal rubella infection. Amniotic fluid may be collected for the RT-PCR test.

Congenital infection may be confirmed in infants by isolation of the virus in neonatal urine or nasopharyngeal secretions, detection of IgM antibody to rubella virus in blood or the persistence of IgG antibody to rubella virus beyond the age of 6 months, at which time maternally acquired antibodies usually wane.

Contact the nearest regional virology laboratory for the availability and applicability of the various diagnostic methods for rubella.

Selected references

Best JM, Banatvala JE. Rubella. In: Zuckerman AJ (editor). *Principles and practice of clinical virology*, 5th edition. John Wiley and Sons, 2004.

Best JM, O'Shea S, Tipples G et al. *Interpretation of rubella serology in pregnancy – pitfalls and problems*. British Medical Journal 2002;325(7356):147-48.

Bottiger M, Forsgren M. *Twenty years' experience of rubella vaccination in Sweden: 10 years of selective vaccination (of 12-year-old girls and of women postpartum) and 13 years of a general two-dose vaccination*. Vaccine 1997;15(14):1538-44.

Centers for Disease Control and Prevention. *Control and prevention of rubella: evaluation and management of suspected outbreaks, rubella in pregnant women, and surveillance for congenital rubella syndrome*. Morbidity and Mortality Weekly Report 2001;50(RR-12):1-23.

Charbonneau S, Valiquette L, Bédard L et al. *Survey of postpartum rubella vaccination, Montreal, Laval, and Montérégie, Quebec, 1992*. Canada Communicable Disease Report 1996;22(5):38-40.

Furesz J, Varughese P, Acres SE et al. *Rubella immunization strategies in Canada.* Reviews of Infectious Diseases 1985;7(Suppl 1):S191-93.

Gyorkos TW, Tannenbaum TN, Abrahamowicz M et al. *Evaluation of rubella screening in pregnant women.* Canadian Medical Association Journal 1998;159(9):1091-97.

Health Canada. *Proceedings of a meeting of the Expert Advisory Group on Rubella in Canada.* Canada Communicable Disease Report 2002;28(Suppl 4):1-24.

Johnson CE, Kumar ML, Whitwell JK et al. *Antibody persistence after primary measles-mumps-rubella vaccine and response to a second dose given at four to six vs. eleven to thirteen years.* Pediatric Infectious Disease Journal 1996;15(8):687-92.

Macdonald A, Petaski K. *Outbreak of rubella originating among high-school students – Selkirk, Manitoba.* Canada Communicable Disease Report 1997;23(13):97-101.

Mitchell LA, Tingle AJ, Grace M et al. *Rubella virus vaccine associated arthropathy in post-partum immunized women: influence of preimmunization serologic status on development of joint manifestations.* Journal of Rheumatology 2000;27(2):418-23.

Pebody RG, Gay NJ, Hesketh LM et al. *Immunogenicity of second dose measles-mumps-rubella (MMR) vaccine and implications for serosurveillance.* Vaccine 2002;20(7-8):1134-40.

Plotkin SA. *Rubella eradication.* Vaccine 2001;19:3311-19.

Reef SE, Frey TK, Theall K et al. *The changing epidemiology of rubella in the 1990s: on the verge of elimination and new challenges for control and prevention.* Journal of the American Medical Association 2002;287(4):464-72.

Tingle AJ, Mitchell LA, Grace M et al. *Randomised double-blind placebo-controlled study on adverse effects of rubella immunization in seronegative women.* Lancet 1997;349(9061):1277-81.

Tipples GA, Hamkar R, Mohktari-Azad T et al. *Evaluation of rubella IgM enzyme immunoassays.* Journal of Clinical Virology 2004;30(3):233-38.

Tookey PA, Peckham CS. *Surveillance of congenital rubella in Great Britain, 1971-96.* British Medical Journal 1999;318(7186):769-70.

World Health Organization. *Standardization of the nomenclature for genetic characteristics of wild-type rubella viruses.* Weekly Epidemiology Report 2005;80(14):126-32.

Smallpox Vaccine

The last known case of naturally occurring smallpox occurred in Somalia in 1977. Three years later the World Heath Organization (WHO) published the Declaration of the Global Eradication of Smallpox. Immunization programs were terminated shortly afterwards. Eradication of this dreaded disease was one of the most significant advances in public health in the 20th century.

The occurrence of a single case of smallpox anywhere in the world is a global emergency. WHO's Executive Board has endorsed a commitment by all countries to provide mutual assistance in the event of the identification of a case.

For research purposes, remaining virus stocks are kept in two WHO reference laboratories in the United States and Russia. There are concerns that other countries may have access to the virus, particularly in the light of previous terrorist events.

There is currently no evidence to support routine smallpox immunization of the general Canadian population. The threat of dissemination of smallpox virus as a biological weapon is unknown but is believed to be very small. In the current environment groups at greatest potential risk include laboratory workers who may handle orthopox viruses and first responders to a suspected case or outbreak, such as ambulance attendants, hospital emergency room staff and other health care workers. Laboratories wishing to vaccinate their staff should contact the Director of the Office of Public Health Security, Centre of Emergency Preparedness and Response (CEPR), Public Health Agency of Canada (PHAC) at tel: (613) 941-6195 to obtain additional information and/or to request the necessary forms.

The Canadian Smallpox Contingency Plan is updated as necessary by the Office of Emergency Preparedness (OEP), CEPR, PHAC, in consultation with the provinces and territories. The plan includes recommendations for action to be taken if a case of smallpox occurs in Canada or elsewhere in the world. Copies of the plan can be requested by contacting the Director of OEP at tel: (613) 946-7003.

For further information on smallpox vaccine, please see the *Statement on Smallpox Vaccination* published in the Canada Communicable Disease Report (15 January, 2002, volume 28, ACS-1) or available at <http://www.naci.gc.ca>.

Tetanus Toxoid

Tetanus is an acute and often fatal disease caused by an extremely potent neurotoxin produced by *Clostridium tetani*. The organism is ubiquitous in soil but has also been detected in the intestines of animals and humans. Wounds that are contaminated with soil or animal/human feces and that are associated with tissue injury and necrosis are most frequently associated with tetanus. Cases related to injection drug use, animal bites and lacerations have been reported as well as rare cases occurring after bowel surgery or bronchoaspiration of soil and feces. In North America, approximately 27% of cases occur in people who do not report any antecedent injury.

Since the publication of the 2002 *Canadian Immunization Guide* changes include 1) recommendation for adolescents aged 14-16 years of age to be vaccinated with tetanus toxoid, diphtheria toxoid and acellular pertussis (Tdap); 2) a new notation that there is no evidence of increased risk of severe adverse events for Canadian adolescents after receiving diphtheria and tetanus toxoid-containing vaccines at intervals of < 5 years; and 3) a new recommendation for subsequent vaccination of persons known to have developed Guillain-Barré syndrome (GBS) within 8 weeks of a previous tetanus vaccine dose.

Epidemiology

Tetanus is rare in Canada. During the 1920s and 1930s, 40 to 50 deaths from tetanus were reported annually. With the introduction of tetanus toxoid in Canada in 1940, morbidity and mortality rapidly declined (see Figure 15). Between 1980 and 2004, the number of cases reported annually ranged from 1 to 10, with an average of 4 per year. During this period, person $\geq$ 60 years of age accounted for 49% of the cases, and 57% were males. No cases were reported among neonates. The immunization status of most of the reported cases was not known. Birth in a foreign country was indicated for 11% of 53 cases with known data. Only five deaths have been reported since 1980, the last in 1997.

Tetanus immunization programs are highly effective, provide long-lasting protection and are recommended for the whole population. However, sero-surveys suggest that a substantial proportion of Canadians have nonprotective tetanus antitoxin levels. Factors associated with lack of immunity to tetanus include increasing age, birth outside Canada and absence of immunization records. Continued attention should be given to improving tetanus immunization in these groups.

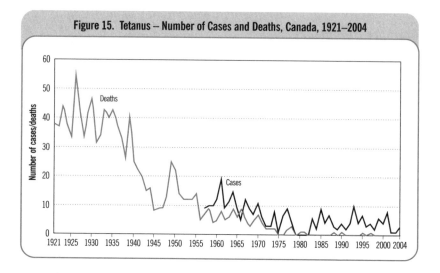

Figure 15. Tetanus – Number of Cases and Deaths, Canada, 1921–2004

Preparations approved for use in Canada

This chapter will deal only with products that are currently marketed in Canada.

◆ Adacel® (tetanus and diphtheria toxoids adsorbed combined with component pertussis vaccine, [Tdap]), Sanofi Pasteur Ltd

◆ DT Polio Adsorbed (diphtheria and tetanus toxoids adsorbed and poliomyelitis vaccine), Sanofi Pasteur Ltd.

◆ Pentacel® (Act-HIB [*Haemophilus* b conjugate vaccine (tetanus protein conjugate)] reconstituted with Quadracel®, [DTaP-IPV-Hib]), Sanofi Pasteur Ltd.

◆ Quadracel® (component pertussis vaccine and diphtheria and tetanus toxoids adsorbed combined with inactivated poliomyelitis vaccine, [DTaP-IPV]), Sanofi Pasteur Ltd.

◆ Td Adsorbed (tetanus and diphtheria), Sanofi Pasteur Ltd.

◆ Td Polio Adsorbed (tetanus and diphtheria toxoids and inactivated poliomyelitis vaccine, [Td-IPV]), Sanofi Pasteur Ltd.

◆ Tetanus Toxoid Adsorbed, Sanofi Pasteur Ltd.

◆ Tripacel® (component pertussis vaccine combined with diphtheria and tetanus toxoids adsorbed, [DTaP]), Sanofi Pasteur Ltd.

Tetanus toxoid is prepared by detoxification of tetanus toxin with formalin. It is combined with aluminum salts, generally aluminum phosphate, in an adsorbed form. Tetanus toxoid is available alone or in various combinations with diphtheria toxoid, acellular pertussis, inactivated poliomyelitis, hepatitis B and *Haemophilus influenzae* type b vaccines. All preparations contain comparable amounts of tetanus toxoid. Preparations that also contain inactivated polio vaccine may contain trace amounts of polymyxin B and neomycin from the cell growth medium.

For a list of all approved products in Canada, please refer to Table 1 in the *General Considerations* chapter, page 7.

Efficacy and immunogenicity

Tests for measuring the immune response to tetanus toxoid include the serum toxin neutralization bioassay performed in mice and serologic tests, which include enzyme immunoassays (EIA) as well as other assays. Because the bioassay is expensive and time-consuming, the EIA is more widely used. The definition of protective antibody level depends on the precise type of assay used. Correlation of serologic test results with the toxin bioassay is useful, as the latter assesses actual neutralization *in vivo*.

Protective antitoxin levels occur in virtually all healthy infants and children who receive primary immunization. A double-blind, randomized controlled trial in rural South America demonstrated that two or three doses of tetanus toxoid administered to previously unvaccinated women of childbearing age protected their infants. Efficacy in standard pre-exposure and post-wound booster immunization regimens in adults has not been assessed in randomized trials but was demonstrated by observational studies during World War II.

Most children who are perinatally infected with human immunodeficiency virus (HIV) develop adequate antitoxin antibody responses following immunization with vaccines containing tetanus toxoid. The antibody response to boosters given to adults with HIV or other humoral immune deficiencies is suboptimal. Tetanus immunity is lost in approximately half of patients undergoing chemotherapy for lymphoma or leukemia. Patients undergoing bone marrow or stem cell transplantation should be re-immunized. Please refer to the chapter on *Immunization of Immunocompromised Persons*, page 117.

Very rare cases of tetanus have been reported despite full immunization and the presence of toxin-neutralizing antibody. These cases may present with a clinical spectrum ranging from mild or localized to severe disease. Explanatory theories include the "overwhelming" of host defences by large quantities of toxin, selective suppression of the immune response or antigenic differences between toxin and toxoid.

Part 4 — Active Immunizing Agents – Tetanus Toxoid

311

Recommended usage

It is recommended that all Canadians receive a primary immunizing course of tetanus toxoid in childhood followed by routine booster doses every 10 years. Adults who have not previously received a primary tetanus toxoid series require three doses as part of an adult primary immunization regimen (see *Schedule and Dosage*).

Active immunization against tetanus should be undertaken for patients who have recovered from this disease, because infection does not confer protective immunity.

Schedule and dosage

The dose of the various forms of tetanus toxoid licensed in Canada is 0.5 mL. For children < 7 years of age, routine vaccine formulations contain tetanus toxoid in combination with diphtheria toxoid, acellular pertussis, inactivated polio and *H. influenzae* type b antigens. For adolescents aged 14-16 years of age, vaccination with tetanus toxoid, diphtheria toxoid and acellular pertussis (Tdap) is recommended. This preparation contains less diphtheria toxoid than the preparation given to younger children. Adults may receive tetanus vaccination using tetanus toxoid, in combination with diphtheria toxoid, or combined with diphtheria toxoid and acellular pertussis. Please refer to the chapters on *Diphtheria Toxoid Vaccine* and *Pertussis Vaccine*, pages 166 and 257, for more information.

For children commencing immunization in early infancy, the primary immunizing series of adsorbed tetanus toxoid consists of a dose at 2, 4 and 6 months of age, a fourth dose at 18 months and a fifth dose at 4 to 6 years of age (school entry). Among children who receive the fourth dose after the fourth birthday, the dose at 4 to 6 years of age is not required. For information on immunization schedules for children not vaccinated in early infancy, please refer to the *Recommended Immunization Schedules* chapter, page 94.

In adults requiring a primary immunization series, the first two doses of tetanus toxoid should be given 4 to 8 weeks apart and the third 6 to 12 months later (given as Td with one of the doses given as Tdap for pertussis protection).

Please refer to the *Immunization of Immunocompromised Persons* chapter, page 117, for recommendations on hematopoietic stem cell and solid organ transplant recipients.

Route of administration

Tetanus toxoid is administered intramuscularly.

Booster doses and re-immunization

To maintain immunity to tetanus after completion of primary immunization, booster doses administered as Td are recommended at 10-year intervals. More frequent boosters may lead to severe local and systemic reactions. Some experts have suggested that booster doses may be given less frequently. Although tetanus cases are uncommon in people who received a primary immunization series but did not receive subsequent boosters every 10 years, cases have occurred in such circumstances. The National Advisory Committee on Immunization (NACI) continues to recommend tetanus boosters every 10 years based on concern regarding the decline of antibody levels with age and potential failure of single booster doses to produce protective levels in older individuals. Periodic health examinations of adults should be used as opportunities to review the need for recommended vaccines, including tetanus booster doses.

Serologic testing

There is no indication for pre- or post-immunization serology.

Storage requirements

Toxoid preparations should be stored in the refrigerator, at a temperature between +2° C and +8° C. They should not be frozen, and any that have been frozen should not be used.

Simultaneous administration with other vaccines

Tetanus toxoid-containing preparations may be given concurrently with other vaccines, using separate needles and syringes.

Adverse reactions

Serious adverse events are rare following immunization and, in most cases, data are insufficient to determine a causal association.

Adverse reactions to primary immunization with tetanus toxoid are rare, especially in children. Their incidence in adults increases with age. Following booster doses, local erythema and swelling are not uncommon. Severe local reactions occur rarely and may be associated with high levels of circulating antitoxin. Lymphadenopathy and fever may occasionally occur. Serum sickness, brachial plexus neuropathy, encephalomyelitis and transverse myelitis have rarely been reported in association with tetanus vaccination. Attribution of adverse reactions to tetanus toxoid may be confounded if other antigens are present in the preparation. Anaphylactic reactions to tetanus toxoid may rarely occur. However, in one study, 94 out of 95 persons who gave a history of anaphylactic symptoms following previous vaccination with tetanus toxoid were nonreactive following intradermal testing and tolerated a further tetanus toxoid challenge without reaction. In consultation with an allergy specialist, a search for IgE antibodies to tetanus toxoid (and other components of the administered vaccine) should be initiated in suspected cases of anaphylaxis.

Trismus associated with tetanus toxoid immunization has rarely been reported. The pathogenesis is unexplained. However, outcomes have been favourable.

Contraindications and precautions

Tetanus toxoid should not be given if a severe systemic reaction, including severe hypersensitivity or a neurologic event, followed a previous dose. People who experience a major local reaction or high fever following a dose of tetanus toxoid should not be given another dose for at least 10 years. In those who have experienced severe local reactions or fever after tetanus toxoid, plain toxoid may be considered for subsequent booster doses, since it is reported to cause fewer reactions than adsorbed toxoid. When a contraindication to tetanus toxoid exists and a patient sustains a major or unclean wound, tetanus immune globulin should be given.

Although a causal association has not been established between tetanus vaccine and GBS, at the present time it is prudent to withhold subsequent vaccinations in children and adults who developed GBS within 8 weeks of a previous tetanus vaccine dose. Those who develop GBS outside this interval or have an alternative cause identified (e.g., *Campylobacter jejuni* infection) may receive subsequent tetanus vaccinations.

Before a combined vaccine is given, it is most important to ensure that there are no contraindications to the administration of any of the components.

There is no evidence that tetanus toxoid is teratogenic. In the event of a tetanus-prone wound during pregnancy the recommendations in Table 13 should be followed. Neonatal tetanus may occur in infants born to unimmunized mothers under unhygienic conditions.

NACI has concluded that there is no evidence of increased risk of severe adverse events for Canadian adolescents after receiving diphtheria and tetanus toxoid-containing vaccines at intervals of < 5 years (please refer to the *Pertussis Vaccine* chapter, page 257, for more information).

Other considerations

Post-exposure prevention of tetanus in the context of wound management

Table 13 summarizes the recommended use of immunizing agents in wound management. It is important to ascertain the number of doses of toxoid previously given and the interval since the last dose. When a tetanus booster dose is required, the combined preparation of tetanus and diphtheria toxoid (Td) is used for adults. For adolescents and adults who have not already received a pertussis booster vaccine dose, the combined preparation of diphtheria, tetanus and acellular pertussis (Tdap) is preferred.

Appropriate cleansing and debridement of wounds is imperative, and use of antibiotics may be considered.

Some individuals with humoral immune deficiency, including those with HIV infection, may not respond adequately to tetanus toxoid. Therefore, tetanus immune globulin (TIg) should be used in addition to tetanus toxoid in individuals with humoral immune deficiency who have wounds that are not clean, regardless of the time elapsed since the last booster.

Table 13. Guide to Tetanus Prophylaxis in Wound Management

History of tetanus immunization	Clean, minor wounds		All other wounds	
	Td or Tdap*	TIg**	Td or Tdap*	TIg
Uncertain or < 3 doses of an immunization series†	Yes	No	Yes	Yes
≥ 3 doses received in an immunization series†	No‡	No	No§	No¶

* Adult-type combined tetanus and diphtheria toxoids or a combined preparation of diphtheria, tetanus and acellular pertussis. If the patient is < 7 years old, a tetanus toxoid-containing vaccine is given as part of the routine childhood immunization.

** Tetanus immune globulin, given at a separate site from Td (or Tdap)

† The immunization series for tetanus is described in the text (see Schedule and Dosage).

‡ Yes, if > 10 years since last booster.

§ Yes, if > 5 years since last booster. More frequent boosters not required and can be associated with increased adverse events. The bivalent toxoid, Td, is not considered to be significantly more reactogenic than T alone and is recommended for use in this circumstance. The patient should be informed that Td (or Tdap) has been given.

¶ Yes, if individuals are known to have a significant humoral immune deficiency state (e.g., HIV, agammaglobulinemia), since immune response to tetanus toxoid may be suboptimal.

Part 4 — Active Immunizing Agents – Tetanus Toxoid

Selected references

David ST, Hemsley C, Pasquali PE et al. *Enhanced surveillance for vaccine-associated adverse events: dTap catch-up of high school students in Yukon.* Canada Communicable Disease Report 2005;31(11):117-26.

Fiorillo L, Robinson JL. *Localized tetanus in a child.* Annals of Emergency Medicine 1999;33(4):460-63.

Jacobs RL, Lowe RS, Lanier BQ. *Adverse reactions to tetanus toxoid.* Journal of the American Medical Association 1982;247(1):40-2.

Katz KC, Walmsley SL. *Postoperative tetanus: a case report.* Canadian Medical Association Journal 2000;163(5):571-73.

Martin-Munoz MR, Pereira MJ, Posadas S et al. *Anaphylactic reaction to diphtheria-tetanus vaccine in a child: specific IgE/IgG determinations and cross-reactivity studies.* Vaccine 2002;20(27-28):3409-12.

Mayaud C, Loupi E, Charara O et al. *Trismus et vaccination antitétanique.* Archives of Pediatrics 1999;6(7):752-54.

McQuillan GM, Kruszon-Moran D, Deforest A et al. *Serologic immunity to diphtheria and tetanus in the United States.* Annals of Internal Medicine 2002;136(9):660-66.

National Advisory Committee on Immunization. *Interval between administration of vaccines against diphtheria, tetanus, and pertussis.* Canada Communicable Disease Report 2005;31(ACS-9):17-22.

Pascual FB, McGinley EL, Zanardi LR et al. *Tetanus surveillance – United States, 1998-2000.* Morbidity and Mortality Weekly Report Surveillance Summaries 2003;52(3):1-8.

Shimoni Z, Dobrousin A, Cohen J et al. *Tetanus in an immunised patient.* British Medical Journal 1999;319(7216):1049.

Shin DH, Park JH, Jung PJ et al. *A case of maternal tetanus in Korea.* Journal of Korean Medical Science 2002;17(2):260-62.

Wassilak SGF, Roper MH, Murphy TV et al. *Tetanus toxoid.* In: Plotkin SA, Orenstein WA, eds. *Vaccines.* 4th edition. Philadelphia: W.B. Saunders 2004;745-81.

Yuan L, Lau W, Thipphawong J et al. *Diphtheria and tetanus immunity among blood donors in Toronto.* Canadian Medical Association Journal 1997;156(7):985-90.

Typhoid Vaccine

Typhoid fever is caused by *Salmonella typhi*, which differs from most other *Salmonella* species in that it infects only humans and frequently causes severe systemic illness. The organism is generally transmitted through food contaminated with the feces or urine of people with the disease or those who are *S. typhi* carriers. The fatality rate is approximately 16% for untreated cases and 1% for those given appropriate antibiotic therapy. Between 2% and 5% of typhoid cases become chronic carriers, sometimes shedding bacteria in stool for years. The risk of severe illness is increased in people with depressed immunity (e.g., due to HIV) or decreased gastric acid levels.

There are no key changes in the recommendations for typhoid immunization since the publication of the 2002 *Canadian Immunization Guide*. A second *Salmonella typhi* Vi (virulence) capsular polysaccharide vaccine is now available in Canada. A combined Vi capsular polysaccharide typhoid vaccine and inactivated hepatitis A vaccine became available in September 2005. Increasingly, strains of *S. typhi* are found to be resistant to one or more of the antibiotics routinely used in treatment, particularly for infections acquired in the Indian subcontinent.

Epidemiology

In endemic areas (such as Africa [with the exception of South Africa], Asia [except for Singapore and Japan], the Middle East [except Israel and Kuwait], Central and South America, the Dominican Republic and Haiti in the Caribbean) typhoid fever has long been considered a disease that has its greatest impact in individuals 5 to 19 years of age. Age-specific incidence rates vary from one country to another, however, and significant illness and numbers of deaths have been reported in children < 5 years of age in some settings. Several factors may contribute to an apparently lower risk in very young children, including age-specific changes in the immune response, atypical or milder disease in this population and under-reporting. Whatever the cause(s), the observation is important in light of our incomplete knowledge of vaccine immunogenicity and efficacy in this age group.

The incidence of typhoid fever is very low in the industrialized world. An average of 70 cases have been reported annually in Canada over the past 5 years. The low incidence rate in industrialized countries is attributable to overall good living conditions, in particular the high quality of drinking water and sewage treatment. The rates were achieved without vaccines, and vaccination has no ongoing role in disease control.

317

The greatest risk of typhoid infection for Canadians occurs while they are travelling in countries where sanitation is likely to be poor. However, not all travellers in these countries are at markedly increased risk. Indeed, the risk of suffering from typhoid fever in many settings in developing countries is minimal (e.g., business-class hotels, conference centres and resort hotels). The greatest risk appears to be associated with exposures to food and water in uncontrolled settings (e.g., market stalls, street vendors, home restaurants and family settings). Even relatively short visits with friends and family can put Canadian travellers (the so-called "visiting friends and relatives" or VFR group) at substantial risk of typhoid in some areas.

Regardless of the setting, typhoid immunization is not a substitute for careful selection and handling of food and water. The available vaccines provide only 50% to 55% protection and do not prevent disease in those who ingest a large number of organisms. However, immunization may reasonably be expected to reduce the risk of typhoid fever among otherwise healthy travellers in areas where this disease is either endemic or epidemic.

Preparations approved for use in Canada

This chapter will deal only with vaccines that are currently marketed in Canada

Three types of typhoid vaccine are currently available for protection against typhoid fever.

Parenteral, capsular polysaccharide vaccines (Typh-I)

- Typhim Vi®, produced by Sanofi Pasteur Ltd. Each 0.5 mL dose of vaccine contains 25 µg of purified polysaccharide.

- Typherix®, produced by GlaxoSmithKline Inc. Available as a single dose of 0.5 mL containing 25 µg of the Vi polysaccharide of *Salmonella typhi*.

Each is an injectable solution of Vi antigen prepared from the capsular polysaccharide of *S. typhi* strain TY2.

Combined vaccine

- ViVaxim™, produced by Sanofi Pasteur Ltd, combines purified Vi polysaccharide typhoid vaccine in solution (25 µg of the Vi polysaccharide typhoid vaccine) and inactivated hepatitis A vaccine in suspension (160 antigen units) in a single-dose, dual chamber syringe.

Oral, live attenuated vaccines (Typh-O)

- Vivotil®, produced by Berna Biotech. Enteric-coated capsules (four doses containing lyophilized bacteria).

- Vivotif L®, produced by Berna Biotech. Foil sachets (three doses of lyophilized bacteria).

318

Both oral formulations contain buffer to enhance passage of the attenuated bacteria through the gastric acid barrier. The vaccines contain the attenuated strain *S. typhi* Ty21a, which was produced by chemical mutagenesis. This bacterium has lost some virulence factors and replicates for only a limited period of time in human hosts.

For a list of all approved products in Canada, please refer to Table 1 in the *General Considerations* chapter, page 7.

Efficacy and immunogenicity

Typh-I Vaccines

The parenteral vaccine stimulates a specific antibody response (i.e., ≥ 4-fold rise in antibody titre) in about 93% of healthy adults. Controlled trials have demonstrated that the serologic response to vaccine is correlated with protective efficacy. Two randomized, double-blind, controlled field trials of Typh-I in disease-endemic areas have demonstrated protective efficacy rates of 55% (95% confidence interval [CI] 30%-71%). The efficacy of immunization with Typh-I has not been systematically studied in people from industrialized countries who travel to disease-endemic regions or in children < 5 years of age. Typh-I has not been tested among children < 1 year of age. Its protective efficacy in people previously immunized with earlier parenteral formulations or the oral vaccine is unknown. Although antibody titres fall with time after vaccination, immunity following Typh-I is thought to last for 2 to 3 years.

In some regions of the world, virulent but Vi-negative strains of *S. typhi* have been reported. Typh-I would not be expected to protect against these rare isolates.

Typh-O Vaccines

Live, attenuated Typh-O vaccines stimulate a cell-mediated immune response, as well as inducing both secretory and humoral antibody. Healthy subjects do not shed vaccine-strain organisms in their stool. As a result, secondary transmission to contacts does not occur. Despite the limited capacity of the vaccine-strain organism to replicate, individuals who are immunocompromised should not receive Typh-O vaccines. In studies delivering at least three doses of the enteric-coated capsular form of the vaccine in typhoid endemic regions, a protective efficacy of 51% (95% CI 35%-63%) can be expected. Although less information is available from field trials about the oral formulation supplied in sachets, the available data suggest that three doses of this formulation are at least as effective as four doses of the capsular form. The oral vaccines appear to be less effective for disease prevention in children 5 to 9 years of age (17%-19%) than in older children and adults (54%-72% among 10- to 19-year-olds). Protective antibodies after the administration of three doses of vaccine are detectable for 3 to 4 years and may persist for longer periods in some individuals.

There are no data on the efficacy or duration of protection in travellers from industrialized countries, or in children < 5 years (capsular formulation) or < 3 years of age (liquid formulation). Neither are there reports regarding the protective efficacy of the oral formulations in people previously immunized with parenteral vaccines. The activity of the Typh-O vaccines against the rare Vi-negative isolates is unknown.

Recommended usage

Routine typhoid immunization is not recommended in Canada. However, selective immunization should be considered in the following groups:

♦ Travellers who will have prolonged (> 4 weeks) exposure to potentially contaminated food and water, especially those travelling to or working in small cities, villages or rural areas in countries with a high incidence of disease. Individuals billeted with or visiting families in such areas may be at particularly high risk. Immunization is not routinely recommended for business travel or short-term (< 4 weeks) holidays in resort hotels in such countries.

♦ Travellers with reduced or absent gastric acid secretion.

♦ People with ongoing household or intimate exposure to an *S. typhi* carrier.

♦ Laboratory workers who frequently handle cultures of *S. typhi*. Technicians working in routine microbiology laboratories do not need to receive this vaccine.

Typhoid immunization is not routinely recommended for workers in sewage plants, for controlling common-source outbreaks, for people attending rural summer or work camps or for people in non-endemic areas experiencing natural disasters such as floods. It is not recommended for the control or containment of typhoid outbreaks in Canada. Typhoid vaccine does not confer complete protection against disease, and immunity may be overwhelmed by a large inoculum of *S. typhi*. Therefore, it is necessary to warn travellers that immunization is only an additional preventive measure against typhoid fever in high-risk situations and that care in the selection of food and water remains of primary importance.

Schedule and dosage

Table 14. Comparison of Typh-O, Typh-I and Combined Vi and Hepatitis A Vaccines

Vaccine type	Route of administration	Schedule	Interactions	Minimum age of recipient
Typh-O* live attenuated	Oral	Alternate days 3 doses (sachet) 4 doses (capsules)	Antibiotics, antimalarials (mefloquine, chloroquine, proguanil)	3 years for sachet (suspension product) > 5 years for capsules
Typh-I** polysaccharide	Intramuscular	Single dose	None	2 years
Combined Vi polysaccharide and inactivated hepatitis A vaccine†	Intramuscular	Single dose	None	16 years

*   Vivotif ® Berna (capsule), Vivotif ® Berna L (sachet)

**   Typhim Vi ®, Typherix ™

†   ViVaxim ™

Route of administration

Typhoid vaccine is available in two formats. The live vaccine is taken orally in a series of doses. The Vi capsular polysaccharide vaccine is administered as a single 0.5 mL intramuscular injection.

Typh-I vaccines

Adults and children ≥ 2 years of age should receive a single dose of 0.5 mL (25 µg) intramuscularly.

Combined purified VI polysaccharide typhoid and inactivated hepatitis A vaccine

Persons ≥ 16 years of age should receive a single dose of 1.0 mL of the mixed vaccine administered intramuscularly.

Part 4 — Active Immunizing Agents – Typhoid Vaccine

Typh-O vaccine, capsular formulation

For adults and children > 5 years of age, one enteric-coated capsule (Vivotil®, Berna vaccine) should be taken on alternate days to a total of four capsules. Each capsule should be taken on an empty stomach with a liquid no warmer than 37° C. All four capsules must be taken for optimal protection.

Typh-O vaccine suspension, supplied in double-chambered foil sachets

The suspension packaged in a double-chambered foil sachet (Vivotif L®, Berna vaccine) is approved for use in adults and children ≥ 3 years of age. Each package contains three double-chambered foil sachets with lyophilized vaccine in one half and buffer in the other half. The contents of both halves of one sachet must be mixed with liquid no warmer than 37° C; it must not be mixed in milk, juice or in a carbonated beverage.

The sachet contents should be re-suspended by gently mixing for 5 to10 seconds and then should be swallowed as soon after mixing as possible. The diluted vaccine-buffer mix should be taken on an empty stomach (e.g., 1 hour before a meal). This procedure is repeated on alternate days for a total of three doses. All three doses must be taken for optimal protection.

Comments applicable to both oral formulations

Antibiotics with activity against *S. typhi* or other *Salmonella* (e.g., broad-spectrum penicillins or cephalosporins, fluoroquinolones, trimethoprim-sulfamethoxazole) may interfere with replication of the vaccine-strain bacterium. For people receiving therapy with such antibiotics, immunization must be deferred until at least 48 hours after the antibiotic course has been completed. Typh-O is killed in vitro by mefloquine at levels achievable in the gut and to a lesser extent by chloroquine and proguanil. Ideally, typhoid immunization should be completed before anti-malarial prophylaxis is initiated. If immunization must occur while one or another of these antimalarials is being taken, at least 8 hours should separate the administration of oral vaccine and the antimalarial.

Booster doses and re-immunization

Relatively few data are available to guide recommendations for either the frequency or timing of booster doses in Canadians residing abroad and in travellers. Nonetheless, periodic booster doses in those at continued risk is reasonable and may be expected to increase antibody titres and protection. Administer every 2-3 years for the parenteral formulation and every 7 years for the oral formulations. Although there are no data regarding the interchangeability of typhoid vaccines, it is presumed that boosting can be performed with any of the available formulations regardless of the vaccine used initially.

Minor variations in dosing schedule are not expected to affect the efficacy of either of the oral typhoid formulations. However, if it is deemed necessary to repeat the series because of long intervals between doses (> 4 days), the administration of an additional full course of vaccine would not be harmful. Although compliance can be an issue with these products because they are self-administered, recent evidence suggests that most travellers take the vaccines competently if properly instructed.

Serologic testing

There is no indication for pre- or post-immunization serology.

Storage requirements

All typhoid vaccines should be maintained at a temperature of $+2^{\circ}$ C to $+8^{\circ}$ C until used.

Simultaneous administration with other vaccines

Although all possible combinations have not been specifically studied, there is no known interaction between the Typh-I vaccines and a number of other relevant travel vaccines, such as hepatitis A vaccine, yellow fever vaccine and hepatitis B vaccine. The concomitant administration of yellow fever vaccine does not suppress the immune response elicited by Typh-O vaccines.

Adverse reactions

The Typh-I vaccines are far less reactogenic than the previous parenteral (whole bacterium) product. A meta-analysis suggests that local reactions (e.g., pain, redness, swelling) can be expected in approximately 4% of vaccinees (95% CI 1.3%-10%), whereas only about 1% report systemic effects such as fever (95% CI 0.1%-12.3%). Virtually all of the available data regarding adverse events following immunization with the Vi polysaccharide vaccine have been acquired in studies of children and young adults (age < 25 years).

The reported adverse events following oral immunization are also relatively rare and mild. Local reactions, such as vomiting (2.1%: 95% CI 0.6%-7.8%) and diarrhea (5.1%: 95% CI 1.7%-14.5%) seldom prevent completion of the course of immunization. Low-grade fever can be expected in approximately 2% of vaccinees (95% CI 0.7%-5.3%). Recent case reports raise the possibility that the Ty21a vaccines may, very rarely, predispose vaccinees to reactive arthritis.

Contraindications and precautions

Contraindications

The only contraindication to administration of the Typh-I vaccines is a history of a severe local or systemic reaction to a previous dose of the vaccine. Similarly, the Typh-O vaccines are contraindicated in individuals with hypersensitivity to any component of the vaccine or the enteric-coated capsule. The oral vaccines should not be given to anyone with an acute gastrointestinal condition or inflammatory bowel disease. Typh-O vaccines should also not be administered to persons with phagocytic function disorders, including chronic granulomatous disease, leukocyte adhesion defect and myeloperoxidase deficiency.

Precautions

◆ **Pediatric use:**

The Typh-I vaccines can be used in children ≥ 2 years. The combined (Vi polysaccharide typhoid and inactivated hepatitis A vaccine) may be administered to those ≥ 16 years. The Typh-O vaccine in capsular format can be administered to children > 5 years of age, and the Typh-O vaccine in sachet (suspension) format may be administered to children aged ≥ 3 years.

◆ **Immunization in pregnant women and nursing mothers:**

Although the Typh-I vaccines would not be expected to have any adverse effects, their safety in pregnancy has not been directly studied. Therefore, the benefits of vaccine must be carefully weighed against any potential adverse effects before Typh-I injectable vaccine is given to pregnant women. The Typh-O live attenuated vaccines should not be given to pregnant women. Although there are no data, it is reasonable to assume that either vaccine could be used safely in nursing mothers.

◆ **Immunization of immunocompromised persons:**

The Typh-O vaccines should not be given to immunocompromised or immunosuppressed people, including those with known HIV infection. Note that these concerns for immunocompromised persons are purely theoretical, and no case of disseminated infection with the attenuated bacterium has been reported. The limited capacity of the attenuated strain to replicate in the human host is primarily due to the degree of its attenuation rather than the host's immune status.

Other considerations

◆ Individuals with decreased gastric acid barriers (e.g., due to achlorhydria, medications that reduce gastric acidity, antacid abuse) who travel to typhoid endemic regions should be offered either parenteral or oral immunization.

◆ Typhoid immunization may also be considered in a control program to limit a typhoid fever epidemic (e.g., in closed communities, refugee settings).

◆ Typhoid immunization in non-travelling Canadians is ONLY recommended for individuals regularly working with this organism in clinical or research laboratories and in family members and close contacts of a chronic carrier of *S. typhi*.

Selected references

Acharya IL, Lowe CU, Thapa R et al. *Prevention of typhoid fever in Nepal with the Vi capsular polysaccharide of Salmonella typhi.* New England Journal of Medicine 1987;317(18):1101-4.

Barnett ED, Chen R. *Children and international travel: immunizations.* Pediatric Infectious Disease Journal 1995;14(11):982-92.

Beeching NJ, Clarke PD, Kitchin NR et al. *Comparison of two combined vaccines against typhoid fever and hepatitis A in healthy adults.* Vaccine 2004;23(1):29-35.

Begier EM, Burwen DR, Haber P, Ball R, the Vaccine Adverse Event Reporting System Working Group. *Postmarketing safety surveillance for typhoid fever vaccines from the Vaccine Adverse Event Reporting System, July 1990 through June 2002.* Clinical Infectious Diseases 2004;38(6):771-79.

Cambell JD, Levine MM. Typhoid and cholera vaccines. In: Jong EC, Zuckerman JN, eds. *Travelers' vaccines.* Hamilton, Ontario: Decker Inc, 2004:162-84.

Centers for Disease Control and Prevention. *Health information for international travel.* U.S. Department of Health and Human Services, 2005:291-307.

Committee to Advise on Tropical Medicine and Travel (CATMAT). *Statement on overseas travellers and typhoid.* Canada Communicable Disease Report 1994;20(8):61-2. URL: <http://www.phac-aspc.gc.ca/publicat/ccdr-rmtc/94pdf/cdr2008.pdf>.

Cryz SJ Jr. *Post-marketing experience with live oral Ty21a vaccine.* Lancet 1993;341(8836):49-50.

Cryz SJ Jr. *Patient compliance in the use of Vivitif Berna™ vaccine, typhoid vaccine, live oral Ty21a.* Journal of Travel Medicine 1998;5(1):14-7.

Engels EA, Falagas ME, Lau J et al. *Typhoid fever vaccines: a meta-analysis of studies on efficacy and toxicity.* British Medical Journal 1998;316(7125):110-16.

Engels EA, Lau J. *Vaccines for preventing typhoid fever.* Cochrane Database of Systematic Reviews 2000;2:CD001261.

Horowitz H, Carbonaro CA. *Inhibition of the Salmonella typhi oral vaccine strain, TY21a, by mefloquine and chloroquine.* Journal of Infectious Diseases 1992;166(6):1462-64.

Ivanoff B, Levine MM, Lambert PH. *Vaccination against typhoid fever: present status.* Bulletin of the World Health Organization 1994;72(6):957-71.

Keitel WA, Bond NL, Zahradnik JM et al. *Clinical and serological responses following primary and booster immunization with Salmonella typhi Vi capsular polysaccharide vaccines.* Vaccine 1994;12(3):155-59.

Keystone JS, Kozarsky PE, Freedman DO et al. *Travel medicine.* Elsevier, 2004.

Klugman KP, Gilbertson IT, Koornhof HJ et al. *Protective activity of Vi capsular polysaccharide vaccine against typhoid fever.* Lancet 1987;2(8569):1165-69.

Levine MM, Ferreccio C, Abrego P et al. *Duration of efficacy of Ty21a, attenuated Salmonella typhi live oral vaccine.* Vaccine 1999;17(Suppl 2):S22-27.

Levine MM, Ferreccio C, Black RE et al. *Large scale field trial of Ty21a live oral typhoid vaccine in enteric-coated capsule formulation.* Lancet 1987;1(8541):1049-52.

Levine MM, Ferreccio C, Cryz S et al. *Comparison of enteric-coated capsules and liquid formulation of Ty21a typhoid vaccine in randomized controlled field trial.* Lancet 1990;336(8720):891-94.

Levine MM, Taylor DN, Ferreccio C. *Typhoid vaccines come of age.* Pediatric Infectious Disease Journal 1989;8(6):374-81.

Lin FY, Ho VA, Khiem HB et al. *The efficacy of a Salmonella typhi Vi conjugate vaccine in two-to-five year old children.* New England Journal of Medicine 2001;344(17):1263-69.

Loebermann M, Kollaritsch H, Ziegler T. *A randomized, open-label study of the immunogenicity and reactogenicity of three lots of a combined typhoid fever/hepatitis A vaccine in healthy adults.* Clinical Therapeutics 2004;26(7):1084-91.

Mahle WT, Levine MM. *Salmonella typhi infection in children younger than 5 years of age.* Pediatric Infectious Disease Journal 1993;12(8):627-31.

Parry CM, Hien TT, Dougan G et al. *Typhoid fever.* New England Journal of Medicine 2002;347(22):1770-82.

Sinha A, Sazawal S, Kumar R et al. *Typhoid fever in children aged less than 5 years.* Lancet 1999;354(9180):734-37.

Steinberg EB, Bishop R, Haber P et al. *Typhoid fever in travelers: Who should be targeted for prevention?* Clinical Infectious Diseases 2004;39(2):186-91.

Taylor DN, Levine MM, Kuppens L et al. *Why are typhoid vaccines not recommended for epidemic typhoid fever?* Journal of Infectious Diseases 1999;180(6):2089-90.

World Health Organization. *Immunizations, vaccines and biologicals – typhoid vaccine.* URL: <http://www.who.int/vaccines/en/typhoid.shtml>.

Varicella Vaccine

Varicella-zoster virus (VZV) is a DNA virus of the herpesvirus family. VZV causes a primary illness (varicella or chickenpox) and establishes latency in the sensory nerve ganglia, which may be reactivated later as herpes zoster (shingles). VZV is spread by the airborne route as well as by direct contact with the virus shed from skin lesions. The incubation period is from 10 to 21 days, usually in the range of 14 to 16 days. Infectiousness begins 1 to 2 days before onset of the rash and lasts until the last lesion has crusted. The attack rate among susceptible contacts in household settings is estimated at 65%-87%.

The changes since the previous edition of the *Guide* include (a) the availability of two refrigerator-stable vaccines in Canada; (b) the development of guidelines for vaccine use in children with select immunodeficiency disorders; (c) updated information on vaccine effectiveness; and (d) a change in terminology to designate cases of varicella occurring in individuals with a history of being immunized with varicella vaccine as "vaccine-modified disease" rather than the previously used term "breakthrough disease". Vaccine-modified disease is the preferred term because it more accurately reflects the fact that cases of varicella occurring more than 6 weeks after varicella vaccination are much less severe than cases occurring in non-immune individuals.

Epidemiology

Varicella is mainly a disease of childhood, developing in 50% of children by the age of 5 years and 90% by the age of 12 years. People from the tropics are less likely to acquire immunity in childhood and therefore have higher rates of susceptibility as adults.

Varicella has been considered to be a benign disease in otherwise healthy children aged up to 12 years. However, this group accounts for 80% to 85% of varicella-associated physician visits, 85% to 90% of hospitalizations and nearly 50% of fatal cases. The complications of chickenpox include secondary bacterial skin and soft tissue infections, otitis media, bacteremia, pneumonia, osteomyelitis, septic arthritis, endocarditis, necrotizing fasciitis, toxic shock-like syndrome, hepatitis, thrombocytopenia, cerebellar ataxia, stroke and encephalitis. Varicella increases the risk of severe invasive group A streptococcal infection in previously healthy children by 40- to 60-fold. Complications are more common in adolescents, adults and immunocompromised people, who have higher rates of pneumonia, encephalitis and death.

Varicella case fatality rates are highest among adults (30 deaths/100,000 cases), followed by infants under 1 year of age (7 deaths/100,000 cases) and then those aged 1 to 19 years (1-1.5 deaths/100,000 cases). Since 2000, a total of six pediatric deaths due to varicella were reported by the the Immunization Monitoring Program ACTive (IMPACT) system, with a range of 0-3 deaths per year. In the pre-vaccine era in the United States, adults accounted for only 5% of cases but 55% of the approximately 100 chickenpox deaths each year. In Canada, 70% of the 59 chickenpox-related deaths in the pre-vaccine years (1987 to 1997) occurred in those over 15 years of age.

Congenital varicella syndrome is rare when infection occurs before the 13th or after the 20th week of gestation. The risk is approximately 2% when infection occurs at 13-19 weeks of gestation. Congenital infection results in a wide clinical spectrum, which may include low birth weight, ophthalmic abnormalities, skin scarring, limb atrophy, cerebral atrophy and a variety of other anomalies. Almost one-third of affected infants die by early in the second year of life. Maternal varicella occurring in the 5 days before to 2 days after birth is associated with severe neonatal varicella in 17% to 30% of infants, with high case fatality for the newborn.

Before varicella vaccine became available, approximately 350,000 varicella cases were estimated to occur each year in Canada. However, assessing the effect of varicella immunization programs on the incidence of varicella and zoster disease is difficult because varicella infections are significantly under-reported, less than 10% of the expected cases being reported through the national Notifiable Diseases Reporting System (NDRS) annually. Furthermore, zoster is not a nationally notifiable disease. Given that the risk of having at least one reactivation to herpes zoster is 15% to 20%, there are likely a significant number of zoster cases occurring each year in Canada. Post-herpetic neuralgia lasting longer than 6 months is more frequent at older ages, occurring in 35% of those aged $\geq$ 50 years.

A review of data from the Canadian Institute for Health Information for 1994 to 2000 showed that over 1,550 varicella hospitalizations occur annually for all age groups. Information on pediatric hospitalized cases and deaths are available from the IMPACT system for the periods 1990 to 1996 and 1999 to 2004. These data indicate that the majority of hospitalizations occur in previously healthy children. For the most recent period, 1999 to 2004, a total of 2,058 pediatric hospitalizations due to varicella or herpes zoster were reported from 12 sites across Canada, averaging 343 hospitalizations annually. Of these cases, just over half were males, and the most affected age groups were children 1 to 4 years old (accounting for 45% of hospitalizations) and those 5-9 years old (30% of hospitalizations).

The total medical and societal costs of varicella in Canada were estimated in a multicentre study to be $122.4 million yearly or $353.00 per individual case. Eighty-one percent of this amount went toward personal expenses and productivity costs, 9% toward the cost of ambulatory medical care and 10% toward hospital-based medical care.

Benefits from varicella immunization have been seen in the United States after varicella vaccine was licensed in 1995. From 1995 to 2005, the United States recommended that children 12-18 months of age receive a single dose of varicella vaccine, with catch-up vaccination of older, susceptible children and adults. Varicella disease incidence in children 19-35 months old declined by 70%-85% in three U.S. communities that had achieved vaccine coverage levels of 75%-85%. Varicella-related hospitalizations in the United States decreased from 2.3-5 per 100,000 population in the pre-vaccine era (1993-1995) to 0.3-1.3 per 100,000 population in 2001-02. Ambulatory care visits for varicella also declined, by 59%. In 2000, the number of varicella-related deaths in the United States had declined by 78% in the < 20 year age group and by 63% in the 20-49 year age group, as compared with the pre-vaccine years, 1990-94.

Preparations approved for use in Canada

This chapter will deal only with vaccines that are currently marketed in Canada.

◆ Varivax® III (varicella virus vaccine, live attenuated, [Oka/Merck]), Merck Frosst Canada Ltd.

◆ Varilrix® (varicella virus vaccine, live, attenuated, [Oka-strain]), GlaxoSmithKline Inc.

Each consists of lyophilized, live, attenuated varicella virus designated the Oka strain, which was developed in Japan in the mid-1970s.

For a list of all approved products in Canada, please refer to Table 1 in the *General Considerations* chapter, page 7.

Efficacy and immunogenicity

In healthy children 12 months to 12 years of age, a single vaccine dose has resulted in a seroconversion rate of 98% at 4 to 6 weeks after vaccination with antibodies persisting in 98% at 5 years and 96% at 7 years after vaccination. In adults and adolescents ≥ 13 years of age, two vaccine doses administered 4 to 8 weeks apart gave seroconversion rates of 99% at 4 to 6 weeks after the second dose with persistence of antibodies in 97% 5 years later.

In a prospective study, children who received a single dose of varicella vaccine between 1 and 12 years of age experienced a cumulative vaccine-modified disease rate of 7.2% over a 10-year follow-up period. Retrospective varicella outbreak studies in the United States revealed an overall vaccine effectiveness of 70% to 90% in preventing varicella disease of any severity and 95% protection against severe varicella for at least 7 to 10 years after immunization. Vaccine-modified disease was classified as mild in 80% of the cases, associated with little or no fever and with a significantly reduced number of lesions (fewer than 50, as compared with several hundred among unvaccinated people).

Recommended usage

Unlike the United States, Canada does not currently have as a goal the elimination of varicella, and NACI continues to recommend a single-dose vaccine strategy for children (two doses for adults and adolescents $\geq$ 13 years of age). The United States adopted a varicella elimination goal in 2005, initially recommending that children receive a second dose of varicella vaccine to control outbreaks. In 2006, after varicella vaccine combined with MMR (MMRV) was licensed in the United States, a routine two-dose MMRV schedule was recommended for children. MMRV is currently not available in Canada.

A. Healthy children, adolescents and adults (see Figure 16)

1. Children between 12 and 18 months of age as a part of routine immunization, preferably at the same visit as MMR vaccination. If varicella vaccine is given at the same visit as MMR, it should be given with a separate syringe and needle at a separate site; if not given at the same visit there should be at least 28 days between the administration of the two vaccines.

   Children with a history of varicella illness occurring at < 1 year of age may receive the recommended vaccination at 12-18 months. Since maternally acquired antibody could modify the clinical presentation of varicella during the first year of life, it may be difficult to ascertain that infection did occur. Furthermore, there is also some evidence that children who acquire wild-type varicella in the first year of life may not develop long-term immunity and could be predisposed to recurrent varicella infection later in life. There are no safety reasons to avoid immunizing such children.

2. Susceptible older children, adolescents and adults, of whom the following groups are considered a priority for immunization:

   * Women of childbearing age. Note that varicella vaccine should *not* be given during pregnancy.

   * Household contacts of immunocompromised people.

   * Health care workers.

   * Adults who may be exposed occupationally to varicella (e.g., teachers of young children, day care workers).

   * Immigrants and refugees from tropical climates who are more likely to be susceptible to varicella.

- Children and adolescents undergoing chronic salicylic acid therapy, because of the associated theoretical risk of Reye syndrome (see *Precautions* section).

- People with cystic fibrosis, because varicella may cause a transient worsening of lung function.

B. Susceptible immunocompromised people (see Figure 17)

A specialist with expertise in varicella vaccination should be consulted when the immunization of people with immunodeficiency diseases is being considered. There are limited safety and effectiveness data in this population. Data on the duration of immunity after vaccination are also lacking. In Canada, only Varilrix® has received approval for the vaccination of select groups of immunocompromised people; however, Varivax® III may also be used under study conditions.

Groups for whom varicella vaccination is recommended

1. People with isolated immunodeficiency diseases and known intact T-cell systems may be vaccinated following the same age-appropriate dosage schedule as for healthy persons:

   - Isolated humoral (immunoglobulin [IG]) deficiency diseases.

   - Neutrophil deficiency disorders.

   - Complement deficiency diseases.

   - Asplenia – either congenital absence, surgical removal or functional (e.g., sickle cell disease).

2. People receiving inhaled or topical steroids.

Groups for whom varicella vaccination may be considered, if the prerequisite conditions allow

- Acute lymphocytic leukemia (ALL) – persons with ALL may be vaccinated provided that the disease has been in remission for ≥ 12 months, the patient's total lymphocyte count is $\geq 1.2 \times 10^9$/L, the patient is not receiving radiation therapy, and maintenance chemotherapy can be withheld for at least 1 week before to 1 week after immunization. Two doses of vaccine are recommended, 1-3 months apart, since North American studies suggest that two doses are more immunogenic than a single dose in these patients.

- HIV infection – persons ≥ 12 months of age with asymptomatic or mildly symptomatic HIV infection (CDC class N1 or A1) and with age-specific CD4 percentages of $\geq 25\%$ may be vaccinated with two doses given 3 months apart.

- People with chronic inflammatory diseases whose long-term immuno-suppressive therapy has been discontinued for at least 6 to 12 weeks.

- Before solid organ transplantation – persons awaiting renal and liver transplantation may be immunized with one to two doses of varicella vaccine, the last dose being given at least 4-6 weeks prior to transplantation. They should not be receiving immunosuppressive treatment at the time of vaccination. The suggested wait period makes vaccination practical mainly in the context of elective transplantation. As there is currently insufficient information regarding varicella immunization of cardiac and lung transplant candidates, no firm recommendations can be made at this time for these patients.

- After solid organ transplantation – immunization may be considered ≥ 2 years after transplantation, when the patient is deemed to be receiving minimal immunosuppressive therapy. Until further data are available, the same age-appropriate dosage schedule as for healthy children or adults may be followed.

- After bone marrow transplantation (BMT) or stem cell transplantation (SCT) – vaccination of recipients at ≥ 2 years after transplantation may be considered, provided there is minimal immunosuppression and no graft-versus-host disease. Until further data are available, the same age-appropriate dosage schedule as for healthy children or adults may be followed.

C. Post-exposure immunization

Varicella vaccine has been shown to be effective in preventing or reducing the severity of varicella if given to a susceptible individual within 3 to 5 days after exposure. Post-exposure immunization would be particularly useful in preventing illness in susceptible immunocompetent individuals who are at higher risk of complications (e.g., adults) and in preventing or limiting outbreaks in hospitals, child care facilities and homeless shelters.

For susceptible pregnant women or immunosuppressed persons who have been exposed to an infectious varicella case, vaccine should *not* be used; instead varicella zoster immune globulin (VarIg) may be given within 96 hours of the exposure to reduce potential maternal morbidity; when given to the pregnant woman, it is currently unknown whether VarIg influences fetal outcome (see the section on varicella-zoster immune globulin in the *Passive Immunizing Agents* chapter, page 353).

Figure 16. Varicella Vaccination Algorithm for Individuals ≥ 12 Months of Age

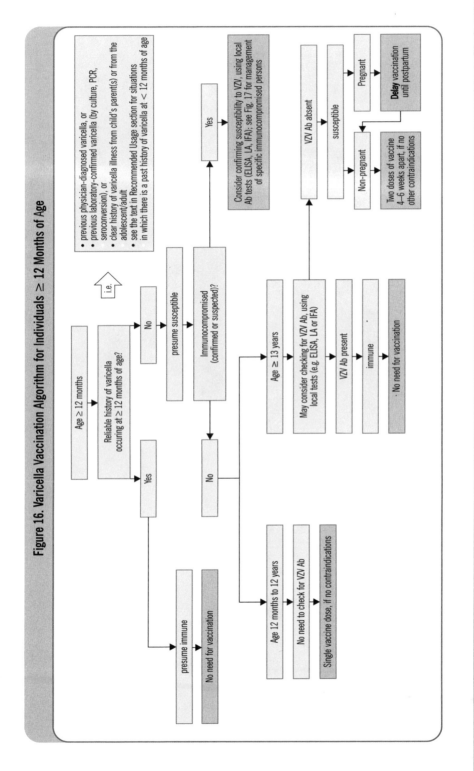

Part 4 — Active Immunizing Agents – Varicella Vaccine

Figure 17. Varicella Vaccination Algorithm for Immunocompromised Individuals

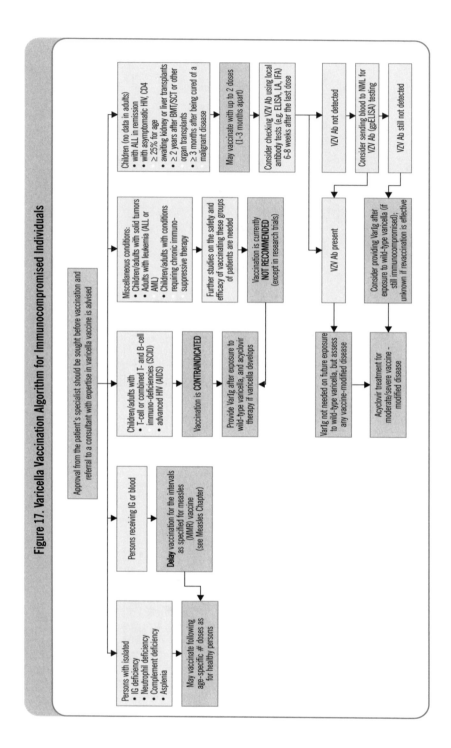

334

AIDS – acquired immunodeficiency syndrome;

ALL/AML – acute lymphocytic leukemia/acute myelogenous leukemia;

BMT/SCT – bone marrow transplant/stem cell transplant;

ELISA - enzyme-linked immunosorbent assay;

gpELISA – glycoprotein enzyme-linked immunosorbent assay;

HIV – human immunodeficiency virus;

IFA – indirect immunofluorescent assay;

IG – immunoglobulin;

LA – latex agglutination;

NML – National Microbiology Laboratory, Winnipeg;

PCR – polymerase chain reaction;

SCID – severe combined immune deficiency;

VarIg – varicella zoster immune globulin;

VZV Ab – varicella-zoster virus antibody

Schedule and dosage

Children aged 12 months to 12 years: a single dose given after the first birthday.

Persons aged ≥ 13 years: two doses given at least 4 weeks (28 days) apart. There is no need to re-start the schedule if administration of the second dose has been delayed. The same vaccine should be used to complete the vaccination series.

The dose is 0.5 mL, containing at least 1,350 plaque-forming units (PFU) of VZV for Varivax III® and not less than 1,995 PFU for Varilrix®.

Route of administration

The lyophilized varicella vaccine should be reconstituted with the diluent provided for this purpose immediately before administration and given subcutaneously. Although the intramuscular route is not recommended, there is some evidence that a dose that is inadvertently given in this way need not be repeated.

Booster doses and re-immunization

NACI does not recommend any booster dose(s) after the age-appropriate primary immunization (see earlier schedule). Follow-up evaluation of children immunized during pre-licensure clinical trials in the United States revealed protection for at least 14 years in most vaccinated children, and studies in Japan indicate protection for at least 20 years.

Serologic testing

Since a history of varicella is highly reliable, serologic testing for proof of susceptibility before immunization in young children is unnecessary (Figure 16). However, testing may be cost-effective in adolescents and adults without a history of varicella, in whom two vaccine doses would be indicated.

Women of childbearing age should be asked about a history of varicella disease and those with a negative history offered serologic testing, as up to 85% may be immune as a result of subclinical varicella during childhood. Susceptible non-pregnant women should be vaccinated using the standard two-dose series.

Post-immunization serologic testing for immunity is not recommended for healthy children and adults, because of the high level of immunity conferred by the vaccine. Commercially available varicella antibody tests, such as the enzyme-linked immunosorbant assay (ELISA), indirect immunofluorescent antibody (IFA) and latex agglutination (LA) do not have sufficient sensitivity to detect antibody after vaccination, although they are useful for establishing immunity after wild-type infection. Wild-type varicella infection induces antibody levels that are up to 10-fold higher than that obtained after vaccination. Cell-mediated immunity testing after immunization is also not recommended, as the test is not available in most laboratories and the results are difficult to interpret.

Adults who previously received two doses of vaccine and who are inadvertently tested are likely to be immune to varicella if there is no detectable antibody by ELISA, IFA or LA tests. There are no studies to indicate whether VarIg prophylaxis is necessary on future exposure to wild-type varicella in these individuals, and VarIg use in this situation is not recommended.

Immunocompromised people who are vaccinated may have antibody testing performed 6-8 weeks after the last dose (Figure 17). If commercially available antibody tests do not detect antibody after immunization, the more sensitive glycoprotein ELISA (gpELISA) test may be requested. This test is available through the National Microbiology Laboratory in Winnipeg, tel: (204)-789-6085. If antibody is not detectable by gpELISA, the patient should be offered VarIg on subsequent exposures to wild-type varicella with further consideration of acyclovir treatment should vaccine-modified disease occur (see varicella-zoster immune globulin section in the *Passive Immunizing Agents* chapter, page 360).

Storage requirements

Varicella vaccine and the corresponding diluent for reconstitution should be stored in the refrigerator at +2° to +8° C. The vaccine and diluent should not be stored in a freezer.

Simultaneous administration with other vaccines

Varicella vaccine may be administered during the same visit but at a separate injection site as MMR vaccine, DTaP-IPV-Hib vaccines, adolescent/adult diphtheria-tetanus-acellular pertussis (Tdap), pneumococcal conjugate, meningococcal conjugate, hepatitis B and influenza vaccines. If not given during the same visit as other live virus vaccines (e.g., MMR), administration of the two live vaccines should be separated by at least 4 weeks.

Adverse reactions

Varicella vaccine is very safe. Reactions are generally mild and include local pain, swelling and redness in 10%-20% of recipients. A low-grade fever has been documented in 10%-15%. A varicella-like rash occurs at the injection site in 3%-5% of vaccinees after the first dose and 1% after a second dose. In a similar proportion of vaccinees (5% after the first dose and 1% after a second dose) a small number of generalized varicella-like papules or vesicles will develop. Lesions usually appear within 5 to 26 days after immunization.

Most varicella-like rashes that occur within the first 2 weeks after immunization are due to wild-type virus. Health care workers with a post-vaccine rash at the injection site may continue to work if the rash is covered. Those with a varicella-like rash not confined to the injection site should be excluded from work in high-risk patient care areas (e.g., where there are premature infants and immunocompromised patients) until lesions are crusted.

Zoster has been reported to occur after varicella immunization and can be due to reactivation of either the vaccine-derived or wild-type strain. However, the risk of zoster developing is lower in vaccinated (estimated at 2.6/100,000 vaccine doses) as compared with unvaccinated children (68/100,000 under 20 years of age).

Serious adverse events are rare following immunization and, in most cases, data are insufficient to determine a causal association.

Vaccine providers are requested to report the following using the Canadian Adverse Event Following Immunization Surveillance System report form: (a) any adverse events occurring within 6 weeks of vaccination, (b) vaccine-modified varicella that is moderate (50-500 vesicular lesions) or severe (with any one of the following: > 500 vesicular lesions, associated complications or admission to hospital) and (c) any persons who develop vaccine-strain varicella within 6 weeks of being in contact with a vaccinee.

Contraindications and precautions

Contraindications

People with a prior history of anaphylaxis to the vaccine or a component of it (including gelatin or neomycin) should not receive further doses. The vaccine does not contain egg proteins, thimerosal or aluminum.

While varicella vaccination may be considered for patients with select immunodeficiency disorders, it is contraindicated in persons with T-cell immunodeficiency. Inadvertent varicella vaccination of patients with unsuspected T-cell immunodeficiency disorders has led to disseminated or prolonged disease with the vaccine strain.

The immunocompromised people for whom varicella vaccination is contraindicated include the following:

* People with immunodeficiency diseases affecting T-cell function, such as SCID and AIDS. Disseminated or prolonged disease with the vaccine strain has been reported after inadvertent vaccination. Therefore, people who have a suspicious medical history for immunodeficiency disorders (e.g., positive family history for congenital immunodeficiency disorder or HIV infection, or history of failure to thrive and recurrent infections) should not be immunized until they have been fully investigated and T-cell dysfunction ruled out.

* People undergoing immunosuppressive treatment for acute myelogenous leukemia or for any malignant solid tumors and adults undergoing treatment for ALL. Data on vaccine safety and effectiveness are limited or non-existent for these people.

* People with chronic inflammatory diseases (e.g., inflammatory bowel disease, collagen-vascular disease, nephrotic syndrome) already taking long-term immunosuppressive therapy (e.g., with high-dose steroids, methotrexate, azathioprine) or whose immunosuppressive therapy was stopped less than 6-12 weeks previously. High-dose steroid therapy is defined as $\geq$ 2 mg/kg of prednisone daily or $\geq$ 20 mg/day for $\geq$ 2 weeks.

* After solid organ transplantation – people who have received solid organ transplants should not be immunized for a period of at least 2 years after transplantation, since they are treated with anti-rejection drugs such as prednisone, cyclosporine, tacrolimus, sirolimus, mycophenolate, OKT3, etc.

* Before BMT or SCT – people awaiting BMT or SCT should not receive varicella vaccine, as they will undergo myeloablative treatment that will likely cancel the benefit of vaccination. The vaccination of the donors immediately before bone marrow or stem cell harvest is also not recommended, as there are currently no safety data and there is no proof that immunity can be transferred from the donor to the recipient.

Pregnant women should not be immunized with varicella vaccine because the effects on fetal development are unknown. Women should postpone pregnancy for 1 month after immunization with the two-dose series. Incidents of inadvertent varicella immunization during pregnancy or of pregnancy occurring within 3 months after immunization with Varivax® III should be reported to the registry maintained by Merck Frosst Canada, Medical Services (tel: 1-800-684-6686). From 1995-2002, there were 58 seronegative women in this registry who were vaccinated in the first or second trimester; among these women there were 56 live births, two spontaneous abortions and no cases of congenital varicella syndrome. Inadvertent vaccination during pregnancy does not constitute a reason for termination of the pregnancy.

GlaxoSmithKline does not maintain a similar pregnancy outcome registry for Varilrix®.

Breast-feeding is not a contraindication to varicella immunization of the mother or child. Varicella vaccine may be given to individuals in households where there is a newborn.

Precautions

Vaccinees with a post-vaccination varicella-like rash rarely transmit the vaccine-associated virus. Data from the United States indicate that after more than 20 million varicella vaccine doses distributed, only three cases have been identified in which vaccine-associated virus was transmitted to close contacts; all contacts experienced a mild rash.

The vaccines approved for prevention of varicella in Canada (Varivax® III and Varilrix®) are not indicated for the prevention of herpes zoster (shingles) in adults. A placebo-controlled study of zoster prevention using a varicella vaccine of higher potency has been published, but this zoster vaccine is currently not available in Canada.

For people undergoing chronic salicylic acid therapy, the manufacturer recommends avoidance of salicylate use for 6 weeks after varicella immunization because of an association between wild-type varicella, salicylate therapy and Reye syndrome. Physicians should weigh the theoretical risks associated with varicella vaccine against the known risks associated with wild varicella. Adverse events have so far not been reported with the use of salicylates after varicella immunization. Consequently, children and adolescents with conditions requiring chronic salicylate therapy should be considered for immunization, with close subsequent monitoring.

The concurrent use of antiviral drugs such as acyclovir, valacyclovir or famciclovir that are active against herpesviruses may reduce the efficacy of varicella vaccine during the period in which the live attenuated vaccine virus is expected to replicate. In the absence of published studies and on the basis of expert opinion, NACI recommends that people taking long-term antiviral therapy should discontinue these drugs, if possible from at least 24 hours before administration of varicella vaccine and up to 4 weeks after vaccination.

Other considerations

Passive immunization

For recommendations on the use of VarIg, please refer to the varicella-zoster immune globulin section of the *Passive Immunizing Agents* chapter, page 353.

For recommendations on the use and timing of passive immunizing agents before or after varicella immunization, refer to the *Recent Administration of Human Immune Globulin Products* chapter, page 53. Because it is a live vaccine, the immune response may be blunted if the vaccine is given after transfusion of plasma, blood (except washed red blood cells), immune globulin (Ig) and VarIg. Although theoretically possible, it is currently unknown whether administration of Rh immune globulin (RhIg) to Rh-negative women in the post-partum period will interfere with the immune response to varicella vaccination. Until further data are available, varicella vaccination of susceptible post-partum women should be delayed for 2 months after they have received RhIg.

Surveillance

Surveillance systems are currently inadequate to assess the impact of varicella immunization in Canada. Varicella cases are under-reported, and herpes zoster is not a reportable disease in most jurisdictions. Varicella-related hospitalizations in children are captured through the IMPACT system, which has provided baseline data from before the introduction of provincial and territorial immunization programs.

Virus identification from clinical specimens (e.g., vesicle scraping) by laboratory methods in order to differentiate wild-type from vaccine-derived VZV should be considered when (a) a severe post-vaccination rash occurs, (b) vaccine-modified varicella requires admission to hospital, (c) herpes zoster occurs in a previously immunized (especially immunocompromised) individual, (d) a varicella-like illness occurs in an immunized health care worker with subsequent spread in the health care setting and (e) a varicella-like illness develops in a pregnant or immunocompromised contact of a vaccinee with a varicella-like rash. Polymerase chain reaction testing to differentiate vaccine-derived from wild-type varicella virus can be performed by the National Microbiology Laboratory in Winnipeg, tel: (204)-789-6085.

Selected references

Arbeter AM, Starr SE, Plotkin SA. *Varicella vaccine studies in healthy children and adults.* Pediatrics 1986;78(4 pt 2):748-56.

Asano Y, Suga S, Yoshikawa T et al. *Experience and reason: twenty year follow-up of protective immunity of the Oka strain live varicella vaccine.* Pediatrics 1994;94(4 Pt 1):524-26.

Brisson M, Gay NJ, Edmunds WJ et al. *Exposure to varicella boosts immunity to herpes-zoster: implications for mass vaccination against chickenpox.* Vaccine 2002;20(19-20):2500-7.

Davies HD, McGeer A, Schwartz B et al. *Invasive group A streptococcal infections in Ontario, Canada. Ontario Group A Streptococcal Study Group.* New England Journal of Medicine 1996;335(8):547-54.

Furth SL, Arbus GS, Hogg R et al. *Varicella vaccination in children with nephrotic syndrome: a report of the Southwest Pediatric Nephrology Study Group.* Journal of Pediatrics 2003;142(2):145-48.

Galil K, Lee B, Strine T et al. *Outbreak of varicella at a day-care center despite vaccination.* New England Journal of Medicine 2002;347(24):1909-15.

Gershon AA, Steinberg SP. *Live attenuated varicella vaccine: protection in healthy adults compared with leukemic children.* Journal of Infectious Diseases 1990;161(4):661-66.

Health Canada. *Proceedings of the National Varicella Consensus Conference: Montreal, Quebec, May 5-7, 1999.* Canada Communicable Disease Report 1999;25(S5).

Kuter B, Matthews H, Shinefield H et al. *Ten year follow-up of healthy children who received one or two injections of varicella vaccine.* Pediatric Infectious Disease Journal 2004;23(2):132-37.

LaRussa P, Steinberg S, Gershon AA. *Varicella vaccine for immunocompromised children: results of collaborative studies in the United States and Canada.* Journal of Infectious Diseases 1996;174(Suppl 3):S320-23.

Law B, Scheifele D, MacDonald N et al. *The Immunization Monitoring Program ACTtive (IMPACT) prospective surveillance of varicella zoster infections among hospitalized Canadian children: 1991-1996.* Canada Communicable Disease Report 2000;26(15):125-31.

Lee BR, Feaver SL, Miller CA et al. *An elementary school outbreak of varicella attributed to vaccine failure: policy implications.* Journal of Infectious Diseases 2004;190(3):477-83.

Levin MJ, Gershon AA, Weinberg A et al. and the AIDS Clinical Trials Group 265 Team. *Immunization of HIV-infected children with varicella vaccine.* Journal of Pediatrics 2001;139(2):305-10.

Levy O, Orange JS, Hibberd P et al. *Disseminated varicella infection due to the vaccine strain of varicella-zoster virus, in a patient with a novel deficiency in natural killer T-cells.* Journal of Infectious Diseases 2003;188(7):948-53.

Mandal BK, Mukherjee PP, Murphy C et al. *Adult susceptibility to varicella in the tropics is a rural phenomenon due to the lack of previous exposure.* Journal of Infectious Diseases 1998;178(Suppl 1):S52-54.

Mullooly J, Black S. *Simultaneous administration of varicella vaccine and other recommended childhood vaccines – United States, 1995 to 1999.* Morbidity and Mortality Weekly Report 2001;50(47):1058-61.

National Advisory Committee on Immunization. *NACI update to statement on varicella vaccine.* Canada Communicable Disease Report 2002;28(ACS-3):1-8.

National Advisory Committee on Immunization. *Statement on recommended use of varicella virus vaccine.* Canada Communicable Disease Report 1999;25(ACS-1):1-16.

National Advisory Committee on Immunization. *Update to the statement on varicella vaccine.* Canada Communicable Disease Report 2004;30(ACS-1):1-26.

Ndumbe PM, Cradock-Watson J, Levinsky RJ. *Natural and artificial immunity to varicella zoster virus.* Journal of Medical Virology 1988;25(2):171-78.

Oxman MN, Levin MJ, Johnson GR et al. *A vaccine to prevent herpes zoster and postherpetic neuralgia in older adults.* New England Journal of Medicine 2005;352(22):2271-84.

Preblud SR. *Age-specific risks of varicella complications.* Pediatrics 1981;68(1):14-7.

Salzman MB, Garcia C. *Postexposure varicella vaccination in siblings of children with active varicella.* Pediatric Infectious Disease Journal 1998;17(3):256-57.

Scheifele DW, Halperin SA, Diaz-Mitoma F. *Three-year follow-up of protection rates in children given varicella vaccine.* Canadian Journal of Infectious Diseases 2002;13(6):382-86.

Seward JF, Watson BM, Peterson CL et al. *Varicella disease after introduction of varicella vaccine in the United States, 1995-2000.* Journal of the American Medical Association 2002;287(5):606-11.

Sharrar RG, LaRussa P, Galea SA et al. *The postmarketing safety profile of varicella vaccine.* Vaccine 2000;19(7-8):916-23.

Shields KE, Galil K, Seward J et al. *Varicella vaccine exposure during pregnancy: data from the first 5 years of the pregnancy registry.* Obstetrics and Gynecology 2001;98(1):14-9.

Shinefield HR, Black SB, Staehle BO et al. *Vaccination with measles, mumps and rubella vaccine and varicella vaccine: safety, tolerability, immunogenicity, persistence of antibody and duration of protection against varicella in healthy children.* Pediatric Infectious Disease Journal 2002;21(6):555-61.

Takashi M, Gershon AA. *Varicella vaccine.* In: Plotkin SA, Mortimer EA, eds. *Vaccines,* 2nd edition. WB Saunders Co, 1994:387-419.

The Immunization Monitoring Program-ACTive (IMPACT) prospective surveillance of varicella zoster infections among hospitalized Canadian children: 1991-1996. Canada Communicable Disease Report 2000;26(15):125-32.

Vazquez M, LaRussa PS, Gershon AA et al. *The effectiveness of the varicella vaccine in clinical practice.* New England Journal of Medicine 2001;344(13):955-60.

Vessey SJ, Chan CY, Kuter BJ et al. *Childhood vaccination against varicella: persistence of antibody, duration of protection, and vaccine efficacy.* Journal of Pediatrics 2001;139(2):297-304.

Watson B, Seward J, Yang A et al. *Postexposure effectiveness of varicella vaccine.* Pediatrics 2000;105(1 Pt1):85-8.

Weibel RE, Neff BJ, Kuter BJ et al. *Live attenuated varicella virus vaccine. Efficacy trial in healthy children.* New England Journal of Medicine 1984;310(22):1409-15.

Wise RP, Salive ME, Braun MM et al. *Postlicensure safety surveillance for varicella vaccine.* Journal of the American Medical Association 2000;284(10):1271-79.

Zhou F, Harpaz R, Jumaan AO et al. *Impact of varicella vaccination on health care utilization.* Journal of the American Medical Association 2005;294(7):797-802.

Yellow Fever Vaccine

Yellow fever (YF) is a zoonotic hemorrhagic fever caused by a flavivirus transmitted by *Aedes aegypti* mosquitoes. YF evolves though a spectrum of three periods of illness, from a non-specific febrile illness with headache, malaise, weakness, nausea and vomiting, through a brief period of remission, to a hemorrhagic fever with gastrointestinal tract bleeding and hematemesis, jaundice, hemorrhage, cardiovascular instability, albuminuria, oliguria and myocarditis. There is a 20% to 30% case fatality rate.

YF is a quarantinable disease subject to international health regulations. It must be reported to the World Health Organization (WHO) within 24 hours through the Travel Medicine Program of the Public Health Agency of Canada (PHAC). The Program must be contacted immediately in the event of a suspected YF case, at telephone number: (613) 941-6195. After hours, contact the PHAC duty officer on call, at telephone number: 1-800-545-7661.

Key changes since the publication of the 2002 *Canadian Immunization Guide* include a change in the age at which infants can be immunized, the addition of a contraindication to vaccine for persons with thymus disease and a precaution for immunizing older persons, aged $\geq$ 60 years. Yellow fever vaccine associated viscerotropic disease (YFV-AVD) and yellow fever vaccine associated neurotropic disease (YFV-AND) are new terms for adverse reactions to immunization previously referred to as post-vaccinal multiple organ system failure and post-vaccinal encephalitis respectively. YFV-AVD is a recently described adverse reaction and clinically resembles YF disease.

Epidemiology

YF is endemic in the tropical areas of equatorial sub-Saharan Africa, Panama in Central America and the tropical region of South America (see Figures 18 and 19). It does not occur in Asia, although the vector, *Aedes aegypti,* is present there. Many countries have endemic *Aedes* mosquitoes but do not have the virus. They are able, by means of the international health regulations, to request proof of YF immunization as a requirement of entry.

Worldwide, 90% of YF cases occur in Africa and 10% in the Americas. The disease manifests itself in two epidemiologic forms, the urban and the sylvatic or jungle, both forms caused by the same virus. Urban outbreaks occur as a result of transmission by *A. aegypti*, which is widely distributed throughout the tropics. Urban disease is a particular problem in Africa and a potential problem in South America. Jungle YF is a disease transmitted by tree-hole breeding mosquitoes (*Haemogogus* mosquitos) to monkeys in the forests of South America and Africa, and can be transmitted to humans.

A recent resurgence of YF in certain countries prompted the WHO to include YF vaccine routinely within the Expanded Program on Immunization.

Disease control includes protection from *Aedes* mosquitoes, which are primarily day-biting, elimination of *A. aegypti* from urban areas and immunization of those at risk of exposure. Unimmunized Canadians can acquire YF when travelling abroad but cannot transmit the disease on their return to Canada, since the recognized mosquito vectors are not present in this country.

Since 1996 there have been reports of YF occurring in American and European travellers visiting YF endemic areas of Africa and South America. Notably, none of these tourists had received YF vaccine. There have been no cases of YF reported to the PHAC since surveillance began in 1924.

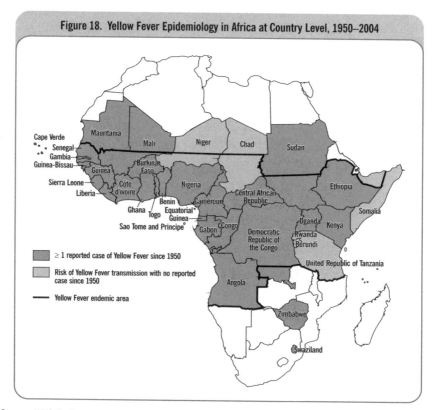

Figure 18. Yellow Fever Epidemiology in Africa at Country Level, 1950–2004

Source: WHO. On-line map at http://www.who.int/csr/disease/yellowfev/impact1/en/. Reprinted with permission.

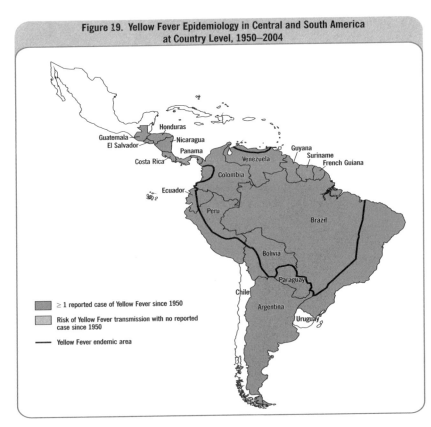

Figure 19. Yellow Fever Epidemiology in Central and South America at Country Level, 1950–2004

Honduras
Guatemala
El Salvador
Panama
Costa Rica
Nicaragua
Guyana
Suriname
French Guiana
Venezuela
Colombia
Ecuador
Peru
Brazil
Bolivia
Paraguay
Chile
Argentina
Uruguay

■ ≥ 1 reported case of Yellow Fever since 1950

■ Risk of Yellow Fever transmission with no reported case since 1950

— Yellow Fever endemic area

Source: WHO. On-line map at http://www.who.int/csr/disease/yellowfev/impact1/en/. Reprinted with permission.

Preparations approved for use in Canada

This chapter will deal only with vaccines that are currently marketed in Canada.

◆ YF-VAX®, Sanofi Pasteur Ltd

YF-VAX®, a live virus vaccine, is prepared in chick embryos from the attenuated 17D strain, is lyophilized and contains sorbitol and gelatin as stabilizers. There is no preservative in the vaccine or the accompanying diluent.

For a list of all approved products in Canada, please refer to Table 1 in the *General Considerations* chapter, page 7.

Efficacy and immunogenicity

Immunity develops 10 days after primary immunization and persists for more than 10 years. More than 90% of persons immunized develop neutralizing antibodies.

Recommended usage

The vaccine is recommended for all travellers ≥ 9 months of age passing through or living in countries in Africa, Central America and South America where YF infection is officially reported or YF immunization is required. It is also recommended for travel outside of urban areas of countries that do not officially report YF but lie in the YF endemic zones (see Figures 18 and 19). Immunization is also recommended for laboratory personnel who work with YF virus.

Pregnant women, immunocompromised people and those aged ≥ 60 years should be considered for immunization only if they are travelling to high-risk areas, if travel cannot be postponed and if a high level of prevention against mosquito exposure is not feasible. Infants < 9 months of age should not be given YF vaccine.

Immunization is required by law upon entry to certain countries irrespective of the traveller's country of origin and in other countries when travellers have passed through endemic areas. In some cases, immunization against YF is recommended, even though not required by law, e.g., if the disease has been reported in the country of destination. In some Asian and other tropical countries where YF does not exist but the transmitting mosquito is present, immunization is required for arrivals from an endemic country to prevent importation of the disease. Current information on the countries for which an International Certificate of Vaccination is required can be obtained from local health departments or from the PHAC Travel Medicine Program through the Internet at http://www.phac-aspc.gc.ca/tmp-pmv/info/yf_fj_e.html.

Only designated Yellow Fever Vaccination Centre clinics approved by the PHAC carry out YF immunization, which is then recorded on an appropriately validated International Certificate of Vaccination. A list of centres can be obtained from the PHAC's Travel Medicine Program Web site, http://www.travelhealth.gc.ca, or by telephone at: (613) 957-8739. The period of validity of the International Certificate of Vaccination for YF is 10 years, beginning 10 days after primary immunization and immediately after re-immunization.

Travellers requiring the certificate but in whom the YF vaccine is contraindicated (see *Contraindications and Precautions*) should be provided an exemption from a designated Yellow Fever Vaccination Centre after completion of an individual risk assessment. Health care providers should note that travellers without a valid International Certificate of Vaccination may be denied entry into a country requiring such documentation or reasons for exemption. It is also possible that they may be offered immunization at the point of entry (e.g., at the airport), where immunization practices fall below Canadian standards.

Schedule and dosage

The vaccine is given as a single dose of 0.5 mL of reconstituted vaccine.

Route of administration

The vaccine is administered subcutaneously. Care should be taken to avoid exposure of the vaccine to disinfectants, allowing the skin to dry after antiseptic preparation before YF vaccine is administered.

Booster doses and re-immunization

Re-immunization is recommended every 10 years, if indicated. Re-immunization boosts antibody titre, although evidence from several studies suggests that immunity persists for at least 30 to 35 years after a single dose and probably for life.

Serologic testing

There is no indication for pre- or post-immunization serology.

Storage requirements

The lyophilized preparation should be maintained continuously at +5° to –30° C until reconstituted for use. Given that it is difficult to guarantee refrigerated temperatures between 1° C and 5° C, YF vaccine is most commonly stored in the frozen state in Canada. Once thawed, **do not refreeze vaccine**. The diluent (sodium chloride injection – contains no preservative) should not be allowed to freeze. Any unused reconstituted vaccine must be discarded 1 hour after reconstitution.

Simultaneous administration with other vaccines

Concurrent administration of other live vaccines does not inhibit the serologic response to YF vaccine. If live vaccines are not given concurrently, they should be spaced at least 4 weeks apart. Inactivated vaccines may be given concurrently or at any interval after YF vaccine.

Adverse reactions

Overall, the vaccine has proved to be very safe and effective. Local reactions have been reported after administration, and 2% to 5% of vaccinees have mild headache, myalgia, low-grade fever or other minor symptoms 5 to 10 days after immunization. Less than 0.2% of vaccinees curtail regular activities. Immediate hypersensitivity reactions, characterized by rash, urticaria and reactive airways, are rare (estimated incidence of 1/130,000 to 1/250,000) and occur principally in people with a history of egg or other allergies. Recently, gelatin stabilizers have been implicated as a cause of allergic reactions in other vaccines.

In 2001, a syndrome of fever and multisystem organ failure was first described in recipients of YF vaccine and is now referred to as vaccine associated neurotropic disease (YFV-AND). All affected persons have required care in an intensive care unit, and the associated mortality rate is estimated to be between 70% and 80%. YFV-AND has previously been reported in young infants but has now also been reported in older adults. The risk of YFV-AND increases with age: the rate is estimated to be 1.1 per 100,000 doses in persons ≥ 60 years and 3.2 per 100,000 doses in those ≥ 70 years. From data collected through a passive surveillance system for adverse events following immunization in the United States, the reporting rate of any serious adverse event following YF immunization was higher among those ≥ 60 years than younger adults (4.2 per 100,000 doses compared with 0.7 per 100,000 doses, respectively). For YFV-AND specifically, the rate was 1.6 per 100,000 doses in persons ≥ 60 years.

Other serious adverse events are rare following immunization and, in most cases, data are insufficient to determine a causal association.

Contraindications and precautions

Allergy to any vaccine component or previous anaphylactic reaction to the YF vaccine is a contraindication to immunization. Because YF vaccine is prepared from chick embryos, it should not be given to individuals with known anaphylactic hypersensitivity to hens' eggs, manifested as urticaria, swelling of the mouth and throat, difficulty breathing or hypotension. A referral to an allergist should be made for those with a questionable history of egg hypersensitivity who are at high risk of exposure to the YF virus. Persons who have an anaphylactic allergic reaction to chicken or gelatin should not receive YF vaccine or should first be evaluated by an allergist to determine whether they can safely receive it.

Recent evidence suggests that persons with thymus disease, including thymoma, thymectomy or myasthenia gravis, are at increased risk of adverse outcomes and should not be immunized with YF vaccine.

Use in infants and seniors

Infants < 9 months of age are more susceptible to serious adverse reactions (encephalitis) to YF vaccine than older children. The risk of this complication appears to be age related and, for this reason, YF vaccine should not be given to infants < 9 months of age. YF vaccine should be used with caution in persons ≥ 60 years of age.

Use in pregnant women and nursing mothers

As the effects of YF vaccine in pregnancy are not well documented, it should not be administered to pregnant women if possible. If a pregnant woman must travel to an endemic area, however, the risk of disease far outweighs the potential risk to the mother or fetus. Historically, many pregnant women have received YF vaccine without significant adverse events. One small study demonstrated that the vaccine virus can infect the developing fetus, but the potential risk of adverse events associated with congenital infection is unknown. Inadvertent immunization of women in pregnancy is not an indication for termination of pregnancy. Seroconversion rates for pregnant women who are immunized have been shown to be lower.

There is a theoretical risk of transmission of the live virus in breast milk, therefore, vaccination of nursing mothers should also be avoided. If travel to an endemic area is required then vaccination with YF vaccine is a lesser risk than that of acquiring the disease.

Use in immunocompromised persons

Generally, YF vaccine should not be given to immunosuppressed individuals. When the primary reason for vaccination is a local vaccine requirement rather than significant risk, a waiver letter should be provided. Immunocompromised travelers should be made aware of the risk of visiting areas of active YF transmission. Travellers thought to have a mild to moderate degree of immunosuppression, e.g., HIV infection with CD4 count > 200 cells/mm^3, who will be at risk of acquiring YF, for example travelling to an area of documented recent activity, should be offered the vaccine and advised of the theoretical risks. WHO advises withholding YF vaccine in children with symptomatic HIV infection. For more information on the use of live virus vaccines in immunocompromised travellers, please refer to the chapter on *Immunization of Immunocompromised Persons*, page 117.

On the basis of the recent reports of adverse events in older travellers, already discussed, immunization in those $\geq$ 60 years of age should be carried out only after an individual risk assessment.

Selected references

Barnett ED, Chen R. *Children and international travel: immunizations.* Pediatric Infectious Disease Journal 1995;14(11):982-92.

Barwick Eidex R, for the Yellow Fever Vaccine Safety Working Group. *History of thymoma and yellow fever vaccination.* Lancet 2004;364(9438):936.

Centers for Disease Control and Prevention. *Fatal yellow fever in a traveler returning from Venezuela, 1999.* Morbidity and Mortality Weekly Report 2000;49(14):303-5.

Centers for Disease Control and Prevention. *Fever, jaundice and multiple organ system failure associated with 17D-derived yellow fever vaccination, 1996-2001.* Morbidity and Mortality Weekly Report 2001;50(30):643-45.

Centers for Disease Control and Prevention. *Health information for international travel 2005-2006.* U.S. Department of Health and Human Services, 2005:308-24.

Choudri Y, Walop W. *Review of adverse events reported following use of yellow fever vaccine – Canada, 1987-2000.* Canada Communicable Disease Report 2002;28(2):9-15.

Keystone JS, Kozarsky PE, Freedman DO et al. *Travel medicine.* Elsevier, 2004.

Khromava AY, Barwick Eidex R, Weld LH et al. *Yellow fever vaccine: an updated assessment of advanced age as a risk factor for serious adverse events.* Vaccine 2005;23(25):3256-63.

Lawrence GL, Burgess MA, Kass RB. *Age-related risk of adverse events following yellow fever vaccination in Australia.* Communicable Diseases Intelligence 2004;28(2):244-48.

Marfin AA, Barwick Eidex RS, Kozarsky PE et al. *Yellow fever and Japanese encephalitis vaccines: indications and complications.* Infectious Disease Clinics of North America. 2005;19(1):151-68.

Martin M, Tsai TF, Cropp B et al. *Fever and multisystem organ failure associated with 17D-204 yellow fever vaccination: a report of four cases.* Lancet 2001;358(9276):98-104.

McFarland JM, Baddour LM, Nelson JE et al. *Imported yellow fever in a United States citizen.* Clinical Infectious Diseases 1997; 25(5):1143-47.

Monath TP. Yellow fever. In: Plotkin SA, Orenstein WA, eds. *Vaccine*, 4th edition. Philadelphia, Pennsylvania: WB Saunders, 1095-1176.

Struchiner CJ, Luz PM, Dourado I et al. *Risk of fatal adverse events associated with 17DD yellow fever vaccine.* Epidemiology and Infection 2004;132(5):939-46.

Tsai TF, Paul R, Lynberg MC et al. *Congenital yellow fever virus infection after immunization in pregnancy.* Journal of Infectious Diseases 1993;168(6):1520-23.

World Health Organization. *International travel and health: vaccination requirements and health advice.* Geneva: World Health Organization, 2005.

Part 5

Passive
Immunization

Passive Immunizing Agents

Three significant changes have been made related to passive immunizing agents since the publication of the 2002 *Canadian Immunization Guide*. Recommendations for the use of palivizumab have replaced those made for respiratory syncytial virus (RSV) immune globulin, which is no longer available in Canada. Recommendations for the interval of time that should elapse from the use of immune globulin preparations and measles vaccine have been generalized to include ALL live viral vaccines with the exception of yellow fever vaccine. Finally, recommendations have been made for the varicella-zoster immune globulin preparation VariZIG™, which has replaced the previously available varicella-zoster immune globulin product.

Protection against certain infections or a reduction in the severity of the illness they cause can be achieved by administration of preformed antibodies derived from humans or animals. The preparations available are of two types: standard immune globulin (Ig) of human origin, sometimes referred to as "immune serum globulin" or "gamma globulin", and special preparations of either human or animal sera containing high titres of specific antibodies to a particular microorganism or its toxin. Products of human origin are preferred over those of animal origin because of the high incidence of adverse reactions to animal sera and the longer lasting protection conferred by human immune globulins.

Passive immunization should be considered when vaccines for active immunization are not available or are contraindicated, or in certain instances when vaccines have not been used before exposure to the infective agent. Passive immunization may also have a role in the management of immunosuppressed people unable to respond to a vaccine. The duration of the beneficial effects provided by passive immunizing agents is relatively short. Protection may be incomplete.

In these guidelines, emphasis is on the prophylactic use of immune sera, and only brief reference is made to their use as therapeutic agents in established infections.

As with all immunizing agents, the risks and benefits of passive immunizing agents need to be explained before administration. The lot number of the product should be recorded in the patient's medical record.

Part 5 — Passive Immunization

Immune globulin (human)

Ig is a sterile, concentrated solution containing between 100 g/L and 180 g/L (10% to 18%) of protein and the preservative thimerosal. It is obtained from pooled human plasma and contains mainly IgG with small amounts of IgA and IgM. The potency of each lot of final product of immune globulin is tested against international standards or reference preparations for at least two different antibodies, one viral and one bacterial. Ig is stable for prolonged periods when stored between +2° and +8° C. Maximum plasma levels are reached approximately 2 days after intramuscular injection, and the half-life in the recipient's circulation ranges from 21 to 27 days.

Intravenous immune globulin (IVIg) is a preparation that contains 50 g/L (5%) of protein with maltose, sucrose or glycine as a stabilizing agent. It is used for continuous passive immunization for patients with selected congenital or acquired immunoglobulin deficiency states and certain diseases. Detailed discussion of IVIg is beyond the scope of this document. Consult appropriate sources and the manufacturer's package insert instructions.

Recommended usage

Prophylactic use of Ig has been shown to be effective in a limited number of clinical situations, which include exposure to measles, hepatitis A and rubella. The commonly recommended doses are given as follows. The dose may vary by manufacturer, and recommendations in the package inserts should be followed.

1. Measles

Ig can be given to prevent or modify measles in susceptible people within 6 days after exposure. To prevent disease, it should be given as soon as possible after exposure, preferably within 3 days. The recommended dose is 0.25 mL/kg body weight with a maximum dose of 15 mL. The dose of Ig for exposed individuals who have underlying malignant disease or who are otherwise immunologically deficient is 0.5 mL/kg or 15 mL maximum.

Ig should be considered for susceptible contacts of measles, particularly all children < 1 year of age and immunologically compromised individuals for whom measles vaccine is contraindicated. Susceptible immunocompetent people who present more than 72 hours but less than 1 week after exposure, i.e., too late for vaccine, can also be considered for Ig. When clinical measles does not develop in a person given Ig, measles vaccine should be given 5 or 6 months later, depending on the Ig dose used, provided the individual is ≥ 1 year of age and there are no contraindications to the vaccine (see Table 4 in *Recent Administration of Human Immune Globulin Products* chapter, page 54 and the *Measles Vaccine* chapter, page 228).

Ig should not be used in an attempt to control measles outbreaks.

2. Hepatitis A

Hepatitis A vaccine is the preferred agent for pre-exposure prophylaxis against hepatitis A. Ig will provide protection against hepatitis A when administered intramuscularly before exposure or during the incubation period. Its relative effectiveness depends upon both the timing of administration and the dose given. Ig may be indicated if the vaccine is unavailable or unaffordable, as well as for infants < 1 year of age, immunocompromised people who may not respond to the vaccine and people for whom the vaccine is contraindicated (please refer to the *Hepatitis A Vaccine* chapter, page 179, for more information).

The recommended dose of Ig varies according to the duration of required protection. It also varies with the manufacturer, so the package insert should be consulted prior to administration. In general, for protection lasting < 3 months the dose is 0.02 mL/kg; for ≥ 3 months, 0.06 mL/kg should be administered; for > 5 months, 0.06 mL/kg should be repeated every 5 months. For post-exposure prophylaxis, the dose of Ig is usually 0.02 mL/kg. Ig prophylaxis should be given as soon as possible after an exposure.

3. Rubella

Ig given soon after exposure to rubella may modify or suppress symptoms but is not certain to prevent infection, including congenital infection. Therefore, the routine use of Ig in susceptible women exposed to rubella early in pregnancy is not recommended.

4. Hepatitis C

Ig is not efficacious in preventing or treating hepatitis C and should not be used for this indication.

Safety of immunoglobulin preparations

Human Ig preparations are among the safest blood-derived products available. Plasma found to be positive for hepatitis B surface antigen, human immunodeficiency virus (HIV) antibody or hepatitis C is excluded from donor pools. As is the case for other blood or organ donations, individuals with known risks for other blood-borne pathogens are excluded from donating plasma for Ig preparation. The method of preparation includes one or more steps that exclude or inactivate hepatitis B and C viruses, and HIV. There are no known reports of transmission of hepatitis B, hepatitis C, HIV, West Nile virus, new variant Creutzfeld-Jakob disease or other infectious agents after the intramuscular injection of Ig. There have been rare reports of transmission of hepatitis B or hepatitis C following the use of certain intravenous Ig preparations that did not undergo the currently required inactivation steps during the manufacturing process.

Part 5 — Passive Immunization

Adverse reactions

Reactions at the site of injection include tenderness, erythema and stiffness of local muscles, which may persist for several hours. Mild fever or malaise may occasionally occur. Less common side effects include flushing, headache, chills and nausea. Anaphylactic reactions may occur rarely with repeat administration.

Contraindications and precautions

Ig should not be given to people with known isolated IgA deficiency or with a known allergy to the preservative thimerosal, a mercury derivative. Pregnancy is not a contraindication to the use of Ig.

Currently available preparations, with the exception of IVIg, must not be given intravenously because of the risk of rare anaphylactic reactions.

Large volumes for intramuscular injection should be divided and injected at two or more sites.

People with severe thrombocytopenia or coagulation disorders that contraindicate intramuscular injections should not be given intramuscular Ig unless the expected benefits outweigh the risks (please refer to *Immunization of Persons with Bleeding Disorders* chapter, page 134).

Ig administration may interfere transiently with the subsequent immune response to measles, mumps, rubella (MMR) and varicella vaccines. Please refer to Table 4, page 54, in the *Recent Administration of Human Immune Globulin Products* chapter for specific recommendations regarding the interval between the administration of Ig and these vaccines.

There are no data to indicate that Ig administration interferes with the response to inactivated vaccines, toxoids or the following live vaccines: yellow fever or the oral preparations of typhoid or cholera.

Specific immune globulins

Specific immune globulins (Ig) are derived from the pooled sera of people with antibody to the specific infectious agents. Antisera from animals, usually horses that are hyperimmunized against a specific organism, are used when human products are not available. Because of the relatively high risk of serum sickness following the use of animal products, human Ig should be used whenever possible. *Before antisera of animal origin are injected, testing for hypersensitivity to the preparation should be carried out in accordance with the manufacturer's recommendation.*

Many of the following products are not readily available and, in some instances, their use may require special access applications. In those situations, local and provincial public health departments should be contacted to facilitate their acquisition.

1. Botulism antitoxin (equine)

Trivalent (type A, B and E) and monovalent (type E) antitoxin preparations, both containing phenol as a preservative, are available on an emergency basis with the assistance of local public health authorities. These products are used therapeutically in people with established or suspected botulism as well as prophylactically in asymptomatic people strongly suspected of having eaten food contaminated with botulism toxin. Type E botulism is most likely to be associated with the consumption of uncooked fish or fish products, or the flesh of marine mammals, including whales and seals. The monovalent type E antitoxin should be used only if such foodstuffs are considered the most likely vehicle of disease or if laboratory tests have established that the toxin involved is type E.

In populations at risk of repeated exposures to botulism toxin because of particular food habits, the repeated use of prophylactic antitoxin can lead to an increased risk of adverse reactions.

2. Diphtheria antitoxin (equine)

This preparation, which also contains phenol as a preservative, is available on an emergency basis with the assistance of local public health authorities for treatment of the disease. Antitoxin should be administered before bacteriologic confirmation when there is clinical suspicion of diphtheria. The method of testing for sensitivity to equine serum, as well as the dose and route of administration, are indicated in the manufacturer's package insert. Intramuscular administration usually suffices, but intravenous administration may be necessary in some cases. If sensitivity tests are positive, desensitization must be undertaken according to the manufacturer's recommendations.

Diphtheria antitoxin is not recommended for prophylaxis of close, unimmunized contacts of diphtheria cases, given the substantial risk of allergic reaction to horse serum and no evidence of additional benefit of antitoxin for contacts who have received antimicrobial prophylaxis.

3. Hepatitis B immune globulin (HBIg)

HBIg is prepared from pooled human plasma from selected donors with a high level of antibody to hepatitis B surface antigen. HBIg provides immediate and effective short-term passive immunity. HBIg administered concurrently with vaccine, but at a different site, does not interfere with the antibody response to the vaccine. The indications for use in susceptible individuals are percutaneous or mucosal exposure to blood containing hepatitis B virus, sexual contact with an acute case of hepatitis B, and birth of an infant to a mother with acute or chronic hepatitis B infection. All infants born to infected mothers should be given an intramuscular dose of 0.5 mL HBIg immediately after birth in addition to the first dose of the three-dose course of hepatitis B vaccine. It is important that HBIg be given within the first 12 hours of birth, since its efficacy decreases sharply after 48 hours. The dose of HBIg for older children and adults is 0.06 mL/kg given intramuscularly. In general, it should be administered to susceptible individuals within 48 hours of exposure. The exception to this is prophylaxis of sexual contacts of an infected individual, when HBIg may be given up to 2 weeks after the last known contact. Please refer to the *Hepatitis B Vaccine* chapter, page 189, for further details concerning prevention of hepatitis B.

4. Rabies immune globulin (RabIg)

Passive immunization with this product is undertaken as part of post-exposure prophylaxis against rabies in unimmunized individuals. Rabies immune globulin (RabIg) provides rapid protection that persists for only a short period of time (half-life about 21 days). Vaccine and RabIg can be administered concurrently **but under no circumstances should the vaccine be administered in the same syringe or at the same site as RabIg**. Please refer to the *Rabies Vaccine* chapter, page 285, for more information on the use of RabIg for post-exposure prophylaxis in unimmunized individuals.

5. Palivizumab (RSVAb)

Respiratory syncytial virus immune globulin (RSVIg) is an intravenous Ig derived from pools of human plasma with high concentrations of protective antibodies that neutralize RSV. RSVIg was approved in August 1997 for prevention of RSV infection in children aged < 2 years old with bronchopulmonary dysplasia (BPD) or a history of premature birth (< 35 weeks' gestation). It is no longer available in Canada.

Palivizumab is a humanized, mouse monoclonal antibody directed against the F protein of RSV. It is effective against both types of RSV. It is 50 to 100 times more potent than RSVIg. Palivizumab is given monthly at a dose of 15 mg/kg of body weight during the period in which the patient is expected to be at high risk of exposure to RSV. Palivizumab is given by the intramuscular route only. Because it is given predominantly to infants, the preferred site of injection is the anterolateral thigh. If the injection volume is over 1 mL, it should be given as a divided dose. Monthly intramuscular doses of 15 mg/kg in children maintain mean trough serum concentrations above 40 mg/mL. In a major clinical trial, children who received palivizumab had a 55% reduction in RSV hospitalization, 42% reduction in the duration of hospital stay, 40% reduction in the length of time they received oxygen and 57% reduction in admissions to the intensive care unit compared with the control group. There may be erythema and pain at the injection site. Fever may occur in 1% to 3%.

Palivizumab prophylaxis is reserved for children who are at highest risk of severe RSV infection, including children 24 months of age or younger with BPD who required oxygen and/or medical therapy for that illness within the 6 months preceding the RSV season, and infants born at 32 weeks and 0 days' gestation or earlier who are 6 months of age or younger (with or without BPD) at the start of the RSV season. Palivizumab does not affect responses to measles, mumps or rubella vaccines. Infants born between 32 and 35 weeks' gestation in isolated communities where hospital care is not readily accessible may be given special consideration for RSV prophylaxis. The appearance of RSV each year varies across Canada, and clinicians should check with local infectious disease specialists or microbiologists to determine when the RSV season begins in their communities. RSV prophylaxis with palivizumab, if undertaken, should be initiated at the start of the RSV season and continued monthly until the end of the season.

Palivizumab is not indicated for the inpatient *treatment* of established RSV infection.

Children less than 2 years of age with hemodynamically significant cyanotic or acyanotic congenital heart disease (who require corrective surgery or are receiving cardiac medication for hemodynamic considerations) should be considered for monthly palivizumab prophylaxis during the winter season. The decision to provide prophylaxis with palivizumab in this population should be made according to the degree of physiological cardiovascular compromise. Infants greater than 32 weeks' gestation with uncomplicated small atrial or ventricular septal defects, patent ductus arteriosus, mild coarctation of the aorta, pulmonic stenosis, uncomplicated aortic stenosis or mild cardiomyopathy, or infants with lesions adequately corrected by surgery and not needing medications for congestive heart failure, without other risk factors, would not be at increased risk of severe RSV, and therefore palivizumab prophylaxis is not recommended for infants with these conditions. Children who have cardiac bypass during surgery should be given repeat doses of palivizumab in the early post-operative period if they remain at risk of RSV infection.

Palivizumab is expensive and so to minimize product wastage, when an entire vial is not required for a patient, residual product may be used for a second patient if administered within the 6-hour expiry time.

6. Tetanus immune globulin (TIg)

Please refer to the *Tetanus Toxoid* chapter, page 309, for more information on the use of TIg in the management of wounds. When used in the treatment of tetanus, TIg should be administered intramuscularly in an effort to neutralize tetanus toxin in body fluids. It has no effect on toxin already fixed to nerve tissue. The optimal therapeutic dose has not been established.

7. Varicella-zoster immune globulin (VarIg)

The VarIg preparation available in Canada is VariZIG™ (Cangene Corporation, Winnipeg, MB). VariZIG™ is a sterile, freeze-dried gamma globulin preparation containing high titres of antibodies to varicella-zoster virus (anti-VZV). VariZIG™ is available through the Canadian Blood Services and Hema-Quebec distribution centres.

The decision to administer VarIg should be based on all four of the following considerations:

+ the exposed person is susceptible to varicella (non-immune);
+ there has been significant exposure to VZV;
+ the person is at increased risk of severe varicella; and
+ post-exposure immunization with varicella vaccine is contraindicated.

Persons who are considered immune (non-susceptible) to varicella include those with

+ a previous history of varicella illness, from a child's parent or from an adolescent or adult;
+ physician-diagnosed varicella;
+ laboratory-confirmed varicella (by culture, polymerase chain reaction or antibody seroconversion);
+ laboratory evidence of immunity;
+ documented immunization with age-appropriate doses of varicella vaccine.

An exception to this is recipients of allogeneic stem cell transplants who should be considered susceptible in the post-transplantation period regardless of a history of varicella or positive serologic test results. These persons should be offered VarIg after known exposure to varicella.

Persons with varicella (chickenpox) are most contagious from 1 to 2 days before and up to 5 days after onset of the rash. Immunocompromised patients may be infectious until the crusting of all lesions. The skin lesions of zoster (shingles) are considered infectious from the onset of lesions until they have crusted and dried. The following situations are considered significant exposures to varicella zoster virus:

+ continuous household contact (living in the same dwelling) with a person with varicella;
+ being indoors for more than 1 hour with a case of varicella;

- being in the same hospital room for more than 1 hour or having more than 15 minutes of face-to-face contact with a patient with varicella;

- touching the lesions of a person with active varicella or zoster (shingles).

VarIg is recommended for the following susceptible people, provided that significant exposure has occurred.

- Pregnant women.

- Immunocompromised patients, such as those with congenital or acquired immunodeficiency due to disease or those receiving immunosuppressive treatment, including patients receiving high-dose systemic corticosteroid therapy (e.g., a dose of $\geq$ 2 mg/kg per day of prednisone or equivalent or $\geq$ 20 mg per day, particularly when given for more than 2 weeks). However, patients receiving regular monthly infusions of $\geq$ 400 mg/kg of IVIg and whose most recent dose was within 3 weeks before exposure do not require VariZIG™. This monthly infusion of IVIG can maintain sufficient protective serum levels of varicella antibody comparable to that achieved with VarIg.

- Newborn infants of mothers who develop varicella during the 5 days before to 48 hours after delivery.

- For the management of significant varicella exposure in a neonatal or pediatric intensive care setting, consultation with the infectious diseases/ infection control specialist regarding the potential use of VariZIG™ is advised.

VariZIG™ is not indicated in healthy adults. Varicella can be more severe in healthy adults than children, but the risk of varicella pneumonia appears to be lower than was formerly believed. Varicella vaccine within 3-5 days after exposure is the post-exposure management of choice for healthy adults. Acyclovir therapy initiated within 24 hours after onset of the rash is effective in accelerating skin lesion healing and can be used for this population as soon as possible after rash onset.

Dosing of VariZIG™ is based on body weight. The recommended dose is 125 IU for each 10 kg of body weight up to a maximum of 625 IU. The minimum dose is 125 IU. VariZIG™ should be given by the intramuscular route. It is of maximal benefit if administered within 96 hours after first exposure. However, since the exact timing of transmission is unknown it can be used within 96 hours of the most recent exposure. Protection is believed to last for approximately 3 weeks. Subsequent exposures more than 3 weeks after a dose of VariZIG™ would require additional doses if the criteria for VarIg, as specified above, still exist.

Selected references

Buckley RH, Schiff RI. *The use of intravenous immune globulin in immunodeficiency diseases.* New England Journal of Medicine 1991;325(2):110-17.

Canadian Paediatric Society, Committee on Immunization and Infectious Diseases. *Palivizumab and respiratory syncytial virus immune globulin intravenous for the prophylaxis of respiratory syncytial virus infection in high risk infants.* Paediatrics and Child Health 1999;4(7):474-80.

Canadian Paediatric Society, Committee on Immunization and Infectious Diseases. *Use of palivizumab in children with congenital heart disease.* Paediatrics and Child Health 2003;8(10):632-33.

Canadian Paediatric Society. *Statement on varicella prevention.* (in press)

Mclntosh D, Isaacs D. *Varicella zoster virus infection in pregnancy.* Archives of Disease in Childhood 1993;68:1-2.

Miller E, Cradock-Watson JE, Ridehalgh MK. *Outcome in newborn babies given anti-varicella-zoster immunoglobulin after perinatal maternal infection with varicella-zoster virus.* Lancet 1989;2(8659):371-73.

Patou G, Midgley P, Meurisse EV et al. *Immunoglobulin prophylaxis for infants exposed to varicella in a neonatal unit.* Journal of Infection 1990;20(3):207-13.

PREVENT Study Group. *Reduction of respiratory syncytial virus hospitalization among premature infants and infants with bronchopulmonary dysplasia using respiratory syncytial virus immune globulin prophylaxis.* Pediatrics 1997;99(1):93-99.

Siber GR, Werner BC, Halsey NA et al. *Interference of immune globulin with measles and rubella immunization.* Journal of Pediatrics 1993;122(2):204-11.

Appendix

Abbreviations for Products Available in Canada

Active Immunizing Agents

Vaccines	Abbreviations
Bacillus Calmette-Guérin	BCG
Cholera - Oral	Chol-O
Cholera - *E.coli* - *Oral*	Chol-Ecol-O
Diphtheria, Tetanus, Acellular Pertussis - pediatric	DTaP
Diphtheria, Tetanus, Acellular Pertussis, Inactivated Polio - pediatric	DTaP-IPV
Diphtheria, Tetanus, Acellular Pertussis, Inactivated Polio, *Haemophilus influenzae* type b - pediatric	DTaP-IPV-Hib
Diphtheria, Tetanus, Acellular Pertussis, Inactivated Polio, *Haemophilus influenzae* type b, Hepatitis B - pediatric	DTaP-IPV-Hib-HB
Diphtheria, Tetanus, Acellular Pertussis, Inactivated Polio, Hepatitis B - pediatric	DTaP-IPV-HB
Diphtheria, Tetanus, Acellular Pertussis, *Haemophilus influenzae* type b - pediatric	DTaP-Hib
Diphtheria, Tetanus, Polio - pediatric	DT-IPV
Hepatitis A	HA
Hepatitis A and B	HAHB
Hepatitis A and Typhoid - Injection	HA-Typh-I
Hepatitis B	HB
Hepatitis B - Thimerosal free	HBTmf
Haemophilus influenzae type b	Hib
Influenza	Inf
Inactivated Polio	IPV
Japanese Encephalitis	JE
Meningococcal - Conjugate	Men-C
Meningococcal - Polysaccharide	Men-P-AC Men-P-ACWY

Active Immunizing Agents (continued)

Measles, Mumps, Rubella	MMR
Measles, Rubella	MR
Pneumococcal-Conjugate - valent	Pneu-C-7
Pneumococcal-Polysaccharide - valent	Pneu-P-23
Rabies	Rab
Tetanus	T
Tetanus, Diphtheria - adult	Td
Tetanus, Diphtheria, Acellular Pertussis - adult	Tdap
Tetanus, Diphtheria, Inactivated Polio - adult	Td-IPV
Tickborne Encephalitis	TBE
Typhoid - Injection	Typh-I
Typhoid - Oral	Typh-O
Varicella	Var
Yellow Fever	YF

Passive Immunizing Agents

Agents	Abbreviations
Botulism Antitoxin	BAtx
Diphtheria Antitoxin	DAtx
Immune Globulin	Ig
Hepatitis B Immunoglobulin	HBIg
Rabies Immunoglobulin	RabIg
Respiratory Syncytial Virus Immunoglobulin	RSVIg
Tetanus Immunoglobulin	TIg
Varicella Immunoglobulin	VarIg

Index

A

ACCA, see adverse events
additives, 5
adjuvants, 4
administration of vaccines, 38
    simultaneous, 51
    timing of, 51
adverse events, 26, 59, 131
    Advisory Committee on Causality Assessment, 63
    and BCG, 154
    MMR and autism, 71,131, 233
    surveillance/reporting system, 62
    YFV-AND and YFV-AVD, 348
advocacy/opportunities for immunization, 24, 59, 96, 115
allergies
    as contraindication, 73, 74
    potential, 14
    to egg and related antigens, 85
aluminum, 4
anaphylaxis
    as contraindication, 73
    management in non-hospital setting, 80
autism, see MMR
avian influenza, 214

B

bat exposure and rabies, 286
Bacille-Calmette Guérin vaccine, 149
BCG and adverse events, 154
benefits of vaccines, 17, 24
bleeding disorders, 134
bovine reagents, 5
breakthrough varicella disease, see vaccine-modified disease, 327
breast-feeding and immunization, 107

C

Canadian Adverse Event Following Immunization Surveillance System, 62
cholera vaccine, 158
cold chain, 45
combination vaccines, 33
communicating effectively about immunization, 29
   immunization truths, 31
   resources, 32
   risk communication, 29
congenital rubella syndrome, 298
congenital varicella syndrome, 328
consent and counselling, 29, 38
contraindications and precautions, 73
   conditions not contraindications, 25, 75
cost of vaccines/other public health interventions, 20

D

diphtheria toxoid, 166

E

education
   for parents, 24
   providers, 27
egg allergy, see allergy
elderly patients, 115
expiry date of vaccines, 38, 47

G

gelatin, 5
Guillain-Barré syndrome, 74, 131, 218, 314

H

Haemophilus vaccine, see Hib vaccine
health care institutions
   immunization of patients, 115
health care providers
   and advocacy, 59, 96, 115
   and hepatitis B, 193, 197
   and influenza vaccine, 213, 215

occupational risk, immunization against, 102
hepatitis A vaccine, 179
   and universal immunization, 184
Hib vaccine, 172
Hib infection and immune deficiency, 175
HIV, 126, 127
human serum albumin, 5

I

Ig, see immune globulin
immigration
   immigration medical examination, 145
   immunization of persons new to Canada, 144
immune globulin, 53, 353
   interval between Ig and vaccine, 54
   specific immune globulins, 356
immune response, 117
immunization
   of adults, 96
   of patients in health care institutions, 115
   records, 55
   registries, 56
   risk groups for, 102
   routine for adults, 99
   schedules, 93
immunocompromised persons, 74, 117
immunosuppression, 73
inactivated vaccine, 4
incidence, see vaccine-preventable diseases
infants
   born prematurely, 113
   immunization schedule, 93
infection control in immunization, 42
influenza vaccine, 209
   avian influenza and culling operations, 214
   and Guillain-Barré syndrome, 218
   and health care workers, 213
   and oculorespiratory syndrome, 218
   recommended recipients, 215
injection route, 40

interchangeability of vaccines, 36
interval between Ig and vaccine, 54
intravenous Ig, 354

J

Japanese encephalitis vaccine,221

L

live attenuated vaccine, 4

M

measles vaccine, 228
MMR and autism, 131, 233
MMRV, 330
multiple injections, 41, 78
mumps vaccine, 251

N

National Guidelines for Immunization Practices, 22
neurological disorders, 131

O

occupational risk
    immunization against, 102

P

pain, techniques to decrease, 41
palivizumab, see RSV
passive immunization, 353
pertussis vaccine, 257
pneumococcal vaccine, 267
polio vaccine, 277
    global eradication, 278
pregnancy, 73,107
    and hepatitis B, 113, 115, 194
prematurity, see infants born prematurely
preservative, 5
product monograph, 61

R

rabies vaccine, 285
records, immunization, 25, 55
   inadequate, 105
regulatory authority, 59
risk communication, 29
RSV and palivizumab, 54, 114, 358
rubella vaccine, 298
   congenital rubella syndrome, 298
   genotyping, 306
   IgG avidity testing, 305

S

safety of Ig, 355, 356
safety of vaccines, 59
   Advisory Committee on Causality Assessment, 63
   expert overviews, 69
   surveillance and assessment, 62
   vaccine evaluation and regulation, 59
schedules, immunization
   for adults, 96
   for infants and children, 93
self-injectors against anaphylaxis, 83
smallpox vaccine, 308
splenic disorders, 119
storage and handling, 45
subunit vaccine, 4
surveillance, see safety of vaccines
syringe selection, 39

T

tetanus toxoid, 309
thimerosal, 5
timing of vaccines, 51
travelers, recommended immunizations, 100, 136
tuberculin skin testing
   as identification tool, 151
   and measles vaccine, 76, 234
typhoid vaccine, 317

V

VAAESS, see Canadian Adverse Event Following Immunization Surveillance System
vaccination
  opportunities for, 24
  errors, 28
  simultaneous, 51
vaccine-preventable diseases
  incidence of, 18, 31, inside back cover
vaccines
  administration, 38
  approval, 59
  attributable risk, 65
  benefits, 17, 24
  classification, 4
  combinations, 33
  currently approved, 7
  interchangeability, 36
  lyophilized, 46
  management, 27, 45
  multiple, 41, 71
  preparation, 38
  records, 25, 55
  safety, see safety of vaccines
  storage and handling, 45
  type, 4
vaccine-modified disease, 327
varicella vaccine, 327
  congenital varicella syndrome, 328
  and the immunocompromised, 331, 336
  recommended usage algorithms, 333, 334
  US data, 329
VarIg, 360
VariZIG, see VarIg, 360

Y

yellow fever vaccine, 343
  YFV-AND, 348
  YFV-AVD, 348